MW00379976

WORKING WITH TRAUMATIZED YOUTH IN CHILD WELFARE

SOCIAL WORK PRACTICE WITH CHILDREN AND FAMILIES

Nancy Boyd Webb, *Series Editor*

Working with Traumatized Youth in Child Welfare
Nancy Boyd Webb, *Editor*

Group Work with Adolescents: Principles and Practice, Second Edition
Andrew Malekoff

Child Development: A Practitioner's Guide, Second Edition
Douglas Davies

Mass Trauma and Violence: Helping Families and Children Cope
Nancy Boyd Webb, *Editor*

Culturally Competent Practice with Immigrant and Refugee Children and Families
Rowena Fong, *Editor*

Social Work Practice with Children, Second Edition
Nancy Boyd Webb, *Editor*

Complex Adoption and Assisted Reproductive Technology: A Developmental Approach to Clinical Practice
Vivian B. Shapiro, Janet R. Shapiro, and Isabel H. Paret

Working with Traumatized Youth in Child Welfare

edited by NANCY BOYD WEBB

FOREWORD BY JAMES R. DUMPSON

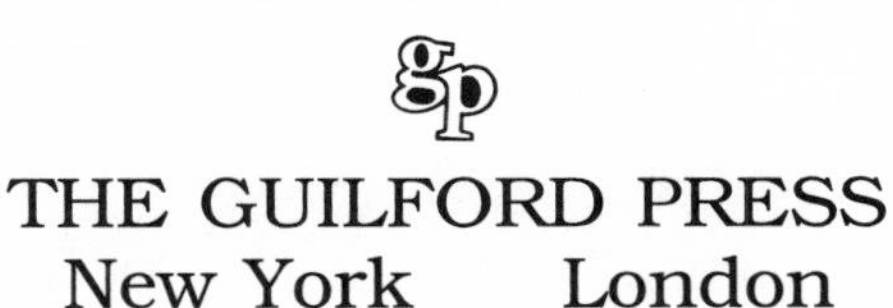

THE GUILFORD PRESS
New York London

A Division of Guilford Publications, Inc.
72 Spring Street, New York, NY 10012
www.guilford.com

Printed in the United States of America

This book is printed on acid-free paper.

Last digit is print number: 9 8 7 6 5 4 3 2 1

Library of Congress Cataloging-in-Publication Data

Working with traumatized youth in child welfare / edited by Nancy Boyd Webb.
p. cm.–(Social work practice with children and families)
Includes bibliographical references and index.
ISBN 1-59385-224-X (cloth)
1. Psychic trauma in children. 2. Child welfare. I. Webb, Nancy Boyd, 1932–
II. Series.
RJ506.P66W67 2006
618.92′8521–dc22

2005015306

In memory of
Dr. Vincent J. Fontana (11/19/1923–7/5/2005)

Medical director and chief pediatrician of New York Foundling Hospital for 43 years, Dr. Vincent J. Fontana was a pioneer in the prevention of child abuse and the care of abused children. For over half a century, Dr. Fontana helped define the problems and magnitude of child neglect in the United States through his books and articles and his dedicated work in the prevention of child maltreatment. The establishment of the Vincent J. Fontana Center for Child Protection at the Foundling Hospital in 2004 appropriately honored a man who devoted his life to helping and protecting children. His work will continue through the Center and his writings.

About the Editor

Nancy Boyd Webb, DSW, BCD, RPT-S, is a leading authority on play therapy with children who have experienced loss and traumatic bereavement. Her bestselling books, which are considered essential references for clinical courses and agencies that work with children, include *Helping Bereaved Children, Second Edition: A Handbook for Practitioners* (Guilford Press), *Mass Trauma and Violence: Helping Families Cope* (Guilford Press), *Play Therapy with Children in Crisis, Second Edition: Individual, Group, and Family Treatment* (Guilford Press), *Culturally Diverse Parent–Child and Family Relationships* (Columbia University Press), and *Social Work Practice with Children, Second Edition* (Guilford Press). In addition, she has published widely in professional journals and produced a video, *Techniques of Play Therapy: A Clinical Demonstration*, which won a bronze medal at the New York Film Festival's International Non-Broadcast Media Competition. Dr. Webb is the editor of The Guilford Press book series Social Work Practice with Children and Families. She is a past board member of the New York Association for Play Therapy.

A board-certified diplomate in clinical social work and a registered play therapy supervisor, Dr. Webb presents frequently at play therapy, social work, and bereavement conferences in the United States and abroad. She has been a professor on the faculty of the Fordham University School of Social Service since 1979, and in October 1997 was named University Distinguished Professor of Social Work. In 1985, she founded Fordham's Post-Master's Certificate Program in Child and Adolescent Therapy to meet the need in the New York metropolitan area for training in play therapy. In April 2000, Dr. Webb appeared as a panelist in a satellite teleconference *Living with Grief: Children, Adolescents, and Loss*, sponsored by the Hospice Foundation of America. Hosted by Cokie Roberts, the conference was beamed to more than 2,100 sites. Dr. Webb was appointed to the endowed James R. Dumpson Chair in Child Welfare Studies at Fordham in 2002, and the same year was honored as Social Work Educator of the Year by the New York State Social Work Education Association. In 2004, Dr. Webb was named Distinguished Scholar by the National Academies of Practice in Social Work, and the same year was presented with the Clinical Practice Award of the Association for Death Education and Counseling. In 2005, she received the Sue Katz Humanitarian Award, presented by the East End (New York) hospice, for her writings and clinical practice with bereaved children.

In addition to teaching, writing, and consulting, Dr. Webb maintains a clinical practice and supervises and consults with schools and agencies. She lectures and conducts workshops throughout the United States, Canada, Australia, Europe, Hong Kong, and Taiwan on play therapy, trauma, and bereavement.

Contributors

Gary R. Anderson, PhD, School of Social Work, Michigan State University, East Lansing, Michigan

Marilyn B. Benoit, MD, American Academy of Child and Adolescent Psychiatry, Washington, DC

Susan M. Brooks, PsyD, Green Chimneys Children's Services, Brewster, New York

Mark Cameron, PhD, Department of Social Work, Southern Connecticut State University, New Haven, Connecticut

David A. Crenshaw, PhD, Rhinebeck Child and Family Center, Rhinebeck, New York

Ruth R. DeRosa, PhD, Division of Child and Adolescent Psychiatry, North Shore University Hospital, Manhasset, New York

Jennifer Elkins, MSSW, School of Social Work, Columbia University, New York, New York

Vincent J. Fontana, MD, [deceased], The Vincent J. Fontana Center for Child Protection, New York Foundling Hospital, New York, New York

Rowena Fong, EdD, School of Social Work, University of Texas at Austin, Austin, Texas

Mayu P. B. Gonzales, MD, Department of Psychiatry and Behavioral Sciences, New York Medical College, and New York Foundling Hospital, New York, New York

Ricky Greenwald, PsyD, Child Trauma Institute, Greenfield, Massachusetts

Neil Guterman, PhD, School of Social Work, Columbia University, New York, New York

Kenneth V. Hardy, PhD, The Eikenberg Institute for Relationships, New York, New York

Carmen Ortiz Hendricks, DSW, Wurzweiler School of Social Work, Yeshiva University, New York, New York

Pamela J. Johnson, MSW, PhD candidate, Mandel School of Applied Social Sciences, Case Western Reserve University, Cleveland, Ohio

Anthony N. Maluccio, DSW, formerly of Boston College Graduate School of Social Work, Boston, Massachusetts, and West Hartford, Connecticut

David Pelcovitz, PhD, Child and Adolescent Psychology, North Shore University Hospital, Manhasset, New York

Bruce D. Perry, MD, The ChildTrauma Academy, Houston, Texas

John Seita, EdD, School of Social Work, Michigan State University, East Lansing, Michigan

Patrick Shannon, PhD, School of Social Work, University at Buffalo, Buffalo, New York

Elizabeth M. Tracy, PhD, Mandel School of Applied Social Sciences, Case Western Reserve University, Cleveland, Ohio

Nancy Boyd Webb, DSW, Fordham University Graduate School of Social Service, Fordham University, Tarrytown, New York

Foreword

The impact of trauma on the mental health of children and youth served by the child welfare system is receiving increased attention in the professional literature. This volume—edited by Nancy Boyd Webb, Distinguished Professor and James R. Dumpson Chair in Child Welfare Studies of the Fordham University Graduate School of Social Service—brings together a multidisciplinary mix of clinicians, researchers, and scholars, who draw upon current findings from the trauma research to offer theoretical and practice perspectives highly useful for practitioners working with this population of children and their families.

Child welfare practitioners have for some time recognized that the trauma associated with child abuse and neglect and with separation from family members, combined with the environmental conditions of poverty, can undermine the healthy development of children and greatly increase their risk for social, behavioral, and psychiatric problems both in youth and in later life. The events of September 11, 2001, served to focus the larger professional community's attention more sharply on the effects of trauma on children and youth using child welfare services, as well as on their caretakers and front-line staff members. These events also underscored the need for a coordinated response from the professional disciplines and from the various other systems working with them in the aftermath of traumatic events.

Moreover, child welfare policy reforms of the last two decades have affirmed the importance of children's attachment relationships with their primary caretakers, and their need for stability and continuity in these relationships. These reforms placed new emphasis on the permanency needs of children. They also acknowledged that some children had actually been further traumatized by past child welfare practices—specifically, the unnecessary severing of their biological bonds and subsequent lingering in foster care. The new aim was to mitigate the harmful effects of these practices when possible, and to prevent them from happening to future generations of children in need of services. This emphasis was reflected in new funding strategies that increased access to mental health services to keep children from being scarred by the experiences of loss and family disruption, which are known to have rippling effects over the life cycle.

The contributing authors to this volume acknowledge the needs of *all* children in foster care for mental health services that address the themes of separation and loss universal to the foster care experience. Some authors offer more nuanced definitions of childhood trauma and implications for clinical practice with what may be a substantial segment of the general population of children served by the child welfare system. The children in this subpopulation are the tragic victims of persistent abuse and chronic neglect at the hands of caretakers who themselves suffer from severe mental health problems or chemical addictions, and/or those who are enmeshed in complex intergenerational networks of family dysfunction and psychopathology. Many such children have not yet benefited from policy reforms that strengthen child safety goals and make it possible for children to be placed in the familiar homes of relatives, who can play a protective role in reducing the additional trauma associated with family disruption and foster care placement.

Drawing on their clinical practice, research, and scholarship, the contributing authors offer the reader a wealth of information that provides new insights into the understanding and treatment of victims of childhood trauma. As a collective effort, this volume makes a significant contribution to the child welfare literature. It does so, first, by increasing sensitivity to the meaning of separation and loss as shared and universal themes in the lives of the general population of children served by the child welfare system; and, second, by offering new insights that support the development of specialized treatment interventions for children and youth suffering from severe and persistent forms of trauma associated with abuse and neglect, as well as from the further trauma caused by poorly planned and monitored substitute care arrangements.

The volume begins by providing a broad theoretical framework for understanding childhood trauma and implications for planning treatment interventions with traumatized children. It then applies these in descriptions of several types of helping interventions with such children in foster care. The volume is rich in case examples and illustrations of practical applications, making it especially useful for direct service practitioners in the planning of innovative treatment interventions for affected children and their families.

I am pleased that this volume has been edited by the current holder of the James R. Dumpson Chair in Child Welfare Studies. The activities of the Chair are devoted to scholarly, interdisciplinary undertakings directed toward building knowledge through research for improving the quality of services to children whose development is jeopardized by conditions in their families and/or in the larger environment. For me, it is both an honor and a humbling experience to have a named chair concerned with the plight of children most in danger of losing their rights because of poverty, discrimination, family disintegration, educational deficits, and substandard housing. This volume, in its application of the best available research to improve mental health outcomes for a population of children traditionally underserved by the mental health system, is very much in keeping with the vision and goals of the Chair. Dr. Webb and her colleagues continue the tradition established in past projects undertaken by holders of the Chair of building on existing knowledge to improve the well-being and outcomes of children.

This important volume appears at a time when the child welfare system is undergoing yet another transformation. This transformation is driven by changes occurring in the larger policy and practice context, which have profound implications for the planning and delivery of clinical services for children and families affected by trauma. The 1997 Adoption and Safe Families Act (ASFA) requires the achieving of the dual and often competing goals of child safety and family preservation. Answers to the difficult questions raised by ASFA–such as how best to ensure the safety of children while preserving family relationships, or how to help children who have experienced traumas associated with abuse and neglect and with foster care placement–are not easily found. Traumatic experiences for children do not occur solely within families, but at the community and society levels as well. Practice trends favoring neighborhood-based services must take this into account and invest in finding solutions to neighborhood and community conditions that increase risk for trauma and child victimization (Carten & Dumpson, 2004). Immigration trends are contributing further to changes in the demographic composition of the foster care caseload, and increasing the number of children and their families who will need help in coping with trauma–in this case, the trauma associated with the immigration and resettlement experience (Carten & Goodman, in press).

As a final word, as one who has devoted much of his professional career to advocating the creation of a caring society where all children can flourish, it is disheartening that although this is well within the realm of possibility, we have yet to make it a reality for all children. This notwithstanding, I am heartened by the ability of the child welfare system to transform and redefine itself in the context of changes in the larger environment, as well as by the resilience of children and families in its care. In the 1980s, when the crack cocaine epidemic was at its height, it was predicted that children exposed to drugs *in utero* would be severely damaged and drain the resources of an already overburdened system. As this social problem continued to unfold–and as a related crisis, the HIV/AIDS epidemic, emerged–it was predicted that hundreds of thousands of children would be either orphaned or otherwise severely affected, and that their needs would far exceed the capacity of the system to respond. With the dismantling of the "safety net" programs for the poor, it was predicted that more children would sink deeper into poverty, and that there would be a corresponding rise in child protective service reports and a swelling of the foster care caseload. None of these dire predictions came to pass, and although there may be considerable disagreement about how well it has done this, the child welfare system has responded to these challenges.

I raise these issues as a final word because this volume–largely based in a medical model for understanding the causes and treatment of childhood trauma–raises many new questions and leaves as many questions unanswered as answered. The *Supplement to the Surgeon General's Report on Mental Health* (U.S. Department of Health and Human Services, 2001) reports deep racial and ethnic disparities in mental health outcomes, and identifies children in foster care as a population about which more research is needed to inform evidence-based practice interventions. The Dumpson Chair also endeavors to promote critical discourse through faculty colloquia, to stimulate innovative research among doctoral students, and to support child welfare curriculum development in schools of social work. This latest publication, edited by the current holder of the Chair, can serve as a catalyst for such endeavors.

JAMES R. DUMPSON, PhD
Former New York City Commissioner of Welfare
Former New York City Human Resources Administrator
Former New York City Health Services Administrator and Chairman of the Health and Hospitals Corporation
Former Dean of the Fordham University Graduate School of Social Service
Former Associate Dean of the Hunter College School of Social Work
Senior Consultant and former Vice President, New York Community Trust

REFERENCES

Carten, A. J., & Dumpson, J. R. (2004). Family preservation and neighborhood based services: An Africentric perspective. In J. E. Everett, S. P. Chipungu, & B. R. Leashore (Eds.), *Child welfare revisited: An Africentric perspective* (pp. 225–241). New Brunswick, NJ: Rutgers University Press.

Carten, A. J., & Goodman, H. (in press). Development of an educational model for child welfare practice with immigrant families. *Child Welfare Journal.*

U.S. Department of Health and Human Services. (2001). *Supplement to the Surgeon General's report on mental health.* Washington, DC: Author.

Preface

In 2002, when I was appointed to the James R. Dumpson Chair in Child Welfare Studies at Fordham University Graduate School of Social Service, I immediately began thinking about how the field in which I was trained—children's mental health services—might begin working more cooperatively and productively with the child welfare field, and vice versa. I soon decided to work on an edited book, with authors from both professions contributing their expertise to enhance knowledge for competent practice.

I chose to focus on traumatized youth because of my own experience with this specialization, in addition to my growing awareness that practitioners in the child welfare field at that time did not appear to acknowledge that the abused and maltreated children in their care were in fact *traumatized* children. Therefore, the title of the book became *Working with Traumatized Youth in Child Welfare.*

In addition to the book, I decided to hold a colloquium on the same topic. Some of the chapter authors participated in the colloquium, and other participants were later recruited to contribute chapters because of their recognized expertise in the area. Thus this volume spans two fields of practice that overlap significantly, despite their histories of working independently. The professions of child welfare and of mental health share a concern for traumatized children, but they operate very differently in their approaches to helping. The purpose of the book is to highlight this shared focus, and to inspire and inform practitioners about working together more effectively for the ultimate benefit of their traumatized young clients.

The child welfare system exists to protect children whose families cannot do so. Some children enter this system as a direct result of recent physical or sexual abuse, whereas many others have endured years of chronic abuse and neglect.

Numerous factors may contribute to a family's inability to care for its children, including parental imprisonment, substance abuse, poverty, and mental illness. These circumstances can lead to neglect, abuse, and/or witnessing of violence; children or adolescents may be traumatized by any of these.

This book focuses on the impact of such traumatization on children and adolescents. It presents a framework for helping that is based on the combined knowledge and experience of mental health and children's services practitioners. The literature on attachment, stress, coping, trauma responses, and risk and resilience serves as a foundation for treatment approaches that include both the individual youth and his or her family when possible. Authors from both child welfare and mental health settings discuss the special challenges of treating traumatized children who have been removed from parental custody and placed in foster homes, residential treatment centers, and other juvenile facilities. They also acknowledge some of the difficulties in attempting to collaborate with practitioners who may have different views of how best to help.

Part I of the book presents an overview of the status of children and adolescents in the child welfare system (Chapter 1), as well as of the impact of trauma on this young population (Chapter 2). Chapter 3 describes the effects of traumatic abuse on the brain, with an emphasis on the implications of trauma and maltreatment for attachment formation and identity development. The topic of trauma assessment is covered in Chapter 4, which includes a review of selected methods of trauma screening, a few of which can be used even by child welfare practitioners without specialized training. Chapter 5 details the family and social factors that contribute to youth traumatization.

Part II of the book offers a variety of treatment approaches with detailed case illustrations. Many of these treatment methods have been specially adapted to deal with the traumatic and loss-laden histories of youth who have been placed out of their homes. Some of the specific topics covered by chapters in Part II include the following:

- Structured time-limited groups
- Individual play and expressive therapy
- Cognitive-behavioral approaches
- Eye movement desensitization and reprocessing
- Animal-assisted therapy

Because the cases described in these chapters have not all had successful outcomes, the authors discuss the particular challenges they have faced because of a child's or adolescent's history, his or her family and social situation, and the difficulties in coordinating mental health and children's services.

Part III of the book discusses challenges and proposals for improved collaboration between mental health services and the child welfare system. The Appendix lists a variety of training and other resources.

There has been a heightened awareness of trauma and its impact since the terrorist events in Oklahoma City on April 19, 1995, and in New York City and Washington, D.C., on September 11, 2001. Similarly, the effects of Hurricane Katrina in 2005 demonstrate how natural disasters can wreak havoc on families that were coping only marginally before the sudden destruction of their homes and communities. Although these acute national traumas differed greatly from chronic, family-based interpersonal trauma, I believe that the increased awareness about the harmful effects of trauma resulting from these events can be applied to children and adolescents in the child welfare system who have histories of either acute or ongoing abuse and trauma.

Child welfare workers have been dealing with traumatized youth for decades without adequate understanding or training in this area. Youth with serious clinical symptoms of depression or posttraumatic stress disorder cannot be helped adequately through a multisystemic approach that employs only family- and community-based interventions. These youth also require individual interventions that are explicitly intended to help them with their distressing and persistent symptoms. As presented in this book, we now have a variety of methods to help alleviate traumatic responses. This book's strong clinical perspective offers a mental health dimension to helping traumatized young people within the child welfare system, thereby strengthening the range of services traditionally offered in child welfare practice.

NANCY BOYD WEBB

Contents

PART I

THEORETICAL FRAMEWORK AND PRACTICE CONTEXT

CHAPTER 1

The Nature and Scope of the Problem

ANTHONY N. MALUCCIO

The field of child welfare in the United States has historically involved three interrelated goals in its mission:

- Protecting children and youth from actual or potential harm, especially child maltreatment;
- Preserving the family unit, including birth family and/or relatives;
- Promoting child well-being and the development of young people into adults who are able to live independently and contribute to their communities.

These goals–and the resulting policies and programs–have evolved in response to the needs of young people coming to the attention of the public or private child welfare system. Many or most of these youth are traumatized or become traumatized following their entry into out-of-home care. This chapter reviews the needs and situations of such youth; examines the response of the service delivery system; suggests required practice transformations; and considers issues in the preparation of adolescents for independent living.

YOUTH COMING TO THE ATTENTION OF THE CHILD WELFARE SYSTEM

We do not have adequate national data about the number of children and families receiving attention of the child welfare system in the United States. This number probably runs over a million at any given time. We know that annually over half a million children and adolescents are placed in some form of out-of-home care. This number has been increasing in recent years–apparently as a result of cuts in federal funds for preventive services, in addition to dramatic increases in parental substance abuse, homelessness, and unemployment, especially among ethnic minority groups.

Youth in out-of-home care placement (either family foster care or group care) represent a major group at risk. According to the most recent data available, there were over 520,000 children in out-of-home care as of March 31, 1998 (U.S. Department of Health and Human Services, 1999). Also, the U.S. Department of Health and Human Services (2003) has estimated that in 2001 there were 1,321 (or 1.81%) child fatalities in foster care. Although precise data are not available, it is reported that most children enter foster care because of the consequences of parent-related problems, largely child abuse or neglect (Berrick, Needell, Barth, & Jonson-Reid, 1998). In addition, increasing proportions of children with special problems are entering care. These include children with special physical or developmental needs; children with HIV infection; infants born with crack cocaine addiction or other effects of exposure to substance use; children from poor or multiproblem families; and/or children with emotional problems (see, e.g., Dore, 1999).

The proportion of adolescents in out-of-home care has increased rapidly since the 1980s, as the permanency planning movement initially resulted in keeping younger children out of care, reuniting them with their biological families following placement, or placing them in adoption or other permanent plans (Maluccio, 1998). Older youth in placement or making the transition out of care are especially vulnerable and require extensive help. Most of them have entered care because of abuse and neglect, including sexual abuse, plus exposure to and involvement in multiple incidents of violence and other traumatic experiences. Many have lived in numerous out-of-home placements or have been returned home and removed repeatedly (Pecora, Whittaker, Maluccio, & Barth, 2000). Moreover, many of them anticipate the future experience of leaving the child welfare system as yet another separation or rejection in their young lives.

A disproportionate and expanding number of children, youth, and families of color are coming to the attention of child welfare services. Unfortunately, there is substantial evidence that minority youth who enter the child welfare system are at greater risk for poor outcomes than their white counterparts (see Jackson & Brissett-Chapman, 1997). In addition, although they are disproportionately represented in foster care and in the child welfare system in general, young people of color receive inadequate as well as differential treatment. Research has found that "children of color and their families experience poorer outcomes and receive fewer services than their [white] counterparts" (Courtney et al., 1996, p. 99).

Another risk factor for young people entering the child welfare system is exposure to substance abuse and/or violence at home and at school, as well as in the community in general. Family violence has a direct impact on the development of attention and conduct problems in both boys and girls (Becker & McCloskey, 2002). In addition to its impact on a young person, violence impedes a parent's ability to meet his or her child's needs. In extreme cases, the result is incarceration of a parent, which provokes further traumatic stress in the child (Smith, Krisman, Strozier, & Marley, 2004).

Young people living with parents who abuse substances are at higher risk for physical abuse and neglect. Over 15 years ago, the National Committee for Prevention of Child Abuse (1989) estimated that 9–10 million children are affected by parental substance abuse, and that 675,000 children are maltreated each year by caretakers addicted to alcohol and other drugs. These numbers have undoubtedly increased since then. Among confirmed cases of child maltreatment nationwide, from 40% to 80% involve substance abuse problems that interfere with parenting (Child Welfare League of America, 1998).

When young people are cared for by parents with substance abuse problems, they are often exposed to a number of risks in addition to child maltreatment, including these (Maluccio & Ainsworth, 2003; Tracy, 1994):

- Chaotic and often dangerous neighborhoods.
- Poverty and homelessness or unstable housing.
- Neglect of the youth's basic needs.
- Lack of an extended family and community support system.
- A parent or parents with poor parenting skills and few or no role models for effective coping.
- Placement in out-of-home care.

RESPONSE BY THE SERVICE DELIVERY SYSTEM

Various programs have evolved in response to the needs of the increasing numbers of youth and their families coming to the attention of child welfare, mental health, and correctional agencies. These include both *traditional* services and *innovative* programs. Traditional services include kinship care, family foster care, residential group care, and adoption. Especially noteworthy is the increase in use of kinship care throughout the country. Although there are obvious advantages to keeping children within the context of their families of origin, we should note that kinship care raises numerous issues that should be considered, including questions about funding, relationships between parents and relatives, and relationships between families and agencies (Hegar & Scannapieco, 1999; Webb, 2003). "Achieving successful outcomes for children in kinship care requires . . . philosophical shifts, policy changes, and practice efforts that support kin caregivers and children" (Lorkovich, Picolla, Groza, Brindo, & Marks, 2004, p. 159). In this regard, it is noteworthy that there are standards and measures for kinship care assessment (Chipman, Wells, & Johnson, 2002).

In addition to such traditional services, innovative programs have evolved in the field of child welfare. These include family preservation, treatment foster care, family reunification, independent living programs, family group decision making, shared family care, and wraparound services. Evaluative studies indicate that these innovations are effective in promoting children's development, especially if the programs are adequately funded and if practitioners and their supervisors are fully trained and supported in their work (Maluccio, Ainsworth, & Thoburn, 2000).

Mental health services have also been developed on behalf of children and families at risk. In situations involving trauma, the fields of child welfare and mental health are becoming much more closely integrated, in contrast to their earlier history; at least, they are collaborating more actively both in provision of services to children and their families, *and* in efforts to influence preventive programs as well as state and federal legislation. We see such collaboration in at least two areas.

First, child welfare and mental health agencies collaborate in planning joint training programs for their staffs, particularly in the area of trauma (such as the trauma of physical and emotional abuse). An innovative feature of some of these programs is the involvement of especially competent and effective workers–and also parents and older adolescents–as trainers or consultants. Such programs also emphasize helping caseworkers to identify children's basic needs, including mental health needs, when they develop case plans and provide services.

Second, in many communities child welfare workers and mental health practitioners participate jointly in case conferences and case planning for parents and/or children with substance abuse, HIV/AIDS, and multiple health or mental health problems. A special feature of these programs is that child welfare and mental health workers build into the service plan the requirement to keep each other informed of progress in each case; in addition, they schedule periodic follow-up conferences to review and revise treatment plans. Moreover, the services are typically provided by one or another of the agencies involved, rather than through referring a case to still another agency that is not known to the clients. The latter approach has contributed to the high dropout rate of child welfare clients referred to mental health clinics; when a family is referred to an unknown agency with a long waiting period, its members lose interest or motivation by the time an appointment becomes available.

Although these innovations are noteworthy, there are other populations for whom greater and better collaboration is required. These include (1) children with developmental disabilities; (2) children with incarcerated parents; and (3) children from families affected by substance abuse.

The occurrence of developmental disabilities in children may be related to trauma caused by accidents or by child abuse, especially during the first year. An estimated 25% of all developmental disabilities are the result of child maltreatment (Maluccio, Pine, & Tracy, 2002). Children with disabilities are at high risk of being abused or neglected and thus experiencing further trauma–partly because their need for special care may be overwhelming for their families or communities. The families, in particular, may be suffering from preexisting environmental problems and life pressures. Practitioners should be aware of the educational rights to which children with disabilities and their families are entitled through the Individuals with Disabilities Education Act, P.L. 101-476 (Altshuler & Kopels, 2003).

In regard to children of incarcerated parents, we need to pay attention to the major rise in the prison population–another serious risk factor for children and families coming to the attention of the child welfare system (Smith et al., 2004). Current estimates are that nearly 2 million children and youth in the United States have an incarcerated parent. Furthermore, the number of women in prison has risen dramatically in recent years. Many of these women abuse substances and have children at home or in foster care. The impact of separation from their mothers often leads to anxiety, low self-esteem, and depression in these children.

Children who witness violence are likely to be overrepresented in families with substance abuse and incarceration. Here again, there are few services for these children–services that could be effectively provided through collaboration among prison, child welfare, and mental health staffs.

Service needs for families with substance abuse extend beyond traditional treatment programs and child welfare services into a variety of additional services in the areas of housing, early childhood intervention, vocational programs, and health and mental health treatment. Especially required–though difficult to implement successfully–are programs enabling mothers or fathers to learn to parent again while simultaneously learning to adopt and maintain a sober lifestyle.

PRACTICE TRANSFORMATIONS

Establishing and maintaining the kinds of programs described in the preceding section require transformations in child welfare as well as mental health practice. Accordingly, as delineated by Pecora et al. (2000, pp. 14–

20), various service reforms have been implemented—or at least initiated—in recent years. The major ones are highlighted in this section.

"Safety planning"—that is, establishing a safe working environment for child, family, and staff members in each case situation—has emerged as a basic practice approach particularly in family situations involving potential risks. The objectives are (1) to protect the child as well as other family members; and (2) to provide every child with a "forever home" through family preservation, reunification, termination of parental rights and adoption, or long-term foster care with guardianship—in that order of priority.

Safety planning is promoted through the use of community-based and neighborhood-based programs, school-based services, wraparound services, youth employment programs, and managed care techniques, thus broadening the mix of service options in many communities. These innovations are noteworthy, as they enable child welfare agencies to become more fully integrated into the community and better positioned to call upon economic, educational, mental health, housing, vocational, education, and other resources for assistance in achieving the shared outcomes they have created for children and parents.

Also evolving are "systems of care" approaches in the field of mental health. Such approaches are intended to organize and deliver services on the basis of three core practice emphases: child- and family-centered, community-based, and culturally competent (Stroul & Friedman, 1996). By implementing these core approaches, agencies can reduce barriers to service, involve parents and children more extensively, and promote the coordination of services. In the field of child welfare, the use of a public–private partnership model of service delivery promotes collaboration and service effectiveness (Lewandowski & GlenMaye, 2002).

In line with the emphasis on service coordination, child welfare agencies are increasingly collaborating with mental health as well as public health agencies. Such systems of care help "to coordinate and integrate mental health services for children and youths, while simultaneously managing existing funding sources more effectively" (Anderson, McIntyre, Rotte, & Robertson, 2002, p. 514). For example, models of child abuse prevention and family support involve public health nurses, social workers, and/or other practitioners (e.g., Olds & Kitzman, 1995). These programs are utilized particularly for families with HIV/AIDS and for children and youth with special needs. They hold promise of more extensive partnerships between child welfare and public health agencies; they also have the potential to strengthen preventive services in the area of child maltreatment in nonstigmatizing ways.

As previously noted, the increase in the numbers of families with substance abuse issues has created a need for additional prevention and treatment programs. Partnerships among child welfare, early childhood, education, mental health, primary health care, and substance abuse treatment services are crucial.

PREPARATION FOR INDEPENDENT LIVING

As noted earlier in this chapter, the proportion of adolescents in family foster care and residential treatment in the United States has increased rapidly since the 1980s. Most of these adolescents are discharged to another plan upon reaching majority age at 18 –typically, to some form of independent living, though it is unrealistic in contemporary society to expect them to be truly independent at such an age.

Evaluative studies regarding the functioning of these young people, in fact, have reported largely negative findings. First, foster parents and social workers have consistently reported that most adolescents approaching emancipation are unprepared for independent living (Maluccio et al., 2000). Second, follow-up studies of young people who grew up in out-of-home placement have pointed to their lack of preparation for life after foster care. Third, it has been found that a high number of homeless persons have a history of foster care placement, with some having been placed in both foster family and residential settings. For instance, Roman and Wolfe (1997) found that persons with a history of foster care placement were overrepresented in the homeless population.

The challenges in preparation for independent living include preparing youth earlier in their placement; offering better vocational assessment and training; providing adequate health care; helping youth to develop life skills; and maintaining supports for young people as they move into adulthood (Nollan et al., 2000). Such a panoply of services is essential, as adolescents in foster care generally have limited supports in their families and social networks and are often emotionally, intellectually, and/or physically delayed from a developmental perspective.

It should also be noted that the very concept of "independent living" has been criticized, especially since it creates unrealistic and unfair expectations of adolescents who have left or are preparing to leave foster care (Maluccio et al., 2000). We have proposed, instead, the concept of "interdependent living" in practice with young people in out-of-home care. Such a concept reflects the assumption that human beings are interdependent, "that is, able to relate to–and function with–others, using community influences and resources, being able to carry out management tasks of daily life and having a productive quality of life through positive interactions with individuals, groups, organizations, and social systems" (Maluccio et al., 2000, p. 88). Practice approaches that emphasize the value of interdependence serve to empower young people who are making the transition from foster care (Propp, Ortega, & NewHeart, 2003).

CONCLUSION

Recent decades have seen a substantial increase in both the number and variety of child welfare services, due in large measure to the contributions of child welfare workers, mental health practitioners, foster parents, child care workers, and other community partners and professionals. As a result, we have considerable knowledge of how traumatized children and youth and their families can be effectively helped at both the treatment and prevention levels. In addition, there are examples of excellent programs that can be adapted in other communities.

We also know that the field of child welfare has for too long been hampered by federal and state funding policies that have rewarded the "wrong" program emphases, such as completing child abuse investigations (rather than preventing the need for new ones) and keeping children in foster care (instead of securing more permanent homes for them). With the renewed emphasis on preserving families for children, agencies are striving to align funding priorities and performance incentive mechanisms to support preventive services along with greater program flexibility.

Such emphasis is leading to decreased use of unnecessary out-of-home care; increased use of services that support preserving families or returning young people to their own homes; and optimized collaboration between the child welfare and mental health service delivery systems. At the same time, it is essential that we continue to persist in working together to meet recurring challenges–especially in regard to funding and politics–in the decision, implementation, and evaluation of such services.[1]

ACKNOWLEDGMENTS

Sections of this chapter have been adapted from Maluccio, Pine, and Tracy (2002) and Maluccio, Ainsworth, and Thoburn (2000). Copyright 2002 by Columbia University Press, and copyright 2000 by the Child Welfare League of America, respectively. Adapted by permission.

REFERENCES

Altshuler, S. J., & Kopels, S. (2003). Advocating in schools for children with disabilities: What's new with IDEA? *Social Work*, *48*, 320–329.

Anderson, J. A., McIntyre, J. S., Rotte, K. I., & Robertson, D. C. (2002).

[1]Following a year of deliberations, the Pew Commission on Children in Foster Care released on May 18, 2004 its recommendations for reforming the nation's child welfare system (see www.socialworkers.org/advocacy/updates/082003_a.asp).

Developing and maintaining collaboration in systems of care for children and youths with emotional and behavioral disabilities and their families. *American Journal of Orthopsychiatry, 72,* 514–525.

Becker, K. B., & McCloskey, L. A. (2002). Attention and conduct problems in children exposed to family violence. *American Journal of Orthopsychiatry, 72,* 83–91.

Berrick, J. D., Needell, B., Barth, R. P., & Jonson-Reid, M. (1998). *The tender years: Toward developmentally sensitive child welfare services for very young children.* New York: Oxford University Press.

Child Welfare League of America. (1998). *Breaking the link between substance abuse and child maltreatment: An issue forum.* Washington, DC: Author.

Chipman, F., Wells, S. J., & Johnson, M. A. (2002). The meaning of quality in kinship foster care: Caregiver, child and worker perspectives. *Families in Society: The Journal of Contemporary Human Services, 83,* 508–520.

Courtney, M. E., Barth, R. P., Berrick, J. D., Brooks, D., Needell, B., & Park, L. (1996). Race and child welfare services: Past research and future directions. *Child Welfare, 75,* 99–137.

Dore, M. (1999). Emotionally and behaviorally disturbed children in the child welfare system: Points of intervention. *Children and Youth Services Review, 66,* 335–348.

Hegar, R. L., & Scannapieco, M. (Eds.). (1999). *Kinship foster care: Policy, practice, and research.* New York: Oxford University Press.

Jackson, S., & Brissett-Chapman, S. (Eds.). (1997). Perspectives in serving African American children, youths, and families [Special issue]. *Child Welfare, 76,* 3–278.

Lewandowski, C. A., & GlenMaye, L. F. (2002). Teams in child welfare settings: Interprofessional and collaborative processes. *Families in Society: The Journal of Contemporary Human Services, 83,* 245–256.

Lorkovich, T. W., Picolla, T., Groza, V., Brindo, M. E., & Marks, J. (2004). Kinship care and permanence: Guiding principles for policy and practice. *Families in Society: The Journal of Contemporary Human Services, 85,* 159–164.

Maluccio, A. N. (1998). Assessing child welfare outcomes: The American perspective. *Children and Society, 12,* 161–168.

Maluccio, A. N., & Ainsworth, F. (2003). Drug use by parents: A challenge for family reunification practice. *Children and Youth Services Review, 25,* 511–533.

Maluccio, A. N., Ainsworth, F., & Thoburn, J. (2000). *Child welfare outcome research in the United States, United Kingdom, and Australia.* Washington, DC: Child Welfare League of America Press.

Maluccio, A. N., Pine, B. A., & Tracy, E. M. (2002). *Social work practice with families and children.* New York: Columbia University Press.

National Committee for Prevention of Child Abuse. (1989). *Fact sheet: Substance abuse and child abuse.* Chicago: Author.

Nollan, K. A., Wolf, M., Ansell, D., Burns, J., Barr, L., Copeland, W., & Paddock, G. (2000). Ready or not: Assessing youths' preparedness for independent living. *Child Welfare, 79,* 159–176.

Olds, D. L., & Kitzman, H. (1995). Review of research on home visiting for pregnant women and parents of young children. *The Future of Children: Home Visiting, 3,* 53–92.

Pecora, P. J., Whittaker, J. K., Maluccio, A. N., & Barth, R. P. (2000). *The child welfare challenge: Policy, practice, and research* (2nd ed.). New York: Aldine de Gruyter.

Propp, J., Ortega, D. M., & NewHeart, R. (2003). Independence and interdependence: Rethinking the transition from "ward of the court" to adulthood. *Families in Society: The Journal of Contemporary Human Services, 84*, 259–266.

Roman, N. P., & Wolfe, P. B. (1997). The relationship between foster care and homelessness. *Public Welfare, 55*, 4–9.

Smith, A., Krisman, K., Strozier, A. L., & Marley, M. (2004). Breaking through the bars: Exploring the experiences of addicted incarcerated parents when children are cared for by relatives. *Families in Society: The Journal of Contemporary Human Services, 85*, 187–195.

Stroul, B. A., & Friedman, R. M. (1996). The system of care concept and philosophy. In B. A. Stroul (Ed.), *Children's mental health: Creating systems of care in a changing society* (pp. 3–22). Baltimore: Brookes.

Tracy, E. M. (1994). Maternal substance abuse: Protecting the child, preserving the family. *Social Work, 39*, 534–540.

U.S. Department of Health and Human Services, Administration for Children and Families. (1999). *The AFCARS report: Current estimates as of January 1999.* Retrieved from www.acf.dhhs.gov/programs/chdata (January 5, 2000).

U.S. Department of Health and Human Services, Administration for Children and Families. (2003). *Child maltreatment–2001.* Washington, DC: U. S. Government Printing Office.

Webb, N. B. (2003). *Social work practice with children* (2nd ed.). New York: Guilford Press.

CHAPTER 2

The Impact of Trauma on Youth and Families in the Child Welfare System

NANCY BOYD WEBB

The occurrence of trauma is usually unpredictable, with effects that can bring lifelong psychological damage and suffering to the unfortunate victims. Traumas come in many shapes and forms–sometimes resulting from deliberate human actions, and at other times occurring as random "acts of God." As an example of the first type, a small boy can be traumatized by a desperate young mother who believes that beating him and locking him in a closet will teach him not to wet his bed. This boy may experience further traumatization at a later time, when a child welfare investigator responding to a neighbor's complaint takes him away suddenly from his mother and siblings, and moves him into a strange home with foster parents and other unknown children. Many youth enter the child welfare system for similar reasons: They are born to poverty-stricken adolescent mothers who lack the knowledge, skills, and/or motivation to care adequately for their infants and dependent young children. The mothers' haphazard parenting often results in periodic or chronic neglect of their children, which may be interspersed with occasional eruptions of abusive behavior when the children cry, misbehave, or otherwise make demands for attention. Sometimes other family members step in to try to assist such a mother by caring for her children. They may take one, several, or all of the children to their homes, where the mother may visit erratically or not at all. This early history of disrupted relationships, chronic neglect, and sporadic abuse is sadly common among children who subsequently end up in foster homes and residential treatment centers, after their family members prove to be unwilling or unable to provide the consistent daily care and emotional support that all children need for their normal development.

This chapter discusses the impact of repeated traumas of various types on the attachment relationships and the developmental course of children and adolescents, and the breakdown of family relationships that culminates in out-of-home placements. Special attention is given to the topics of attachment and loss, and to the cumulative effects of multiple separation experiences on both children/youth and their families.

TRAUMA

The word "trauma" comes from the Greek, meaning "wound," and in an expanded sense it is now used to refer to an emotional wound caused by a frightening and painful experience. Since the terrorist attacks of September 11, 2001, the U.S. general public has become familiar with the term, but not always with its actual meaning; people may use it carelessly to refer to events that are upsetting but not truly traumatic. In contrast, mental health specialists rely on the definition provided in the official criteria for the diagnosis of posttraumatic stress disorder (American Psychiatric Association, 2000, p. 467) as the basis for understanding the circumstances that set the stage for traumatic responses. The first of these criteria defines a "traumatic event" as one that threatens actual death or serious injury to an individual or to others, and in which the individual who is traumatized experiences intense fear, helplessness, or horror. As a result of the terrifying experience, the person develops a variety of symptoms.

The Nature of the Traumatic Event

Lenore Terr (1991) distinguishes between Type I and Type II traumas, with Type I consisting of a single event (e.g., seeing a parent murdered), and Type II consisting of *numerous* frightening events occurring over time (as in many cases of physical or sexual abuse). In most circumstances, Type I traumas do not lead to long-term symptoms, and recovery occurs in more than three-quarters of cases, even after very tragic experiences (McFarlane, 1990; Cohen, 2004). Therefore, the response of a child who is placed in a foster home after his or her mother is murdered in a drive-by shooting will probably be drastically different from that of a child who is placed following repeated experiences of abuse and neglect at the hands of a mother with substance addiction. These examples draw attention to the *source* of the trauma, and particularly to whether it has resulted from an accident or an intentional act. In addition, when the person who inflicts the trauma is a caretaker on whom the child depends and toward whom he or she feels some form of attachment, the child's response will tend to be more complicated and more resistant to treatment than the reactions of a child who was traumatized by a stranger as the result of a random event.

The Tripartite Assessment

Multiple factors influence any individual's response to a trauma. The nature of the overall circumstances in which the trauma occurs, the individual's own history, and the degree of support in the surrounding environment all contribute to the person's specific responses to a traumatic experience. I refer to the assessment of these three sets of factors—individual and family factors, social/environmental factors, and mediating factors in the support system—as the "tripartite assessment" (Webb, 2003). Often youth in the child welfare system have compromised personal histories due to their backgrounds of neglect and abuse, and they may live in an environment of poverty and ongoing danger with few mediating factors to support them. This makes these youth especially vulnerable to the stresses of everyday life, as well as to feelings of terror and anxiety associated with traumatic experiences.

Neurological Effects of Early Trauma

Growing evidence suggests that trauma alters the early development of the right brain, thereby compromising the capacity to cope with emotional stress (Schore, 2003; Perry et al., 2001; see also Perry, Chapter 3, this volume). These early experiences may have a lasting effect, insofar as "responses to early trauma need to be understood as the initial manifestations of long-term risks to the child's unfolding development" (Lieberman & Van Horn, 2004, p. 112). Thus a child who does not begin developing the ability to regulate his or her emotions in the first 2 years of life may fail to develop this ability later; as a result, this child may resort to hostile, aggressive behavior to deal with his or her own overreactivity to stress.

The effects on the brain as a result of trauma early in life occur not only when a child is a victim of abuse, but also when he or she witnesses or otherwise experiences the effects of domestic violence in the home. The child's neurophysiological responses are believed to produce subsequent changes in his or her brain structure and functioning. According to Lieberman and Van Horn (2004, p. 117), "These changes in central nervous system functioning can leave a traumatized child feeling perpetually anxious and on edge, or psychologically numb. They can lead to the child's experiencing persistent and overgeneralized fears." These responses, in turn, may result in a later propensity toward violence and a lack of empathy and disregard for the feelings of others (Schore, 2003).

The implications of this startling evidence should cause practitioners in the child welfare field to commit themselves to early intervention that is family- and caretaker-centered, in order to curtail (as much as possible) the potentially awesome effects of early abuse on a young child. Methods for reversing or ameliorating early brain damage are still being explored and present special challenges for treatment planning.

ATTACHMENT

Infancy and Early Childhood

The developing baby faces two major tasks in the first year of his or her life (Van Horn & Lieberman, 2004). These are (1) to establish a relationship with an adult caretaker, and (2) to learn to modulate his or her feelings so that they are not overwhelming. This modulation process is referred to as "affect regulation" by Schore (2003) and as the "regulation of fearful arousal" by Schuder and Lyons-Ruth (2004). Regardless of the terminology used, the ability to attain a sense of calm after a period of being upset is essential to keep the infant from feeling consistently overstimulated and overwhelmed. Because infants by definition are immature, they all require assistance in calming themselves much of the time. This task requires the active participation of an adult partner who takes the initiative in comforting, protecting, stimulating, and gently encouraging a baby in the process of restoring the infant's sense of stability and well-being. Babies who have the good fortune to receive appropriate and loving attention from caretakers who are attuned to their needs will develop a trusting attachment relationship to these persons, and this attachment produces a sense of protection from danger. When a traumatic event occurs, such as a house fire or an accidental injury, attentive and sensitive caretakers will control their own fears in order to soothe and comfort their infants and to keep the babies' anxiety from escalating. Children who are blessed with these secure relationships with caretakers usually do not end up in the child welfare system, and therefore are not the focus of this book. Rather, this volume concentrates on those babies whose caretakers fail to comfort them when they are upset, and who as a result learn very early that they cannot rely on adults. Sadly, some caretakers not only neglect the babies in their care, but also abuse them by speaking angrily to them or even hitting or shaking them when they cry. This constitutes trauma to the infants, who are helpless and who remain in a state of hyperarousal and fear. In such situations, these traumatized infants do not know from one minute to the next whether they will receive care, or will be ignored or abused. They experience their world as unpredictable and unsafe; their attachment relationships reflect this uncertainty, and therefore are characterized as "anxious" or "insecure."

The nature of the child–caretaker relationship received intense scrutiny in John Bowlby's (1969/1982) seminal work on attachment, which outlined the different forms that this relationship may take. Studies by Ainsworth, Blehar,, Waters,, and Wall (1978) and by Main and Solomon (1990) confirmed and expanded on Bowlby's work, with identification of several subtypes of attachment. As summarized by Davies (2004), these subtypes include the following:

- Secure
- Insecure–avoidant

- Insecure–ambivalent/resistant
- Insecure–disorganized/disoriented

Secure Attachment

The cornerstone of attachment behavior is proximity seeking (Bowlby, 1969/1982). The baby wants to be held close and feels safe in the arms or lap of a protective adult. In situations in which the baby becomes disturbed or alarmed, he or she cries to signal distress and the need for relief through the experience of being picked up and comforted. The infant is biologically programmed to desire closeness to an adult protector, who ideally notices and responds to his or her cries of distress. Similarly, a toddler who is upset approaches and clings to the caretaker, thereby signaling his or her desire for physical reassurance through bodily contact. The ideal form of attuned relationship between baby/child and caretaker (usually the mother) has been labeled "secure attachment." Babies with secure attachment come to expect that their needs will be met, and that their caretakers will protect them from harm. A mother's or other caretaker's response is critical in shaping an infant/child's ability to tolerate stress and other intense emotions. Without this gradual process of learning how to regulate their affect, children grow up at the mercy of their emotions (affect dysregulation), and also without a sense of trust in the ability of adults to help them when they are afraid.

Insecure Attachments

As listed above, there are three different forms of insecure attachment. These stem from different types of inappropriate caretaker–child interactions that result in distinctive behaviors in the child. Insecure attachment occurs when a caretaker is oblivious to, inattentive to, or angry about a child's needs for comfort. This statement may appear to be judgmental and insensitive about the mother's or other caretaker's situation, feelings, and motivation. However, we know that many mothers of insecurely attached children were themselves abused and insecurely attached as children, and their personal backgrounds make them unable to behave sympathetically toward their own children. This review of insecure attachment (as well as the case example later in this chapter, and the content of many other chapters in this book) acknowledges the intergenerational influence of a mother's *own* history as a child on her ability to meet her children's needs. The research on the intergenerational transmission of insecure attachment increasingly supports this conclusion (National Clearinghouse on Child Abuse and Neglect Information, 2002; Pears & Capaldi, 2001; Schore, 2003).

"Insecure–avoidant attachment" occurs in infants who have learned to expect rejection or disapproval from their angry mothers (or other caretakers), and who as a result have developed precocious defenses of appearing self-contained, withdrawn, and expressionless. They do not show their upset in distressing situations, because they have learned that their mothers do not tolerate their negative feelings, and this negative conditioning has led them to fear being punished for expressing them. These babies/toddlers still want contact and manage to stay close to their mothers, but they do not expect any solace from them. As these babies/toddlers grow into preschoolers, they continue their insecure–avoidant behavior with other adults, and this makes them appear distant and withdrawn. In situations where most children would seek help from an adult, these avoidant children tend to sulk and withdraw. Having learned that others will not help them, they develop a hostile, aggressive, and negative attitude with both adults and peers.

"Insecure–ambivalent/resistant attachment" occurs when mothers are inconsistent in their responses to their babies, and the babies become distressed and angry as a result. Sometimes their mothers meet their needs, and at other times they ignore them. The children want close bodily contact with their mothers, but seem very uncertain and insecure about how to approach their mothers. As they grow older and enter preschool, they maintain a similar inhibition and lack of assertiveness in peer and social interactions.

"Insecure–disorganized/disoriented attachment" occurs among babies who live with parents (or other caretakers) who frequently frighten and mistreat them. Because of the parents' abusive behavior, these children never know how the parents will behave and whether they will be sympathetic and comforting or angry and hurtful. As previously mentioned, researchers have found that many parents of children with disorganized/disoriented attachments have histories of unresolved traumas themselves; the parents' own compromised backgrounds prevent them from providing appropriate comforting behaviors toward their children. The parents' ongoing anxieties and fears that originated in their own traumatic pasts become reenacted in their relationships with their children through the intergenerational transmission of disordered attachment (Schore, 2003). The results are often physical and/or sexual abuse and rejection of the children. Therefore the children become traumatized at an early age by their parents, even as the parents years before endured similar pain at their own parents' hands.

Disorganized/disoriented attachment relationships frequently coexist with substance abuse, mental illness, and other risk factors, such as poverty and family disorganization (Ouimette & Brown, 2003; see also Anderson & Seita, Chapter 5, and Tracy & Johnson, Chapter 7, this volume). The multiple factors leading to abuse clearly point to the essential importance of involving the parent/caretaker/family in each child/youth's treatment plan.

Effects of Attachment History on Placement

When children with insecure attachment histories enter the child welfare system, they come with expectations about adult behavior that are based on their own early experience with their adult caretakers. One might speculate that a child with an abusive or neglectful parent might feel relief at being put into a safe environment with adults who are consistent and dependable. But the child who has little or no experience to cause him or her to trust any adult approaches a new relationship in anticipation of further rejection and even abuse. Many such children suffer from low self-esteem and have come to believe that they are as "bad" as their caretakers have accused them of being. Because children with attachment disorders *expect* rejection and hostility from others, they present with personas ranging from guarded to negative to actively hostile and aggressive. Crenshaw and Hardy (Chapter 10, this volume) poignantly refer to these children as "fawns in gorilla suits"! In other words, they may have an underlying sweet, innocent identity like a fawn, but they hide this with the tough exterior of an angry gorilla. Clearly, this is a defensive reaction. Children who have many years of unsatisfactory or hurtful relationships with adults stop expecting anything different. In addition, those who have been abused may have full or partial symptoms of posttraumatic stress disorder, thereby making them unnaturally alert and on guard for the next attack (which they think is inevitable, given their past experience). They tend to overreact in situations they perceive as dangerous, and may misread another person's face as angry when it would be more accurately described as registering mild disapproval. They do not trust others, and their behavior conveys their attitudes of disdain, contempt, and/or remoteness. Needless to say, these youth are very difficult to manage, and often adults give up on them. By the time they reach adolescence, many have assumed a very tough exterior that holds adults at bay and that resists engagement in any kind of trusting relationship.

Impact of Traumatic Experiences on Children/Youth's Development

Using the previous definition of trauma as a guide makes it clear that various forms of abusive behavior at the hands of a parent/caretaker can result in trauma for a child. The earlier discussion has detailed how abuse from a parent/caretaker can contribute to an insecure and disordered attachment relationship; it has also noted how the effects of a disordered attachment relationship early in life tend to persist as the child grows, due to the child/youth's ongoing expectations about the behavior of others. Bowlby (1969/1982) referred to an individual's conclusions about the reactions of others as "internal working models," which serve as templates for interpreting future relationships.

This conceptualization may seem to be overly deterministic, and of course it does not apply rigidly and universally to all children. Schore (2003) reassures us that not *all* emotionally neglected and traumatized children turn into violent adolescents who lack empathy for others. He refers especially to the possibility that a single positive relationship can deter a life trajectory that appeared to be headed for tragedy. Other factors that may contribute to a youth's resilience include a safe haven in the community, and the child's own temperament and intellectual capacity (Van Horn & Lieberman, 2004). However, many youth in the child welfare system have not had the good fortune to have these redeeming factors in their lives; they possess, instead, a bleak and harsh outlook on life that serves to turn other people away from them.

MULTIPLE LOSSES

As already indicated, the entry of a child into the child welfare system generally occurs because of neglect or abuse: An adult caretaker has been found incapable of providing adequately for the child or has been determined to have harmed him or her. Statistics indicate that about 55% of children reported to state child protective service agencies have been victims of neglect; about 25% have suffered physical abuse; and 12% have been victims of sexual abuse (Children's Defense Fund, 2000). The potentially traumatizing effects of these experiences on children have already been discussed in terms of the resulting insecure attachment relationships. Because of society's commitment to ensure safety to helpless and dependent young children, the child protective services agency has the responsibility to make an assessment after a complaint has been filed, and then it has the power to remove a child from his or her family and to place him or her in a safe environment. The child may be placed with extended family members (kinship placement) or in a foster home with strangers. Sometimes youth who are out of control and difficult to manage are placed in emergency shelters or residential facilities.

Regardless of the type of placement, babies/children/youth who are removed from their familiar environments and the daily interactions with their known caretakers suffer losses through this relocation. They must become acquainted with new people, new food, and different beds, in addition to new and different expectations regarding adult rules about appropriate behavior. Besides these necessary home-based adjustments, older children have to get used to new schools, new peers, and new neighborhoods. Dave Pelzer (1995, 1997, 2000), in his three autobiographical accounts of his life in various foster homes, refers to his great discomfort in having to admit to his schoolmates that he did not live with his parents. Children who have grown up anticipating inconsistent or negative responses from others have a lot of difficulty adjusting to different circumstances. They typically expect a continuation of their abusive, neglectful experiences with their new caretakers, and their lack of trust and tendency to overreact create problems for them in adapting to their new environments.

Age considerations may further influence the children's adjustment. For example, toddlers or preschoolers who have been abused often believe that they were somehow to blame for what happened. Young children, who are typically egocentric, do not have the capacity to understand the motivation of others; they cannot comprehend that their parents or caretakers are mentally ill, addicted to substances, or otherwise unable to care for them properly, and that these factors are the real causes of the abusive behavior. Instead, they assume that they themselves caused the abuse or neglect because they were in some way "bad."

Older children or adolescents gradually become aware that their families were deficient and/or destructive, compared to the home lives of less troubled kids. This awareness brings with it a painful sense of loss for the young persons of "what they never had"—families that loved and protected them. This profound realization can bring about a deep and tragic sense of deprivation; some youth respond to this with rage, and others with the beginnings of a deep depression.

The family of a child in placement may experience varying degrees of shame, guilt, or anger about the situation. In an earlier publication (Webb, 2003), I have referred to the placement of an infant or child as a form of public exposure in which one or both parents have been deemed unfit to care for their own child. This "loss of face" constitutes a form of "disenfranchised grief" (Doka, 2002), because the stigma of the placement cannot be openly discussed or mourned. Therefore, whereas the child experiences a loss of his or her familiar environment and relationships, the family suffers the public humiliation of being declared unfit to carry out its parenting roles. Often the family protects itself from feeling inadequate by blaming the system: "What right do *they* have to tell me how to raise my own child?" This angry resistance presents a challenge to child welfare workers who have been advised that they should consider family members as "partners" in the treatment planning for their child.

A CASE OF THREE GENERATIONS IN THE CHILD WELFARE SYSTEM

The award-winning investigative journalism of Nina Bernstein (2001) presented the lives of three generations of a poverty-stricken black family, the Wilders, who were involved with the child welfare system in New York City between 1972 and 2000. Bernstein described the intimate details of these family members' lives, with their permission, and her account is summarized here to serve as an example of the intractable personal and social factors that may perpetuate a family's involvement with this system.

Bernstein's (2001) book, *The Lost Children of Wilder: The Epic Struggle to Change Foster Care*, exposed the operation of New York City's child welfare system and followed the course of a class action suit that revealed deep flaws in the system, even as it presented the gripping personal stories of a mother, her son, and her young grandson. The book gives a thorough portrayal of the system through its detailed accounts of the experiences of the mother, who ran away from an abusive home at age 12, and her son, who grew up in a series of foster homes, failed preadoptive homes, residential treatment centers, and adolescent group homes and shelters. The brief synopsis here focuses primarily on the experiences of insecure attachment, multiple traumas, and repeated losses that permeated the Wilders' stories. These experiences constitute compelling real-life examples of the theoretical concepts discussed in the first part of this chapter.

The Mother: Shirley Wilder

Shirley Wilder's early life was replete with losses and traumatic abuse. Her own mother died of tuberculosis when she was 4 years of age, and she then moved to live with her maternal grandmother, who died when Shirley was 11. She was raped twice when she was only 9 years old. After her grandmother's death, Shirley moved to her father and stepmother's home, where she endured regular beatings at the hands of her alcoholic stepmother. Both adults also accused her of lying and sexual promiscuity, and Shirley finally ran away when she was 12. After her father took out a Person in Need of Supervision (PINS) petition, the girl was placed in a state "training school," where she was brutally sexually assaulted by older girls and then put into solitary confinement when she tried to report this. She repeatedly ran away from the various facilities in which she was placed, and by the age of 14 she became pregnant and gave birth to a son. Shirley voluntarily signed permission for her baby to enter foster care, and initially she visited him sporadically. However, later she lost contact with her child, and her maternal rights were terminated. Throughout her adolescence Shirley continued in various forms of care, where her adjustment was usually marginal at best. When a situation was too difficult for her, the young woman's coping method was to ran away and live on the streets. By age 19 she was addicted to crack cocaine, and she was later imprisoned for selling drugs. She eventually developed both cancer and AIDS, and at age 38 she died. She was alone at the time of her early death, and her family members argued about who could afford to pay for her burial.

The Son: Lamont Wilder

Shirley's baby had the good fortune for his first 4 years of being placed in a foster family that loved and cared for him in a positive way. The foster mother wanted to adopt him, in fact, but there was conflict in the marriage; when the couple divorced, the foster mother decided that she could not raise a child alone. Lamont was then sent to a preadoptive home in the Midwest. This was a white family, and Lamont was the only black child in his preschool. He continued to wet his bed (a problem he had had previously), and the foster father became increasingly upset with him about this and other behaviors. Some problems in school caused the teacher to complain about the boy as well, and after 1 year the family decided not to adopt him. On his 6th birthday, Lamont was moved to another preadoptive home in the Midwest, where he was given a new first name and where his enuresis persisted. This family was extremely strict and punished him severely, and Lamont regressed as a result. He was sent to a psychiatric center for an evaluation and was diagnosed as having schizophrenia; this second preadoptive placement failed soon thereafter. On his 7th birthday, Lamont returned to New York City, where he was placed in a residential treatment center. An evaluation there indicated that the boy had difficulty forming attachments. He was also diagnosed as having conduct disorder and attention deficit disorder, and was put on medication (Thorazine). His continued residence in the treatment center was stormy.

During his adolescence Lamont lived in several group homes, where he got into various kinds of trouble, usually at the instigation of other youth. He never completed high school, worked off and on as a barber, met a woman with whom he fathered a son, and finally reunited briefly with his own mother when he was 19 years old. He also became acquainted with his birth father, his paternal grandmother, and various relatives, many of whom (like his mother) abused substances. Because of Lamont's job instability and their personality clashes, Lamont and his girlfriend had a lot of conflict over his nonsupport of the child. At one time, the baby's mother was responsible for putting Lamont in prison for this. The couple did not live together, but maintained contact in a very conflicted relationship. At age 5, their son tore up his classroom and told his teachers that his mommy put his daddy in jail. The teachers were considering reporting the family to child's protective services.

Discussion

Bernstein's (2001) account shows history repeating itself in a tragic way. Lamont's mother's early experiences of multiple losses and severe abuse seemed to have lasting negative effects on her. Although Shirley was close to her maternal grandmother, who took care of her between the ages of 4 and

11, both this grandmother's death and that of her mother 7 years before could have interfered with the girl's willingness to risk closeness in subsequent relationships. She very much wanted to have a relationship with her father, but he repeatedly rejected her by siding with his wife, who was openly hostile to Shirley. The rape experiences at age 9 and the later traumatic sexual assaults at the hands of peers exposed this girl prematurely to sexuality and created an unfortunate link between sex and aggression for her. She learned very early that adults would not protect her from harm, and this lesson led to a general mistrust of people. In this overall context, it is understandable that this young woman developed inappropriate ways of interacting and receiving attention, such as sexual promiscuity. Later, she used substances to regulate her feelings. Poverty and racial discrimination also played roles in this woman's short and unhappy life.

Similar negative circumstances affected this mother's son. Lamont did have a supportive start in his first foster home, even though he gradually came to notice the difference in skin color between himself and his foster family. The foster parents were Hispanic and appeared to be strongly attached to this boy. But the later series of failed preadoptive placements had a serious impact on this child, who came to believe that he was as "bad" as his preadoptive parents and teachers considered him to be. We see in this example how a child's self-esteem can be eroded by the opinion and treatment of others, and how a child can come to internalize these negative views.

In regard to Lamont's adult adjustment, it is notable that despite his conflicts with his child's mother, Lamont did not resort either to multiple and casual relationships with other women or to physical abuse or violent behavior. Also to his great credit, he did not adopt the reliance on substances that pervaded his community and extended family. He was employed sporadically and appeared to care genuinely for his child. This behavior points to resilience that may have been rooted in Lamont's own early experiences of security. Nonetheless, the serious arguments between Lamont and his girlfriend were having an impact on their child, whose acting-out behavior in school seemed to reflect the boy's fear and sense of insecurity about his parents' relationship. We can only hope that with the publicity about this book and its sympathetic portrayal of the Wilders, outreach services have now been and will continue to be made available to this family, to avoid having the fourth generation also enter the child welfare system.

CONCLUSIONS

The effects of relationships and experiences in early childhood continue well into adulthood. When early experiences are positive, they provide a firm foundation for future relationships that are positive and fulfilling. Conversely, when they are negative, the individual lives with a sense of insecurity and imminent threat about how others will respond. Traumas can occur unexpectedly or can result from abuse, severe neglect, or the witnessing of violence; in any case, they result in a flood of emotions and the need for comfort and security. In particular, a child who is exposed to domestic violence or to physical or sexual abuse during his or her early life carries a burden of mistrust and despair about other people. Although it is possible for these negative perceptions to change as a result of a later favorable relationship and/or a supportive community contact, these factors are not always present.

Our understanding of the extreme importance of the first 2 years of a child's life argues strongly for early intervention that is family-centered and focused on the adult caretaker(s) as well as on the vulnerable child. Many of the chapters in Part II of this book deal with programs that follow this basic principle.

REFERENCES

Ainsworth, M. D. S., Blehar, M. C., Waters, E., & Wall, S. (1978). *Patterns of attachment: A psychological study of the Strange Situation.* Hillsdale, NJ: Erlbaum.

American Psychiatric Association. (2000). *Diagnostic and statistical manual of mental disorders* (4th ed., text rev.). Washington, DC: Author.

Bernstein, N. (2001). *The lost children of Wilder: The epic struggle to change foster care.* New York: Pantheon Books.

Bowlby, J. (1982). *Attachment and loss* (Vol. 1). New York: Basic Books. (Original work published 1969)

Children's Defense Fund. (2000). *State of America's children.* Washington, DC: Author.

Cohen, J. A. (2004). Early mental health interventions for trauma and traumatic loss in children and adolescents. In B. T. Litz (Ed.), *Early intervention for trauma and traumatic loss* (pp. 131–146). New York: Guilford Press.

Davies, D. (2004). *Child development: A practitioner's guide* (2nd ed.). New York: Guilford Press.

Doka, K. J. (Ed.). (2002). *Disenfranchised grief: New directions, challenges, and strategies for practice.* Champaign, IL: Research Press.

Lieberman, A. F., & Van Horn, P. (2004). Assessment and treatment of young children exposed to traumatic events. In J. D. Osofsky (Ed.), *Young children and trauma: Intervention and treatment* (pp. 111–154). New York: Guilford Press.

Main, M., & Solomon, J. (1990). Procedures for identifying infants as disorganized/disoriented during the Ainsworth Strange Situation. In M. T. Greenberg, D. Cicchetti, & E. M. Cummings (Eds.), *Attachment in the preschool years: Theory, research, and intervention* (pp. 121–160). Chicago: University of Chicago Press.

McFarlane, A. C. (1990). Post-traumatic stress syndrome re-visited. In H. J. Parad

& L. J. Parad (Eds.), *Crisis intervention, book 2* (pp. 69–92). Milwaukee, WI: Family Service America.

National Clearinghouse on Child Abuse and Neglect Information. (2002). *In harm's way: Domestic violence and child maltreatment.* Washington, DC: U.S. Department of Health and Human Services.

Ouimette, P., & Brown, P. J. (Eds.). (2003). *Trauma and substance abuse: Causes, consequences, and treatment of comorbid disorders.* Washington, DC: American Psychological Association.

Pears, K. C., & Capaldi, D. M. (2001). Intergenerational transmission of abuse. A two-generational prospective study of an at-risk sample. *Child Abuse and Neglect, 25,* 1439–1461.

Pelzer, D. (1995). *A child called It.* Deerfield Beach, FL: Health Communications.

Pelzer, D. (1997). *The lost boy.* Deerfield Beach, FL: Health Communications.

Pelzer, D. (2000). *A man called Dave: A story of triumph and forgiveness.* New York: Plume/Penguin Putnam.

Perry, R. J., Rosen, H. R., Kramer, J. H., Beer, J. S., Levenson, R. L., & Miller, B. L. (2001). Hemispheric dominance for emotions, empathy and social behaviour: Evidence from right and left handers with frontotemporal dementia. *Neurocase, 7,* 145–160.

Schore, A. N. (2003). Early relational trauma, disorganized attachment and the development of a predisposition to violence. In M. F. Solomon & D. J. Siegel (Eds.), *Healing trauma: Attachment, mind, body, and brain* (pp. 107–167). New York: Norton.

Schuder, M. R., & Lyons-Ruth, K. L. (2004). "Hidden trauma" in infancy: Attachment, fearful arousal, and early dysfunction of the stress response system. In J. D. Osofsky (Ed.), *Young children and trauma: Intervention and treatment* (pp. 69–104). New York: Guilford Press.

Terr, L. C. (1991). Childhood traumas. An outline and overview. *American Journal of Psychiatry, 148,* 10–20.

Van Horn, P., & Lieberman, A. (2004). Early intervention with infants, toddlers, and preschoolers. In B. T. Litz (Ed.), *Early intervention for trauma and traumatic loss* (pp. 112–130). New York: Guilford Press.

Webb, N. B. (2003). *Social work practice with children* (2nd ed.). New York: Guilford Press.

CHAPTER 3

Applying Principles of Neurodevelopment to Clinical Work with Maltreated and Traumatized Children

The Neurosequential Model of Therapeutics

BRUCE D. PERRY

This chapter examines therapeutic work with maltreated children from a neurodevelopmental perspective. The overarching premises of this perspective are that an awareness of human brain development and functioning provides practical insights into the origins of the abnormal functioning seen following adverse developmental experiences (e.g., abuse, neglect, and trauma), and, furthermore, that an understanding of how neural systems change suggests specific therapeutic interventions.

This overview of the key principles related to human brain organization, function, and development provides the rationale for a specific process of assessment, staffing, and intervention that my colleagues and I call the "Neurosequential Model of Therapeutics" (NMT). During the last 20 years, our interdisciplinary group has been involved in the evaluation and treatment of more than 2,500 children ranging from infants to young adults. Most of these children were in the child protective system (CPS), whereas some were in the juvenile justice system, but all of them were traumatized or maltreated in some fashion. The NMT has been used by the ChildTrauma Academy and its clinical partners in various forms for the last 10 years. Most recently, this model has been most systematically implemented and evaluated by Rick Gaskill and his team at a therapeutic preschool program in Kansas, in collaboration with the ChildTrauma Academy (Barfield &, 2004; Barfield & Gaskill, 2005).

Prior to this, our work with maltreated and traumatized children, at least half of whom were in the CPS system, was primarily a medical model. We evaluated and treated children when they were brought to our clinic in a tertiary care academic setting. We conducted evaluations and provided conventional psychopharmacological, individual, group, and family therapies. We had limited success: Some children improved dramatically; most had minor to moderate improvement in primary neuropsychiatric symptoms (e.g., symptoms of posttraumatic stress disorder); and far too many truly did not get better. In parallel with our clinical work, our group was conducting research on the neurodevelopmental impact of trauma and neglect on the developing child. Over time, it became clear that our conventional medical model was essentially ignoring fundamental principles of neurodevelopment, which we now feel are essential to both understanding and helping traumatized or maltreated children and youth in an optimal fashion.

The present chapter is an overview of these principles; it is not a comprehensive description of the specifics of the assessment, staffing, and intervention components of the NMT. Interested readers are encouraged to learn more about the neurodevelopmental rationale and specific implementation of this approach elsewhere (Perry, Pollard, Blakely, Baker, & Vigilante, 1995; Perry & Pollard, 1998; Perry, 1999; Perry, Dobson, Schick, & Runyan, 2000).

CONTEXT: A DESCRIPTION OF THE PROBLEM

We live in strange times. Modern Western society has benefited from advances in technology, communications, transportation, social justice, and economy beyond the dreams of our ancestors. And yet our society seems to be incapable of ensuring that our children grow up in safe, predictable, relationally enriched, and humane environments. Hundreds of thousands of children each year in the United States are terrorized, abused, neglected, or otherwise maltreated in some fashion. Children growing up in chaos, neglect, and threat do not have the fundamental developmental experiences required to express their underlying genetic potential to self-regulate, relate, communicate, and think. These children are undersocialized and at great risk for emotional, behavioral, social, cognitive, and physical health problems. The costs are incalculable (Franey, Geffner, & Falconer, 2001). How can we truly measure the lost potential of millions of children, let alone the astounding economic burdens caused by the needs for special education, therapy, probation, and jail? How "advanced" is our society when we have to create governmental agencies—with budgets in the billions each year—whose primary responsibility is protecting children from their parents?

It is a sad reality that all of our best efforts—all of our governmental programs, our not-for-profits, our public and private institutions, our CPS, and our education, mental health, and juvenile justice systems—fail these highest-risk children. We recreate the chaos, fragmentation, trauma, and neglect these children have experienced in their homes. We fail maltreated children in many ways, not the least of which is an appalling lack of effective therapeutic services for these children. Most of these children have limited access to therapeutic services. Those who do get therapy get too little, too late; how can we possibly expect 45 minutes a week with a therapist to heal a child after 10 years of chaos, threat, humiliation, degradation, and terror?

THE IMPACT OF CHILDHOOD TRAUMA AND MALTREATMENT

Chaos, threat, traumatic stress, abuse, and neglect are bad for children. These adverse experiences alter a developing child's brain in ways that result in enduring emotional, behavioral, cognitive, social, and physical problems. Hundreds of studies in several fields (e.g., child welfare, education, developmental psychology, psychiatry) have documented various aspects of the negative impact of developmental trauma and other adverse childhood experiences (Perry & Pollard, 1998; Bremner & Vermetten, 2001; Read, Perry, Moskowitz, & Connolly, 2001; Teicher, Andersen, Polcari, Anderson, & Navalta, 2002; De Bellis & Thomas, 2003; Bremner, 2003; Anda et al., in press). All of these negative effects are caused by alterations in various neural systems in the brain. Simply stated, traumatic and neglectful experiences during childhood cause abnormal organization and function of important neural systems in the brain, compromising the functional capacities mediated by these systems.

A key question arises: If adverse experiences alter the developing brain and result in negative functional effects, can therapeutic experiences change the brain in ways that allow healing, recovery, and restoration of healthy function? The short answer is yes. The longer answer is also yes, but the nature, pattern, timing, and duration of the therapeutic experiences are very crucial in determining whether a "therapy" is genuinely therapeutic or just an expensive salve for a guilty and indifferent public. Much of what ends up being therapeutic is not in the context of conventional therapy, and much of what we do in conventional therapies is not therapeutic. Matching the correct therapeutic activities to the specific developmental stage and physiological needs of a maltreated or traumatized child is a key to success. Unfortunately, it is very difficult to do this within a conventional medical model. The majority of children who have been traumatized or maltreated do not get the therapeutic services required to help them heal and develop in optimal ways.

There are many reasons for this–not the least of which is that far too many of our intervention models have been developed in ignorance of fundamental principles of neurodevelopment and neurobiology. The primary assumption of the NMT is that the human brain is the organ that mediates all emotional, behavioral, social, motor, and neurophysiological functioning. Therefore, therapeutic interventions seek to change a person by changing the person's brain. Without an appreciation of how the brain is organized and how it changes, therapeutic interventions are likely to be inefficient or, sadly, ineffective. The following section discusses several of the key principles that provide the neurobiological rationale for the NMT.

KEY PRINCIPLES OF NEURODEVELOPMENT AND NEUROBIOLOGY

PRINCIPLE 1. The brain is organized in a hierarchical fashion, such that all incoming sensory input first enters the lower parts of the brain.

The human brain is comprised of billions of neurons and glial cells. These billions of cell divide, move, specialize, connect, interact, and organize during development into a hierarchical group of structures (Figure 3.1). The more simple regulatory functions (e.g., regulation of respiration, heart rate, blood pressure, body temperature) are mediated by the "lower" parts of the brain (the brainstem and diencephalon), and the most complex functions (e.g., language and abstract thinking) are mediated by its most complex cortical structures. Chains of interconnected neurons–neural networks–communicate and interact both within and across these structures, thereby allowing a remarkable range of functions.

The human brain is continually sensing, processing, storing, perceiving and acting in response to information from both the external and internal environments. The five senses of the human body transform forms of energy from the external world into the patterned activity of sensory neurons. The neural patterns of activity created by sensory input first come into the brain separately: Visual input comes into one group of nuclei, auditory another, olfactory another, and so on. The first "stops" for primary sensory input both from the outside environment (e.g., light, sound, taste, touch, smell) and from inside the body (e.g., glucose levels, temperature) are the "lower," regulatory areas of the brain–the brainstem and diencephalon, which are incapable of conscious perception. As this primary sensory input is further processed, these signals are sent to sensory association areas; images, sounds, scents, and touches co-occurring

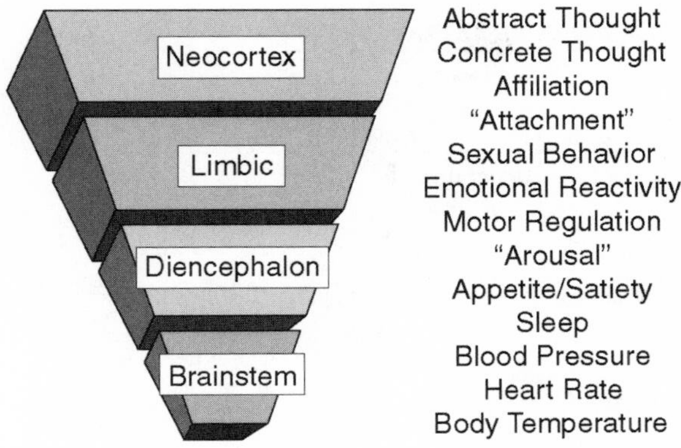

FIGURE 3.1. Hierarchy of brain function. The human brain is organized from the most simple (e.g., fewest cells–brainstem) to most complex (e.g., most cells and most synapses–frontal cortex). The various functions of the brain, from the most simple and reflexive (e.g., regulation of body temperature) to the most complex (e.g., abstract thought), are mediated in parallel with these various areas. These areas organize during development and change in the mature brain in a "use-dependent" fashion. The more a certain neural system is activated, the more it will "build in" this neural state–creating an internal representation of the experience corresponding to this neural activation. This use-dependent capacity to make internal representations of the external or internal world is the basis for learning and memory.

in time become connected. This remarkable biological gift of making associations–the capacity to connect patterns of neural activity that co-occur in time–is what allows us to create a complex, seamless, and dynamic internal representation of the world from a set of separate sensory inputs.

As these waves of neural activity move up the brain into the higher, more complex areas (e.g., limbic and cortical), these patterns of neural activity are matched against previously stored patterns of activation (i.e., stored memories: see Perry, 1999). If a pattern is novel or associated with previous threat (e.g., the pattern of neural activity created by a sudden loud noise), an initial alarm response begins. The internal state of arousal begins to shift, moving along the arousal continuum (see Figure 3.2 and Perry, 1999, 2001). This alarm system activation begins a wave of neuronal activity in key brainstem and diencephalic nuclei, which include neurons containing a variety of neurotransmitters (e.g., norepinephrine, dopamine, and serotonin), neuromodulators, and neuropeptides (e.g. adrenocorticotropic hormone, endorphins, corticotropin-releasing factor, and vasopressin).

Potential threat thus initiates a cascade of patterned neuronal activity in these primitive areas of the brain, which moves up to more complex

Ages	30 ←15	15 ←8	8 ←3	3 ←1	1 ←0
Develop-mental Stage	Adult / Adolescent	Adolescent / Child	Child / Toddler	Toddler / Infant	Infant / Newborn
Primary/ *Secondary* Brain Areas	Neocortex / *Subcortex*	Subcortex / *Limbic*	Limbic / *Midbrain*	Midbrain / *Brainstem*	Brainstem / *Autonomic*
Cognition	Abstract	Concrete	"Emotional"	Reactive	Reflexive
Mental State	Calm	Arousal	Alarm	Fear	Terror

FIGURE 3.2. State-dependent shifts in level of developmental functioning with shifts down the arousal continuum. When threatened, a child is likely to act in an "immature" fashion. Regression, a retreat to a less mature style of functioning and behavior, is commonly observed in all of us when we are physically ill, sleep-deprived, hungry, fatigued, or threatened. As we regress in response to the real or perceived threat, our behaviors are mediated (primarily) by less complex brain areas. If a child has been raised in an environment of persisting threat, the child will have an altered baseline, such that the internal state of calm is rarely obtained (or only artificially obtained via alcohol or drugs). In addition, the traumatized child will have a highly sensitized alarm response, overreading verbal and nonverbal cues as threatening. This increased reactivity will result in dramatic changes in behavior in the face of seemingly minor provocative cues.

Children exposed to significant threat will "reset" their baseline state of arousal, such that even at baseline—when no external threats or demands are present—they will be in a physiological state of persisting alarm. As external stressors are introduced (e.g., a complicated task at school, a disagreement with a peer), the traumatized child will become more reactive, moving into a state of fear or terror in the presence of even minor stressors. The child's cognition and behavior will reflect his or her state of arousal. This increased baseline level of arousal, and increased reactivity in response to a perceived threat, play a major role in the behavioral and cognitive problems exhibited by traumatized children.

parts of the brain. In addition to sending these signals to higher parts of the brain, this cascade of threat-responsive activity initiates a set of brainstem and midbrain responses to the new information from the environment, allowing the individual to react in a near-reflexive fashion. In many instances, the brain's responses to incoming sensory information will take place well before the signals can get to the higher, cortical parts of the brain, where they are "interpreted."

At each level of the brain, as the incoming input is "interpreted" and matched against previous similar patterns of activation, a response is initiated (see Figure 3.3). The brain responds to the potential threat. This immediate response capability is very important for rapid response to potentially threatening sensory signals; classic examples of this include the immediate motor action of withdrawal of a finger after being burned, and the jump that takes place following an unexpected loud sound (startle

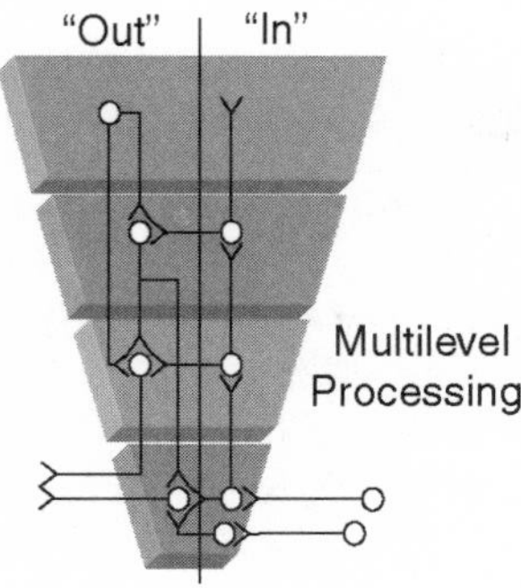

FIGURE 3.3. Precortical association and sequential processing. All incoming sensory information first enters the central nervous system at the level of the spinal cord or brainstem. This means that the first places where patterns of activation are matched against previously stored templates are these lower, more primitive areas. Indeed, the spinal cord and brainstem may process and act on incoming information before the integrated and interpreted signals even get up to the cortex (e.g., reflex withdrawal of a finger from fire).

response). Clearly, in order for the brain to react in this immediate, "uninterpreted" fashion, the more primitive portions of the brain (i.e., the brainstem and the midbrain) must store previous patterns of sensory neuronal input that are associated with threat. In other words, there must be "state" memories—memories of previous patterns of sensory input that were connected with bad experiences. This explains why a child who was sexually abused in early life by the mother's paramour will have an automatic threat reaction later to a friendly touch on the shoulder by a male math teacher.

It is important to understand that *this alarm activation can occur even before complete processing and interpretation of the information.* Activation of these key systems results in patterns of neuronal activation that move from the brainstem through the diencephalon to the thalamic, limbic, and cortical areas. At the level of the brainstem and midbrain, there is very little subjective perception. It is at the level of the thalamus and the limbic areas that the actual affective sensation of fear arises. Only after communication with cortical areas is the individual able to make the more complex cognitive associations that allow interpretation of this internal state of anxiety.

Clinical Implications. The clinical implications of this first neurodevelopmental principle. The brain's remarkable capacity to make associations between patterns of neural activity that co-occur in time is the origin of many trauma-related symptoms. The cue-specific increases in physiological reactivity, distress, fear, and other symptoms are due to the brain's making associations between incoming sensory signals that occurred during the traumatic experiences. A young child growing up in a home with pervasive threat, for example, will create a set of associations–primarily precortical and therefore out of his or her conscious awareness–between a host of neutral cues and threat. For the rest of the child's life, these neutral cues will have the capacity to activate a fear response and therefore to alter emotions, behaviors, and physiology (see Figure 3.2). These fear-inducing cues can range from expressions (e.g., eye contact can become associated with impending threat), to scents (e.g., an abusive father's aftershave), to music, to styles of interpersonal interaction. Among the saddest examples of this occurs when the primary caregiver–the source of food, warmth, comfort, and love for the dependent infant and child–is also the source of episodic, unpredictable threat, rage, and pain. The disorganized attachment that results can impair healthy relational interactions for a lifetime. Again, many if not most of the resulting dysfunctional relational interactions will be beyond the awareness and understanding of the developing child, youth, or adult.

These precortical associations can profoundly interfere with therapeutic work. When a child, youth, or adult is in a high state of fearful arousal, his or her brain will process and function differently (see Figures 3.2 and 3.4). During therapy or in school, if any emotionally charged content is present, the person's state will shift. If this shift is dramatic enough, the person will essentially be so anxious and regressed that his or her functioning will be "brainstem-driven." The individual will think and act in very primitive ways, and therefore will be less accessible to academic or therapeutic interventions using words or therapeutic relationships as the mutative agents of change.

Transference and countertransference are also related to this neurobiological principle. In order to break these inaccurate and false associations, the client must have opportunities for new experiences that will allow the brain either to break false associations or to decrease the overgeneralization of trauma-related associations. For example, the associations in the brain of a girl abused by one male may have generalized to all males. In order to modify this overgeneralization, this child will require many positive experiences with nonabusing males.

PRINCIPLE 2. Neurons and neural systems are designed to change in a "use-dependent" fashion.

Neurons are uniquely designed to change in response to activity. Neural stimulation or lack of stimulation will result in cellular modification; synapses, axons, cell bodies, and dendrites can all be shaped and altered by activity. Therefore, neural networks change in a "use-

Adaptive response	Rest	Vigilance	Freeze	Flight	Fight
Predictable deescalating behaviors *(behaviors of the teacher or caregiver when a child is in various states of arousal)*	Presence Quiet Rocking	Quiet voice Eye contact Confidence Clear, simple directives	Slow, sure physical touch "Invited" touch Quiet, melodic words Singing, humming music	Presence Quiet Confidence Disengagement	Appropriate physical restraint Withdrawal from class TIME!
Predictable escalating behaviors *(behaviors of the teacher or caregiver when a child is in various states of arousal)*	Talking Poking Noise Television	Frustration, anxiety Communicating from distance without eye contact Complex, compound directives Ultimatums	Raised voice Raised hand Shaking finger Tone of voice, yelling, threats Chaos in class	Increased or continued frustration More yelling Chaos Sense of fear	Inappropriate physical restraint Grabbing Shaking Screaming
Regulating brain region	Neocortex Cortex	Cortex Limbic	Limbic Midbrain	Midbrain Brainstem	Brainstem Autonomic
Cognition	Abstract	Concrete	Emotional	Reactive	Reflexive
State	Calm	Arousal Attention	Alarm	Fear	Terror

FIGURE 3.4. Altered functioning with change in state of arousal. As a child experiences some degree of perceived threat, he or she will move along this arousal continuum from a state of calm to a state of terror. In different states of arousal, different parts of the brain become the predominant areas of control. The styles of thinking and of behavioral functioning change. This chart gives some indication of the kinds of interactions between a teacher, clinician, or caregiver and with a traumatized or maltreated child that can influence movement along the arousal continuum. One of the major mistakes we make with maltreated children is misunderstanding their internal states. When these children are in a state of fear, we think they are in a state of attention and capable of understanding our directives—for instance, "Take out the garbage, and then take your backpack upstairs to your room." The children process our simple directives inaccurately, because of the fearful state they are in. When they forget one part of this compound command, we raise our voices and issue an ultimatum: "How many times do I have to tell you? If you don't do what I ask, you will not have any TV this week." The children's fear escalates, and they begin to act in a more hostile, inappropriate, and immature way. We ourselves get confused and frustrated, and can easily escalate the child further; the result may be a full-blown flight or fight reaction.

Knowing where a child is on the arousal continuum—accurately knowing the child's internal state—can help us determine when to talk, and when to stop talking and start using simple, nonthreatening, nonverbal interactions to quiet and contain the escalating child.

dependent" fashion. As the brain is developing, normal organization of any brain area or capability is "use-dependent." If the developing child is spoken to, the neural systems mediating speech and language will receive the sufficient stimulation to organize and function normally. A child who does not hear words will not have this capacity expressed. This is true for any part of the developing brain: All functional capacities in the brain are dependent to some degree upon the presence of appropriately timed, appropriately patterned signals that will specifically stimulate the neural systems mediating that function. Normal motor organization requires the opportunity to crawl, stand, cruise, walk, and run; normal socioemotional development requires attentive, attuned caregiving and a rich array of relational opportunities during development; and so forth. Healthy organization of neural networks depends upon the pattern, frequency, and timing of key experiences during development. Patterned, repetitive activity changes the brain. Chaotic, episodic experiences that are "out of sync" with a child's developmental stage create chaotic, developmentally delayed dysfunctional organization.

Clinical Implications. A child exposed to consistent, predictable, nurturing, and enriched experiences will develop neurobiological capabilities that will increase the child's chance for health, happiness, productivity and creativity. Conversely, neglect, chaotic, and terrorizing environments will increase a child's risk for significant problems in all domains of functioning. The specific symptoms or physical signs a child develops following maltreatment or trauma will reflect the history of neural activation—or, in the case of neglect, the history of inactivation. Neuropsychiatric symptoms and signs present in maltreated or traumatized children are related to the nature, timing, pattern, and duration of their developmental experiences—both adverse and protective.

As the brain organizes and changes as a reflection of the pattern, nature and intensity of experience, fear and chaos, for example, will result in persistent, repeated activation of the stress response systems in the brain. The neurotransmitter networks (including epinephrine, norepinephrine, dopamine, and serotonin) involved in both major patterns of stress responses (the hyperarousal and dissociative responses; see Perry et al., 1995) originate in the lower parts of the brain—the brainstem and diencephalon—and send axonal connections throughout the rest of the brain. This allows these important systems to orchestrate and regulate a host of brain functions important to surviving challenges and overt threat. When these neural networks are altered by chronic stress or extreme traumatic stress, a whole cascade of brain areas and the functions these areas mediate are altered as well. The results are use-dependent alterations in these systems; they become sensitized, overreactive, and dysfunctional. Development threat, then, creates a *persisting* fear state (i.e., the state becomes a "trait"). The specific sets of maladaptive emotional, behavioral, and cognitive problems of a maltreated child are rooted in the original *adaptive* responses to a traumatic event. These symptoms may include hypervigilance, impulsivity, anxiety, affect regulation problems, sleep problems, and a host of other abnormalities related to dysfunctional stress response neural networks and the neurotransmitter systems in these networks (see Perry et al., 1995; De Bellis & Thomas, 2003; Bremner, 2003).

If a child is neglected—if he or she hears fewer words, has fewer relational opportunities, receives less physical comfort, and has less love—the rapidly organizing networks in the brain that mediate language, social affiliation, and attachment will not receive sufficient patterned, repetitive activation to develop normally. The result is a neglect-related set of deficits. The deficit will be in the domains where the neglect occurred (see Perry, 2002a; Smith & Fong, 2004).

The therapeutic implications of this second neurodevelopmental principle cannot be overstated. Repetition, repetition, repetition: Neural systems—and children—change with repetition. Furthermore, the repetition must be in those very neural systems that mediate the symptoms; Parts of the brain cannot be changed if they are not activated. Herein lies a problem with much conventional psychotherapy used with maltreated children. The original fear response will activate systems that are widely distributed in the brain: The threat response neural systems originate in the brainstem and send projections to (and thereby influence) diencephalic, limbic, and cortical functioning. Trauma-related symptoms originate in the lower parts of the brain. Therefore, therapeutic interventions that seek to influence trauma-related symptoms must influence the brainstem. Due to the orchestrating and communicating roles of the brainstem's stress response neural systems, any efforts to treat symptoms related to higher parts of the brain without first regulating the brainstem will be inefficient or unsuccessful.

A primary therapeutic implication for this is the repetitive nature of the replacement experiences that are required to help neglected children recapture normal functioning. If fundamental organizing experiences are missed when key brain areas are organizing, the number of repetitions required to learn or develop any capability is often so frustratingly high that adoptive parents, teachers, and clinicians become discouraged. Neglected children can change; however, the process is long, and it requires patience and an understanding of development. It is often true that these children age but do not develop. Therefore, the replacement (therapeutic) experiences required must be developmentally appropriate, but not completely age-inappropriate. This is a major challenge as these children get older.

Children with fundamental attachment problems due to early childhood neglect need many, many positive nurturing interactions with trustworthy peers, teachers, and caregivers. Unfortunately, the very pathology related to their neglect makes it difficult for them to engage in and benefit from relational interactions even when there are caring adults present. In some cases, beginning the recovery process for relational neglect can start with animals. Dogs have the capacity to provide the unconditional accepting and repetitive nurturing experiences required to help some of these children.

Children with brainstem-mediated hypervigilance, impulsivity, and anxiety require patterned, repetitive brainstem activities to begin to regulate and organize these brainstem systems; talking, or even therapeutic relational interactions, are not particularly effective at providing brainstem-altering experiences. Dance, drumming, music, massage—patterned, repetitive sensory input will begin to provide the kinds of experiences that may influence brainstem neurobiology to reorganize in ways that will lead to smoother functional regulation.

Enrichment or therapeutic services for maltreated children need to be consistent, predictable, patterned, and *frequent*. Clearly, this is not usually true of the fragmented, multiple-transition services that most children in the CPS system experience. If interventions with these children are going to work, the number of repetitions required cannot be provided in weekly therapy. Effective therapeutic and enrichment interventions must recruit other adults in a child's life—caregivers, teachers, parents—to be involved in learning and delivering elements of these interventions, in addition to the specific therapy hours dedicated to them during the week.

PRINCIPLE 3. The brain develops in a sequential fashion.

The brain, at birth, is undeveloped. During its development, it organizes and grows in a sequential fashion—starting from the lowest, most regulatory regions of the brain, and proceeding up through the more complex parts of the brain responsible for more complex functions. Brain development is characterized by (1) sequential development and sensitivity (from the brainstem to the cortex), and (2) use-dependent organization of these various brain areas. The stress response systems originate in the lower parts of the brain and help regulate and organize higher parts of the brain; if they are poorly organized or regulated themselves, they dysregulate and disorganize higher parts of the brain.

Clinical Implications. Traumatic stress will result in patterned, repetitive neuronal activation in a distributed and diverse set of brain systems. Trauma can have an impact on functions mediated by the cortex (e.g., cognition), the limbic system (e.g., affect regulation), the diencephalon (e.g., fine motor regulation, startle response), and the brainstem (e.g., heart rate, blood pressure regulation). *The key to therapeutic intervention is to remember that the stress response systems originate in the brainstem and diencephalon.* As long as these systems are poorly regulated and dysfunctional, they will disrupt and dysregulate the higher parts of the brain.

All the best cognitive-behavioral, insight-oriented, or even affect-based interventions will fail if the brainstem is poorly regulated (see Figures 3.2 and 3.4). Extreme anxiety, hypervigilance, and a persistently activated threat response will undermine academic, therapeutic, and socioemotional learning opportunities. The internal state of arousal can have a profound impact on how individuals think and act. The sensitized stress response system in maltreated children keeps them in a persistent state of high arousal; furthermore, these children will be very labile. When a traumatized child perceives any challenge or threat, he or she will be easily moved along the arousal continuum. The child must feel safe to start to heal. A sense of safety will help keep the child's state of arousal during therapy, school, and other important learning opportunities at a manageable level. Once state regulation has improved, the child can begin to benefit from more traditional therapy. The sequence of providing therapeutic experiences matters. Just as healthy development does, healing following childhood trauma starts from the bottom up.

Accordingly, therapeutic activities will be most effective if they are provided in the sequence that reflects normal development—from the brainstem up. As described above, a poorly regulated brainstem will make most conventional therapeutic interventions ineffective or useless. The major conventional approach to "constraining" the brainstem has been psychopharmacology. The majority of psychotropic medications used with traumatized children (e.g., antidepressants, clonidine, and neuroleptics) influence the key monoamine neurotransmitters involved in the various neural responses to stress and threat. The specificity and efficacy of these agents in children are still not clear, and the effects tend to be nonspecific.

Alternative brainstem-modulating interventions are beginning to emerge—or, rather, are being rediscovered and appreciated for their fundamental therapeutic value. Music and movement activities that provide patterned, repetitive, rhythmic stimulation of the brainstem are very successful in helping modulate brainstem dysregulation (see Miranda, Arthur, Milan, Mahoney, & Perry, 1998; Miranda, Schick, Dobson, Hogan, & Perry, 1999). Several therapeutic approaches, including eye movement desensitization and reprocessing (EMDR), involve patterned, rhythmic activation of the brainstem as part of the intervention. We have hypothesized that EMDR is effective because it can short-circuit the chain of traumatic memory that follows a specific traumatic event by tapping into a much more powerful brainstem–diencephalic memory—the association created *in utero*. Powerful associations are made during the prenatal development of the brainstem and diencephalon between rhythmic auditory, tactile, and motor activity at 80 beats per minute (i.e., the maternal heart rate heard and felt *in utero*) and the neural activation mediating the sensation of being warm, satiated, safe, and soothed. EMDR, dancing, drumming, music, and patterned massage can all "quiet" the brainstem through rhythmic activity that provides brainstem stimulation at 80 bests per minute or subrhythms (40, 60) of this primary "soothing" pattern (Perry, 2002b). Such patterned, repetitive, rhythmic activity has always been a central element of healing and grief rituals in aboriginal cultures. The use of music and movement interventions with traumatized children has been very promising (e.g., Miranda et al., 1999).

Therefore, therapeutic and enrichment experiences must be provided to a child in an appropriate sequence and matched to the child's level of neurodevelopment (see Table 3.1). In turn, this matching process is dependent upon adequate assessment of the child's development in the key areas of physical/motor, behavioral, emotional, social, and cognitive domains (see the later discussion of assessment).

PRINCIPLE 4. The brain develops most rapidly early in life.

The majority of this sequential and use-dependent development of the brain takes place in early childhood. Indeed, by age 4, a child's brain is 90% adult size. The organizing brain is very malleable and responsive to the environment. This means that of all the experiences throughout the life of an individual, the organizing experiences of early childhood have the most powerful and enduring effects on brain organization and functioning! Three years of neglect can cause a lifetime of dysfunction and lost potential. As discussed below, the brain continues to be capable of change, but it is much easier to organize the brain in healthy ways than it is to take a poorly organized neural system and try to reorganize it.

Clinical Implications. The primary clinical implication of this fourth principle is that early childhood trauma or maltreatment has a disproportionate capacity to cause significant dysfunction, in comparison with similar trauma or maltreatment later in life (see Rutter & English and Romanian Adoptees Study Team, 1998; Rutter et al., 1999). In contrast to prevailing bias, children are more vulnerable to trauma and neglect than adolescents and adults. Indeed, the younger a child is, the more likely the child is to have enduring and pervasive problems following trauma. Severe neglect in the first years of life can have a devastating impact even if a child is removed from the neglectful environment (see Figure 3.5; Perry, 2002a). And the longer a child remains in such an environment, the more vulnerable he or she becomes (e.g., Rutter & English and Romanian

TABLE 3.1. Sequential Neurodevelopment and Therapeutic Activity

Age of most active growth	"Sensitive" brain area	Critical functions being organized	Primary developmental goal	Optimizing experiences (examples)	Therapeutic and enrichment activities (samples)
0–9 mo	Brainstem	• Regulation of arousal, sleep, and fear states	• State regulation • Primary attachment • Flexible stress response • Resilience	• Rhythmic and *patterned* sensory input (auditory, tactile, motor) • Attuned, responsive caregiving	• Massage • Rhythm (e.g., drumming) • Reiki touch • EMDR
6 mo–2 yr	Diencephalon	• Integration of multiple sensory inputs • Fine motor control	• Sensory integration • Motor control • Relational flexibility • Attunement	• More complex rhythmic movement • Simple narrative • Emotional and physical warmth	Music and movement • Reiki touch • Therapeutic massage • Equine or canine interactions
1–4 yr	Limbic	• Emotional states • Social language; interpretation of nonverbal information	• Emotional regulation • Empathy • Affiliation • Tolerance	• Complex movement • Narrative • Social experiences	Play and play therapies • Performing and creative arts and therapies • Parallel play
3–6 yr	Cortex	• Abstract cognitive functions • Socioemotional integration	• Abstract reasoning • Creativity • Respect • Moral and spiritual foundations	• Complex conversation • Social interactions • Exploratory play • Solitude, satiety, security	Storytelling • Drama • Exposure to performing arts • Formal education • Traditional insight-oriented or cognitive-behavioral interventions

Note. This table outlines the sequential development of the brain, along with examples of appropriately matched experiences that help organize and influence the respective parts of the brain that are most actively developing at various stages. For maltreated children, developmental "age" rarely matches chronological age; therefore, the sequential provision of therapeutic experiences should be matched to developmental stage and not chronological age.

Adoptees Study Team, 1998; Rutter et al., 1999; O'Connor, Rutter, & English and Romanian Adoptees Study Team, 2000).

This principle informs policy, programming, and practice. The primary policy implication is that even a minimal investment in early childhood surveillance models to find highest-risk children and families will be wise. We do not capitalize on this window of opportunity in early childhood. Indeed, we typically wait until a child is clearly impaired and dysfunctional (e.g., acting out and failing in school) before we initiate services. Those few resources that are dedicated to early childhood tend to be inefficient and unfocused.

Early intervention with high-risk children works (Reynolds, Temple, Robertson, & Mann, 2001). The primary programming implication is that the earlier we can begin to provide appropriate services to children, the more effective we will be. The interventions will cost less, and the children's progress will be more dramatic (see Figure 3.5). A few promising practices demonstrate the powerful impact of proactive interventions; the Rameys' Abecedarian projects (Ramey et al., 2000) and Old's home visitation interventions (Olds, Henderson, & Eckenrode, 2002), for example,

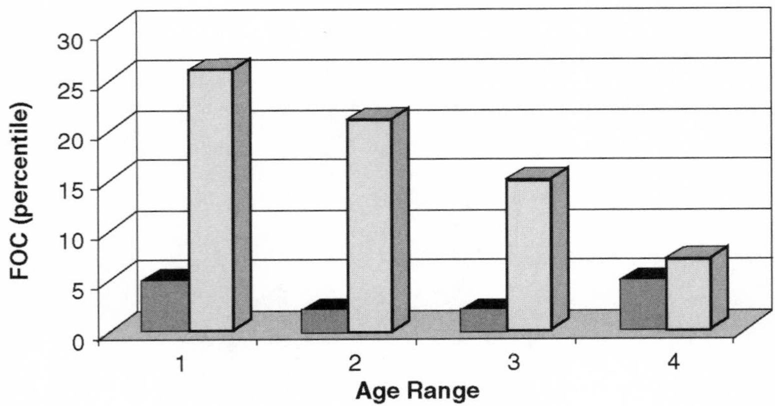

FIGURE 3.5. Sensory deprivation neglect: Effects of early removal on recovery. Children were removed from severely neglectful environments at different ages (ages 8 months to 4 years, 8 months). Their frontal–occipital circumference (FOC; a crude indicator of brain size) was measured (black bars) and compared to same-age norms. Children were placed in foster care and were reevaluated 1 year later . FOC was measured (white bars) and increased in each group; with increasing age, however, the improvement after a year of foster placement started to decrease, such that after 3 years in the neglectful environment (group 4), there was no longer any statistically significant improvement 1 year later. It is interesting to note that 100% of the children in group 4, 74% in group 3, 46% in group 2, and only 27% in group 1 required special educational services when they reached school age.

have a long-term impact on high-risk children when services are provided during the first years of life.

Proactive therapeutic interventions are better than reactive ones. It is easier and more cost-effective to provide enrichment, educational, and therapeutic services earlier than later. The longer we wait to help these children, the more difficult the therapeutic challenge will be.

PRINCIPLE 5. Neural systems can be changed, but some systems are easier to change than others.

The primary assumption of therapy is that a person can change. The parallel assumption is that the person's brain is capable of being changed with therapeutic intervention. As discussed above, the human brain is remarkably malleable while it is being organized during development. Once organized, the brain is still capable of being influenced, modified, and changed. The ease with which the brain's neural networks can be modified, however, changes as the child grows and the brain becomes more organized.

The degree of brain plasticity is related to two main factors—the stage of development, and the area or system of the brain. Once an area of the brain is organized, it is much less responsive to the environment; in other words, it is less plastic. For some brain areas such as the cortex, however, significant plasticity remains throughout life, such that experiences can still easily alter neurophysiological organization and functioning. A critical concept related to memory and brain plasticity is the differential plasticity of various brain systems. Not all parts of the brain are as plastic as others (see Figure 3.6). Once the brain has organized (i.e., after age 3), experience-dependent modifications of the regulatory system are much less likely than experience-dependent modifications of cortically mediated functions such as language development.

Clinical Implications. As described in detail above, trauma-related symptoms are related to dysfunction of neural systems in the lower, less plastic parts of the brain. The number of repetitions required to change brainstem neural organization is far greater than the number required to change the cortical neural organization. In other words, it is easier to change beliefs than feelings. It is not that a child won't change; it is just that change will not occur unless sufficient repetitions are provided. The current medical model does not provide sufficient repetitive, patterned experiences for brainstem-related neural systems to reorganize. We try to modify these symptoms by using medications that alter the functioning of these brainstem neural systems—sometimes with effect. No medication, however, can provide the specific patterns of neural activation required to

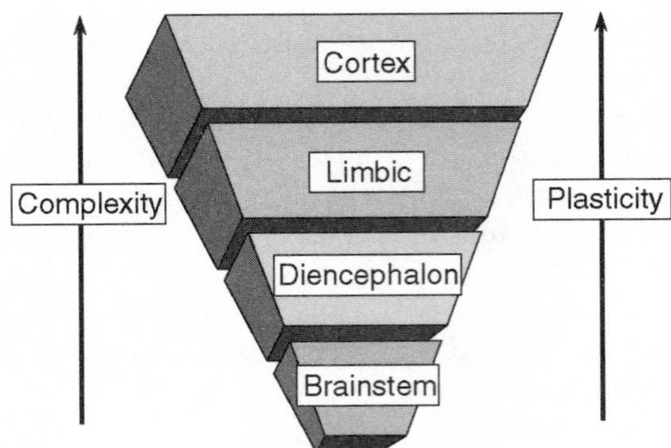

FIGURE 3.6. Differential plasticity across different regions of the organized brain. The malleability of specific human brain areas is different. The most complex area of the brain—the cortex—is the most plastic. Some cortex-related functions can be modified throughout life with minimal effort. For example, even a 90-year-old person can learn a new phone number. The lower parts of the brain—those mediating core regulatory functions—are not very plastic. And this is for good reason: It would be very destructive for these basic and life-sustaining functions to be easily modified by experience once they were organized.

organize and reorganize dysfunctional neural networks. We can contain behavior by regulating emotional dysfunction with medications, but we cannot create new, healthy neural networks. Therefore, medication use alone does not have an enduring positive impact on maltreated children. This is not to say that medications should not be used; medications can be very helpful in containing brainstem dysregulation enough to allow positive, repetitive healing experiences to take place through other therapeutic activities (e.g., individual cognitive-behavioral therapy).

PRINCIPLE 6. The human brain is designed for a different world.

We humans have not always lived the way we do now. Human beings are biological creatures. Of the 250,000 years or so that our species has been on the planet, we spent 245,000 years living in small transgenerational hunter–gatherer bands of 40–50 individuals. The human brain has evolved specific capabilities that are hominid and prehominid adaptations to millions of years of living in the natural world in these transgenerational groups. One of the most important features of this natural world was the relational milieu. We lived in a far richer relational environment in the natural world. For each child under the age of 6, there were four developmentally more mature persons who could protect, educate, enrich, and nurture the developing child—a ratio of 4:1. In contrast, our modern world is defining a caregiver-to-child ratio of 1:4 as a "best-practice" ratio for young children (1/16th the relational ratio the human brain is designed for). Our children also spend many hours each day watching television; they spend very few hours in the socioemotional learning opportunities created by interactions with older children, younger children, aunts, uncles, nephews, grandparents, or neighbors. In contrast to our ancestors, we live in a relationally impoverished world.

The relationally enriched, developmentally heterogeneous environment of our past is what the human brain "prefers." The brain is not well designed for artificial light, pervasive visual overstimulation from television, distracting sounds and images, anonymous social interactions, and numerous other phenomena related to life in the modern Western world. The impact of these changes on the way we live, work, and raise our children has not been completely examined. Many of our current lifestyle choices, though well intended, are probably contributing to emotional, social, cognitive, and physical health problems in our children. The most alarming of these is the relational poverty that many of our children are experiencing. This is most disturbing, because we humans are fundamentally relational creatures.

We are born dependent and grow to be interdependent. We need each other, and we are neurobiologically connected to each other. Indeed, our survival as a species is dependent upon our ability to form and maintain successful relationships with others. The most essential functions that the brain mediates—survival, procreation, and protecting/nurturing offspring—depend upon the capacity to form and maintain relationships. Our human neurobiology reflects our functional interdependence. The most powerful rewards and the most intense pain come from relational experiences. The attention and approval of a loved or respected person stimulates the reward systems in the brain, and disapproval or loss of attention and affection activates pain-mediating neural systems (rejection, humiliation, and loss actually hurt). The neural systems mediating stress response, procreation, reproduction, social affiliation, and communication are all interrelated; indeed, they often share the very same fundamental neurotransmitter networks and brain regions (see Perry, 1999, 2001, 2002a).

Clinical Implications. On average, our child care settings have 1 caregiver for 6–8 children. Our elementary schools have 1 teacher for 30 children. Our children take 6 hours a day to watch television. Fragmented, mobile nuclear families separate children from extended family members. A host of factors combine to produce hundreds of thousands of children growing up in homes and communities that are impoverished in relationships. This poverty of relationships contributes to a host of neuropsychiatric problems. The more isolated physically and socially a family becomes, the more vulnerable a child becomes.

Some children have so few relational experiences that they never fully develop their capacity to be socially appropriate, empathic, self-regulating, and humane. By the time they reach age 10, they have only had the number and quality of social interactions that a typical 5-year old gets. This socioemotional immaturity leads to a mismatch between the expectations of teachers, parents, and peers on the one hand and a child's capacity on the other. The child acts like a 5-year-old, but lives in a world of 10-year-old expectations, challenges, and opportunities. The child falls behind, frustrates teachers, and puzzles peers; as a result, he or she begins to feel inadequate, useless, and stupid. If this socioemotional poverty is significant enough, it can result in a child who is persistently selfish, self-absorbed (but also self-loathing), and incapable of empathic, humane behavior. Such characteristics, in combination with exposure to domestic violence and to violence on the media, place a child at great risk for aggressive or even violent behaviors.

The primary therapeutic implication is the need to increase the number and quality of relational interactions and opportunities for the high-risk child. One therapy session a week will not provide sufficient healthy relational interactions to permit the child to catch up from years of relational poverty. The therapeutic approach must address the process of helping to create a "therapeutic web." Using any healthy and invested people in the child's life—teachers, coaches, foster parents, siblings, extended family, neighbors, youth ministers—can help provide therapeutic opportunities. This simple but powerful fact appears to underlie the efficacy of a host of intervention models with high-risk young children. Increasing the number and quality of relational interactions by bringing more healthy adults into the lives of these children and their parents is a key element of home visitation models, mentoring programs, and after-school programs. The more developmentally delayed the children are, the more desperately they need relational interactions; how often have we heard that a difficult child in a preschool group does just fine one on one? This child is 5, but actually requires the relational richness of the 1:1 interaction typically reserved for infants. A neglected, maltreated child is all too often an infant emotionally. If given this relational attention for a sufficient length of time, the child will begin to "develop" (i.e., to resume a more typical developmental trajectory), and over time will no longer require this level of relational attention. Unfortunately, our systems are rarely capable of providing this level of reparative interaction. We tend to be stingy with our relational attentions in these therapeutic preschool and school settings, choosing to label these children with pejorative diagnostic labels rather than to understand their developmental difficulties as very predictable consequences of their chaotic, relationally distorted, and impoverished early lives.

THE NEUROSEQUENTIAL APPROACH

Each of these principles points to the wisdom of, and need for, a more developmentally informed, biologically respectful approach to working with traumatized children in the CPS system. Through examining the history of success and failure with thousands of maltreated children over a 20-year period, and integrating this with an emerging understanding of fundamental principles of neurobiology (many of which have been discussed above), our group has developed a neurodevelopmental approach to clinical work and program development. This approach continues to be modified for implementation in various settings, such as residential treatment for youthful offenders, conventional mental health outpatient clinical settings, the postremoval CPS assessment process, the special education classroom, and therapeutic preschool and nursery settings (see various descriptions on the ChildTrauma Academy website, www.childtrauma.org).

Clinical application of this neurodevelopmental approach is best demonstrated by NMT. The approach for use in a therapeutic preschool setting has been developed in collaboration with Rick Gaskill and colleagues. In a quasi-experimental study (Barfield & Gaskill, 2005) replicated their findings in a 2003 cohort of children in a therapeutic preschool (Barfield, 2004) in a group of 14 children in a therapeutic preschool setting. The 2004 study used a single-subject, time series design, both individually and aggregated. During the regular school year, the Conscious Discipline (CD) curriculum was used. During the summer program, the NMT was used exclusively along with the other services described (e.g., case management and family therapy). The children served as their own control group. The last 3 weeks of the regular classroom, when the CD model was used, served as the baseline for comparison with the NMT model, which was used exclusively during the summer program. Children showed significantly more improvement in the NMT program on overall social/emotional development, emotion regulation, helpfulness, fair assertiveness, impulse modulation, cooperation, and empathy compared to the CD model ($p = < .006$). Of the 14 children, 13 showed more improvement using the NMT model than CD. Other specific applications will vary, depending upon the age of the child, the involvement of the family, the availability of clinicians and practitioners, and the clinical setting. In all settings, however, three key steps are present: assessment, staffing/training, and therapeutic interventions/activities. An overview of the key elements for each step is presented below.

Assessment: Determining Developmental "Ages"

Children age chronologically at the same rate. Children born on the same day of the same year are exactly the same chronological age. Yet each of these children will develop differently. The rate of physical, emotional, social, cognitive, and behavioral development can vary remarkably from child to child. As discussed above, the rate and nature of development in any given neural system (and therefore function) is related to the nature, pattern, and timing of experience. Children in chaotic, neglectful, relationally deprived, and cognitively impoverished environments will have a much slower rate of development in key functional capabilities. A maltreated 5-year-old boy may only have heard the same number of words that a healthier 3-year-old would have heard; he may have only had the same number of socioemotional learning opportunities as a typical 2-year-old. When this boy enters preschool, he will be 5, but he will think and communicate like a 3-year-old and will relate to peers and teacher like a 2-year-old. The mismatch will result in a host of problems for the child, his peers, and the teacher—most of them related to misunderstandings of the child's developmental "ages."

This becomes a fundamental challenge of caregiving, education, and therapeutic work with maltreated children. Misunderstanding of a child's true "ages" will lead to mismatching expectations and learning/therapeutic activities. A 17-year-old boy in the juvenile justice system may only have the relational skills of a 3-year-old. To expect this boy to function well in a group is unrealistic; such an expectation will only lead to problems in the group, and there will be no true therapeutic impact of the group "therapy." No 3-year-old could manage a complex, insight-oriented group—and neither can the 17-year-old with the relational skills of a toddler.

In order to understand any maltreated child, youth, or adult, then, assessment is crucial. We have developed several multidimensional assessment processes that help us begin to understand a child's multiple "ages" (e.g., chronological, emotional, social, cognitive, physical, moral, spiritual). The specific elements of this assessment process are described in detail elsewhere (Perry et al., 2000). In brief, some objective or psychometric measures in combination with a semistructured subjective interview will yield the necessary information to provide the developmental anchors for the key domains.

The most essential element of assessment is history. The most essential element of assessment is history of primary caregiving during early childhood. And the key to this history is the caregiver's own history of primary caregiving. In general, we humans parent the way we were parented. The brain is a historical organ; as described above, it stores experience. Awareness of the nature, timing, duration, and pattern of developmental trauma and neglect can tell us which systems in the brain are likely to be affected and in what fashion. Furthermore, this history will predict the symptoms and signs the child is likely to express.

As part of the assessment process, we have developed a set of brain-region-specific questions to target the functioning and development of each of the four major regions of the brain. These questions help anchor the child's strengths and vulnerabilities, and suggest clear reparative and therapeutic activities.

Staffing and Training

A primary challenge of the neurosequential model is the need to integrate a fundamental understanding of neurodevelopment and early childhood into the existing working models used by the different professionals collaborating in the interdisciplinary team. The range of educational background, personal history, and experience among these professionals can complicate the process of creating an integrated, developmentally sensitive set of interventions. The most effective way we have found to address this is to provide cross-disciplinary training activities that are "case-based." When possible, all staff members and affiliated collaborating professionals receive both didactic and case-based training in the neurodevelopmental principles and the impact of maltreatment and trauma on children. In addition, an ongoing staffing process is used for the purposes of clinical problem solving and continuing education. This process slowly builds capacity and comfort with the approach, which may often involve intervention approaches that seem counterintuitive or even opposite to an approach suggested by conventional educational or mental interventions.

Interventions

Each child is different and will have a unique set of strengths and vulnerabilities. As indicated above, each maltreated child will have a range of developmental "ages." When clinicians are creating the child's individualized plan of therapeutic activities, the primary objectives are to ensure that the experiences are relevant, relational, repetitive, and rewarding. Activities and interventions are selected that match the child's developmental status in any given domain of function (i.e., social, emotional, cognitive, and physical); in other words, they are relevant. The second key is that the activities are provided in a healthy relational context; this is necessary to provide the sense of safety and predictability necessary for optimal healing and learning. Third, the activities must be provided with sufficient repetition and duration to produce actual change in the target neural systems. Finally, the activities must have some element of reward; therapeutic and learning experiences will generalize and ultimately be most successful if some pleasure is gained from the activities themselves or from the mastery that the activities lead to.

The selection and timing of experiences will depend upon the findings of the assessment. In all cases, it is wisest to start with simple rhythmic and repetitive activities that help the brainstem neural systems become well organized and regulated. As therapy progresses and evidence of brainstem regulation emerges, the activities can begin to target higher, more complex parts of the brain. Over time—once the lower stress response systems in the brainstem and diencephalon become well regulated—the effective use of more conventional individual therapies becomes possible (see Table 3.1).

SUMMARY

A clinical approach to helping maltreated and traumatized children that is informed by principles of neurobiology can provide insights regarding assessment, training, and intervention. The present overview is merely an introduction to some of these principles. The NMT is intended to complement and restructure therapeutic efforts and activities. The central clinical implication of this model is that successful treatment with traumatized children must first regulate the brainstem's sensitized and dysregulated stress response systems. Only after these systems are more regulated can a sequence of developmentally appropriate enrichment and therapeutic activities be successfully provided to help the children heal. More outcome-based studies will be required and are planned to fully document this approach in various clinical settings.

ACKNOWLEDGMENTS

The ChildTrauma Academy's work outlined in this chapter has been supported in part by grants from the Texas Department of Protective and Regulatory Services, the Children's Justice Act, the Court Improvement Act, the Hogg Foundation for Mental Health, and the Brown Foundation. I would like to acknowledge the generous support of the Greater Houston Community Foundation's Richard Weekley Family Fund. I would also like to acknowledge the ongoing collaborative work of Rick Gaskill and his colleagues at the Sumner Mental Health Center in Wellington, Kansas.

REFERENCES

Anda, R. F., Felitti, R. F., Walker, J., Whitfield, C., Bremner, D. J., Perry, B. D., Dube, S. R., & Giles, W. G. (in press). The enduring effects of childhood abuse and related experiences: A convergence of evidence from neurobiology and epidemiology. *European Archives of Clinical Neuroscience.*

Barfield, K. T. (2004). *Best practices in early childhood mental health programs for preschool age children: A report to the Kansas Department of Social and Rehabilitation Services.* Topeka: Division of Health Care Policy, State of Kansas.

Barfield, S., & Gaskill, R. (2005). *Positive impact of the Neurosequential Model of Therapeutics in high-risk children in a therapeutic pre-school setting.* Lawrence, KS: Universty Press of Kansas.

Bremner, J. D. (2003). Long-term effects of childhood abuse on brain and neurobiology. *Child and Adolescent Psychiatric Clinics of North America, 12,* 271–292.

Bremner, J. D., & Vermetten, E. (2001). Stress and development: Behavioral and biological consequences. *Developmental Psychopathology, 13,* 473–489.

De Bellis, M., & Thomas, L. (2003). Biologic findings of post-traumatic stress disorder and child maltreatment. *Current Psychiatry Reports, 5,* 108–117.

Franey, K., Geffner, R., & Falconer, R. (Eds.). (2001). *The cost of maltreatment: Who pays? We all do.* San Diego: Family Violence and Sexual Assault Institute.

Miranda, L., Arthur, A., Milan, T., Mahoney, O., & Perry, B. D. (1998). The art of healing: The Healing Arts Project. *Early Childhood Connections: Journal of Music- and Movement-Based Learning, 4*(4), 35–40.

Miranda, L., Schick, S., Dobson, C., Hogan, L., & Perry, B. D. (1999). *Positive developmental effects of a brief music and movement program at a public preschool: A pilot project* [Abstract]. Available at www.childtrauma.org/ctaServices/neigh_arts.asp

O'Connor, C., Rutter, M., & English and Romanian Adoptees Study Team. (2000). Attachment disorder behavior following early severe deprivation: Extension and longitudinal follow-up. *Journal of the American Academy of Child and Adolescent Psychiatry, 39,* 703–712.

Olds, D., Henderson, C., & Eckenrode, J. (2002). Preventing child abuse and neglect with prenatal and infancy visiting by nurses. In K. Browne, H. Hanks, P. Stratton, & C. Hamilton (Eds.), *Early prediction and prevention of child abuse: A handbook.* Chichester, UK: Wiley.

Perry, B. D. (1999). Memories of fear: How the brain stores and retrieves physiologic states, feelings, behaviors and thoughts from traumatic events. In J. M. Goodwin & R. Attias (Eds.), *Images of the body in trauma* (pp. 26–47). New York: Basic Books.

Perry, B. D. (2001). The neuroarcheology of childhood maltreatment: The neurodevelopmental costs of adverse childhood events. In K. Franey, R. Geffner, & R. Falconer (Eds.), *The cost of maltreatment: Who pays? We all do* (pp. 15–37). San Diego, CA: Family Violence and Sexual Assault Institute.

Perry, B. D. (2002a). Childhood experience and the expression of genetic potential: What childhood neglect tells us about nature and nurture. *Brain and Mind, 3,* 79–100.

Perry, B. D. (2002b). *Traumatic memory and neurodevelopment: A proposed mechanism of action for EMDR.* Plenary paper presented at the annual meeting of the EMDR International Association, San Diego, CA.

Perry, B. D., Dobson, C., Schick, S., & Runyan, D. (2000). *The children's crisis care center model: A proactive, multidimensional child and family assessment process.* Available at www.childtrauma.org/CTAMATERIALS/cccc_paper.asp

Perry, B. D., & Pollard, R. (1998). Homeostasis, stress, trauma, and adaptation: A neurodevelopmental view of childhood trauma. *Child and Adolescent Psychiatric Clinics of North America, 7*(1), 33–51.

Perry, B. D., Pollard, R., Blakely, T., Baker, W., & Vigilante, D. (1995). Childhood trauma, the neurobiology of adaptation and "use-dependent" development of the brain: How "states" become "traits." *Infant Mental Health Journal, 16*(4), 271–291.

Ramey, C. T., Campbell, F. A., Burchinal, M., Skinner, M. L., Gardner, D. M., & Ramey, S. L. (2000). Persistent effects of early childhood education on high-risk children and their mothers. *Applied Developmental Science, 4,* 2–14.

Read, J., Perry, B. D., Moskowitz, A., & Connolly, J. (2001). The contribution of early traumatic events to schizophrenia in some patients: A traumagenic neurodevelopmental model. *Psychiatry, 64*(4), 319–345.

Reynolds, A. J., Temple, J. A., Robertson, D. L., & Mann, E. A. (2001). Long-term effects of an early childhood intervention on educational achievement and juvenile arrest: A 15-year follow-up of low-income children in public schools. *Journal of the American Medical Association, 285*(18), 2339–2346.

Rutter, M., Andersen-Wood, L., Beckett, C., Bredenkamp, D., Castle, J., Grootheus, C., Keppner, J., Keaveny, L., Lord, C., O'Connor, T. G., & English and Romanian Adoptees Study Team. (1999). Quasi-autistic patterns following severe early global privation. *Journal of Child Psychology and Psychiatry, 40,* 537–549.

Rutter, M., & English and Romanian Adoptees Study Team. (1998). Developmental catch-up, and deficit, following adoption after severe global early privation. *Journal of Child Psychology and Psychiatry, 39,* 465–476.

Smith, M. G., & Fong, R. (2004). *The children of neglect: When no one cares.* New York: Brunner-Routledge.

Teicher, M. H., Andersen, S. L., Polcari, A., Anderson, C. M., & Navalta, C. P. (2002). Developmental neurobiology of childhood stress and trauma. *Psychiatric Clinics of North America, 25,* 397–426.

CHAPTER 4

Assessment of Trauma in Children and Youth

MARK CAMERON
JENNIFER ELKINS
NEIL GUTERMAN

By definition, many children and adolescents helped by child welfare services have experienced potentially traumatic actions, conditions, and situations in their lives (see Webb, Chapter 2, this volume). Many of these children suffer with upsetting and disabling symptoms and are at risk for serious developmental problems. Unfortunately, even with the best of care, some children in the child welfare system will also experience trauma as a consequence of out-of-home placements, hospitalizations, loss of family and friends, and other events consequent to intervention. However, although there is minimal research in this area, systematic assessment for trauma among children and youth does not appear to be routine in child welfare practice. Perhaps surprisingly, such assessment also appears to be relatively uncommon among mental health practitioners (Frueh et al., 2002; Guterman & Cameron, 1999; Guterman, Hahm, & Cameron, 2002; Saunders, Kilpatrick, Resnick, & Tidwell, 1989), as well as among professionals in the pediatric health care system (Groves & Augustyn, 2004). This failure to assess for trauma may be costly, because untreated victims of trauma may face dire developmental consequences and may exhibit symptoms that can interfere with and damage the chances for success of child welfare interventions. If child welfare practitioners can be helped to routinely and accurately identify those children and adolescents who may be in need of trauma treatment, their young clients' chances for attaining well-being and healthy development may be substantially improved.

This chapter describes ways in which child welfare practitioners may identify trauma in children and help them to receive the services that they may need. We identify conceptual issues that may challenge practitioners' understanding of trauma in children, describe characteristic childhood trauma symptoms and their relationship to traumatic events, discuss organizational influences on performing trauma assessments in child welfare, and recommend methods and instruments practitioners may use to help these children.

DEFINING TRAUMA

Making clinical trauma assessment a routine part of clinical and child welfare practice may be hindered by problems related to the ways in which the term "trauma" is used and misused (Klapper, Plummer, & Harmon, 2004; Groves & Augustyn, 2004). In the literature, "trauma" has been variously defined as an overwhelming experience that may produce problematic adaptations or symptoms; as a particular type of psychological suffering; as a psychological outcome of an identifiable, traumatizing event (Sparta, 2003); and also as a nonpathological reaction to extreme stressors (Smith, Perrin, & Yule, 1998). Laypersons and clinicians may routinely use the terms "trauma" and "traumatized" to describe all of these phenomena indiscriminately, obscuring a specific and nuanced understanding of trauma (Klapper et al., 2004).

The *Diagnostic and Statistical Manual of Mental Disorders*, fourth edition, text revision (DSM-IV-TR) diagnosis of posttraumatic stress disorder (PTSD) offers a basic definition of trauma: the appearance of characteristic symptoms following exposure to an environmental or interpersonal event or events subjectively experienced with "intense fear, helplessness, or horror" (American Psychiatric Association [APA], 2000, p. 462) as a threat to one's own safety or physical integrity, or as a threat to the safety or physical integrity of others (see Sparta, 2003). Though incomplete and overly abstract, this definition outlines and differentiates the three key elements of trauma: (1) a precipitating event or series of events (2) experienced as a threat and (3) producing characteristic symptoms.

POTENTIALLY TRAUMATIC EVENTS

Defining and classifying potentially traumatic events are also deceptively complex. Traumatic events may be typified by the nature of the particular actions, situations, or conditions to which an individual may be exposed (Kira, 2001). Examples of these potentially traumatizing stressors include physical abuse, sexual abuse, community violent acts (e.g., a mugging or rape), car accidents, natural disasters (e.g., hurricanes and floods), and human-made disasters (e.g., war and violent acts of terrorism). A child may be exposed to one discrete traumatizing episode (acute traumatization, also known as Type I trauma), or to ongoing, repeated episodes (Type II trauma) that may come to be viewed by some victims as common occurrences (Terr, 1981). Traumatizing events may also be categorized as either interpersonal (e.g., physical and sexual abuse) or noninterpersonal (e.g., car accidents and natural disasters) (Sparta, 2003).

Potentially traumatic events may also be defined by the nature of victims' involvement with the actions, situations, and conditions that they face, as well as their relationships with others involved in these incidents. A child's role at the time of a traumatic incident–as direct victim, indirect victim (hearing news that has a traumatic effect), witness, participant, and/or forced participant–helps to determine both the traumatized child's experience and the nature of the sequelae. Interpersonal traumatic events may be distinguished by proximity (the victim's physical closeness to traumatic situations) and immediacy (the role relationship and emotional closeness between the victim and perpetrator[s] of traumatic actions) (Ronen, 2002). Traumatic actions may be perpetrated by family members, friends, community members, others with whom a child is emotionally close but physically distant, or others who are physically close but not emotionally related to the child (Ronen, 2002). Given these factors, potentially traumatic events may most appropriately be considered as the product of the interaction of all these factors: specific actions, situations, and conditions; their chronicity; the presence or absence of others in these incidents; the role played by the exposed individual during the incidents; and the relationship between the exposed individual and others involved (see Nader, 2004).

TRAUMA SYMPTOMS

The particular appearance of trauma symptoms in children is determined by a variety of environmental and intrapersonal factors in children's lives, producing idiosyncratic symptom patterns. Environmental factors include the nature and chronicity of the traumatic event(s), the ways in which parents respond to their children's victimization, the overall social supports available to children, and cultural influences that may promote resilience or increased vulnerability (De Bellis et al., 2001; Ronen, 2002; Sparta, 2003). Webb (2004) proposes a tripartite model to refer to the interactive components of the traumatic event, the individual's response, and factors in the recovery environment. Individually based factors include the victim's age (see Table 4.1), "predisposition for autonomic arousal" (Sparta, 2003, p. 212), problem-solving and coping skills, emotional regulation, understanding of emotion and thinking, cognitive inhibition, memory retrieval, knowledge level, language abilities, previous traumatization, comorbid disorders (if any), and secondary responses to trauma (Cook-Cottone, 2004; Davis & Siegel, 2000; Salmon & Bryant, 2002).

TABLE 4.1. Symptoms of Trauma among Children and Adolescents during Developmental Stages

Infants

Eating and sleeping problems
Persistent crying and upset
Recurrent recollections of the traumatic event(s)
Separation anxiety
Head banging and other self-injuring behaviors
Intense affect
Inability to evoke protective responses from parents
Distressing dreams

Toddlers

All of the symptoms of infancy
Posttraumatic play reenacting some aspect of the traumatic event(s)
Generalized fears
Recklessness
Preemptive and self-protective aggression
Angry disobedience

Preschoolers

All of the symptoms of earlier stages
Preoccupation with body integrity
Power plays in relationships

School-age children

Psychic numbing
Flashbacks
Nightmares
Futurelessness
Avoidance of places, situations, or people associated with the traumatic event(s)
Panic attacks triggered by stimuli simulating the traumatic event(s)
Dissociation
Truancy or sudden decline in academic performance

Adolescents

Psychic numbing
Avoidance of places, situations, or people associated with the traumatic event(s)
Flashbacks
Futurelessness
Dissociation
Sudden decline in academic performance/truancy
Dangerous and reckless behaviors
Delinquency
Suicidal ideation
Running away
Promiscuity
Dating violence

Note. Data from American Psychological Association (2000); Garbarino, Dubrow, Kostelny, and Pardo (1992); and Lieberman and Van Horn (2004).

Symptoms characteristic of trauma in children may be thought of primarily as pertaining to three of the DSM-IV-TR diagnostic criteria for PTSD: the psychological reexperiencing of the traumatic event(s); the avoidance of stimuli associated with the trauma and numbing of general responsiveness; and increased arousal (APA, 2000). Specifically, these include the following:

- *Symptoms related to reexperiencing of traumatic events*: Recurrent, intrusive, and distressing recollections (in young children, repetitive play enacting aspects of the trauma); distressing dreams; flashbacks; intense physiological or psychological distress reactions to "internal or external cues" reminiscent of the traumatic events.
- *Symptoms related to avoidance of stimuli and numbing of responsiveness*: Active avoidance of thoughts, feelings, activities, places, or people related to the event(s); forgetting aspects of the traumatic event(s); estrangement from others; loss of interest in formerly meaningful activities; restricted affect; sense of futurelessness.
- *Symptoms of increased arousal*: Sleep problems; irritability and/or angry outbursts; concentration problems; hypervigilance; exaggerated startle response (APA, 2000).

The DSM-IV-TR PTSD framework is not inclusive of all symptoms demonstrated by traumatized children and does not convey the full complexity of trauma symptom patterns in children. Some may develop symptoms associated with other syndromes, such as attention-deficit/hyperactivity disorder, bipolar disorders, depression, and conduct disorder (Famularo, Kinscherff, & Fenton, 1990; Rutter, 1996; van der Kolk et al., 2002). Less severe symptoms resulting from traumatic experiences may initially be indistinguishable from typical variations in childhood or adolescent behaviors (Perrin, Smith, & Yule, 2000). Some traumatized children may even appear to be asymptomatic but suffer from difficult-to-detect symptoms, such as increased heart rates (Cohen, 1998; Sauter & Franklin, 1998). The appearance of trauma symptoms is also influenced by time. For some children, the onset of symptoms following a traumatizing event or events may be delayed by months or even years (Sparta, 2003). The duration of symptoms can vary considerably as well: For about half of symptomatic traumatized children, their symptoms will last about 3 months (Sparta, 2003).

CHALLENGES AND OBSTACLES IN THE ASSESSMENT OF TRAUMA IN CHILDREN

Child welfare practitioners may be unlikely to assess for trauma in their practices, due to issues related to their agencies, their education and training, and their clients. In the child welfare system, agencies not primarily involved in providing therapeutic services do not routinely assess or diagnose their clients for mental health problems. The paramount tasks of this system—the substantiation of maltreatment and assessment of risk of future harm—frame and constrain practitioners' focus. Maltreatment substantiation primarily requires identification and documentation of observable, behaviorally based forensic evidence. Resources in child welfare agencies are often very limited, and practice that is considered extraneous to the primary mission may not be encouraged.

In addition, many practitioners in child welfare may not have extensive education or training in child development, trauma, or trauma assessment. Some understanding of child development as well as developmental psychopathology may be required to assess adequately for trauma in children (Sparta, 2003). Practitioners may be reluctant to question children about their traumatic experiences, either to avoid evoking symptomatic responses in the youth (Spiers, 2001) or to prevent their own vicarious traumatization, which can result from hearing about clients' traumatic experiences (see Hesse, 2002; Jankowski, 2003; Pynoos, Steinberg, & Goenjian, 1996).

Practitioners may also question the accuracy of children's and parents' reports about traumatic events. Children generally do not discuss traumatic events with adults (Ronen, 2002). When they do, their reports may be distorted, due to a number of factors: They may have cognitive difficulties in understanding what has happened to them (Lieberman & Van Horn, 2004; Weiss, 2004); they may change how they understand things (Nader, 2004; Weissman, 1991); they may cope through diminished awareness (Nader, 2004); they may provide incomplete reports (Carrion, Weems, Ray, & Reiss, 2002; Nader & Fairbanks, 1994); they may have a short attention span or language deficiencies (Ronen, 2002); and/or they may distort events in an effort to please the interviewer or to avoid conflict with parents, especially if the parents are present during the interview (Nader, 1997; Peterson, Prout, & Schwartz, 1991; Yule & Gold, 1993; Yule & Udwin, 1991; Yule & Williams, 1989). Parents may have little knowledge of their children's inner experiences and may underestimate their trauma-related upset (Achenbach & Rescorla, 2001; Peterson et al., 1991; Reynolds & Kamphaus, 1998). This is especially likely if the parents have psychological problems themselves (Ronen, 2002). Collaborative partnerships with parents may be crucial for obtaining accurate information about children's traumatic experiences (Lieberman & Van Horn, 2004), but in child welfare, establishing these partnerships with parents may not always be possible.

Understandably, without adequate organizational training and support, and given the challenges and complexities of the work that they do, child welfare practitioners are limited in their ability and readiness to assess for trauma as an integral part of their practice.

ASSESSMENT APPROACHES AND INSTRUMENTS

If trauma goes undetected, appropriate intervention is not likely to be provided. Early intervention with children exposed to potentially traumatic events may prevent the onset of PTSD as well as other seriously detrimental outcomes (Berliner, 1997; Ozer, Lipsey, & Weiss, 2003). Especially when these outcomes are manifested as externalizing behavior problems, they can threaten the success of child welfare interventions, and may result in multiple failed placements and increasingly discouraged, disconnected children (Ronen, 2002). To ensure the safety and well-being of children receiving child welfare services, and to ensure the success of those services, practitioners need to identify and respond to their traumatized child clients.

Child welfare practitioners concerned about childhood trauma may informally screen for the characteristic symptoms of trauma during their routine work. First, however, practitioners must become knowledgeable about the characteristic symptoms of trauma, and must approach their work with the mindset that trauma is likely to be present in many of their clients. Using observation of children and adolescents, and mindful of the influences of developmental stage, practitioners can easily perform a brief trauma screening. For example, practitioners can observe children at play for reenactment of traumatic events, emotional lability, and aggressiveness with other children. Adolescents may be observed demonstrating reckless behaviors; avoiding places, situations, or others; or evincing signs of dissociation. Follow-up interviews with children and parents can be used to establish the facts and details regarding the traumatization, as other practitioners might routinely do.

For those practitioners who would like to take a more structured approach, semistructured interview guidelines or standardized instruments may be used. Interview guidelines contain suggested areas of focus and/or specific questions for assessing trauma that may be used as a stand-alone interview or incorporated with other protocols. Ronen (2002) has developed a three-part parental interview guideline, with specific questions focusing on the identification of the presence of DSM-IV-TR PTSD symptoms, noticeable changes in the child's behavior, and the influences of the child's age and stage of emotional and cognitive development on the impact of the trauma. For assessing specifically for trauma related to exposure to community violence, an assessment framework has been developed that identifies the nature of the traumatic events, sequelae, ongoing lethality, and the risks and supports available to the child (Guterman & Cameron, 1997). Structured interviews and standardized measures can be used if practitioners have the time and organizational support to incorporate them into their work.

Brief descriptions of the most strongly recommended measures appear in Appendix 4.1.

TRAUMA ASSESSMENT AND INTERVENTION

Systematic trauma assessment in child welfare can be helpful to both children and the professionals serving them. For children who may very recently have experienced a traumatic event or are being subjected routinely to traumatic situations, immediate identification of the traumatization may enable "psychological first aid" (Pynoos & Nader, 1993) to be administered. This immediate response may help to stem further deterioration on the part of the child; may suggest discrete steps that might be taken to inoculate the child from further exposure to traumatic situations and/or relationships; and, not insignificantly, may build trust between the child and the child welfare worker and agency. When referrals to mental health services are available and accessible to families, tentative determinations of trauma help child and family therapists to triage their efforts and develop intervention plans that may help children and avoid inadvertent re-traumatization of young clients. Finally, systematic trauma assessment can help child welfare practitioners understand the ways in which trauma may be a product of the losses and transitional problems created by the services provided; this may allow for modification of intervention plans and methods, and for prevention of further institutional traumatization.

DISCUSSION

Child welfare practitioners' work with challenging situations and clients allows for minimal consideration of clinical factors, which may seriously limit the ultimate success of their efforts. Without additional resources, including training, ongoing supervisory support, and time, formal trauma assessment of trauma will probably not take place. However, dedicated practitioners, mindful of the importance of identifying trauma in their clients and with knowledge of the characteristic symptoms of trauma, can expand the observation and interviewing methods they already use to incorporate a trauma screening. For those who may have additional resources of time and other forms of organizational supports, semi-structured interviews and standardized instruments can be used for more thorough and valid trauma assessments. Use of most of these instruments requires some training, and each is accompanied by a manual that provides directives. For those practitioners without training, the Children's

PTSD (CPTSDI), the Lifetime Incidence of Traumatic Events (LITE), the PTSD-Reaction Index, and the Trauma Symptom Checklist for Children (TSCC) are recommended (see Table 4.2). Ideally, child welfare agencies should include trauma screening as a standard part of their regular intake assessment procedures.

Of course, assessment is only the first step. Practitioners need to have access to clinical services for children that can help their young clients recover and continue to develop. Ultimately, administrators of child welfare agencies must advocate for the necessary resources and for partnerships with mental health organizations, to ensure that traumatized children do not continue to fall into the cracks within and between these systems. When trauma in children in the child welfare system is identified and appropriate help is provided to them, their health and development are supported, and the efforts of professionals serving them are more likely to be successful.

TABLE 4.2. Standardized Trauma Assessment Instruments for Children and Adolescents

Instrument	Young	School-age	Older/ adolescents	Parent version
Anxiety Disorders Interview Schedule–Child (ADIS-C)		×	×	
Children's PTSD Inventory (CPTSDI)	×	×		
Clinician-Administered PTSD Scale for Children (CAPS-CA)			×	
Child Report of Post-Traumatic Symptoms (CROPS) and Parent Report of Post-Traumatic Symptoms (PROPS)		×	×	×
Diagnostic Classification of Mental Health and Developmental Disorders of Infancy and Early Childhood (Diagnostic Classification: 0–3)	×			×
Dissociative Experiences Scale (DES), Child and Adolescent Versions		×	×	
Impact of Event Scale–8 Child Items (IES–8)			×	
Lifetime Incidence of Traumatic Events (LITE)		×	×	
PTSD-Reaction Index		×	×	
Trauma Symptom Checklist for Children (TSCC)		×	×	

APPENDIX 4.1. STRUCTURED CLINICAL INTERVIEWS AND STANDARDIZED MEASURES

For more details about these and other instruments, see Fletcher (n.d.), Greenwald (1999), Sauter and Franklin (1998), Weiss (2004), and Nader (2004).

- *Anxiety Disorders Interview Schedule–Child (ADIS-C)* (Silverman & Nelles, 1988). This semistructured interview survey follows DSM criteria and is designed to identify anxiety disorders in children, including symptoms associated with PTSD.
- *Children's PTSD Inventory (CPTSDI)* (Saigh et al., 2000; Yasik et al., 2001). This child-friendly PTSD inventory requires no expertise to use and taps into children's experiences.
- *Clinician-Administered PTSD Scale for Children (CAPS-CA)* (Nader et al., 2004; Newman & Ribbe, 1996). This interview-based scale conforms to DSM PTSD criteria and is expanded to include other conditions, such as fears, derealization, depersonalization, and changes in attachment. It is best suited for older children.
- *Child Report of Post-Traumatic Symptoms (CROPS) and Parent Report of Post-Traumatic Symptoms (PROPS)* (Greenwald & Rubin, 1999). These 24-item and 28-item self-report surveys cover a wide range of PTSD symptoms.
- *Diagnostic Classification of Mental Health and Developmental Disorders of Infancy and Early Childhood (Diagnostic Classification: 0–3)* (National Center for Clinical Infant Programs, 1994). This parent/caretaker survey was specifically developed for use for infants and younger children.
- *Dissociative Experiences Scale (DES)* (Carlson et al., 1993). A screening checklist, this scale is available in child and adolescent versions.
- *Impact of Event Scale–8 Child Items (IES–8)* (Dyregrov & Yule, 1995). This brief adaptation of a longer scale contains eight items concerning intrusive thoughts and avoidance related to a specific event. It is recommended for use with adolescents (Fletcher, n.d.).
- *Lifetime Incidence of Traumatic Events (LITE)* (Greenwald, 2000). This simple and brief survey covers a wide range of traumatic events and experiences, and examines the emotional impact of events.
- *PTSD-Reaction Index* (McNally, 1991, 1996). This is a popularly used semistructured interview survey measure of PTSD in youth. It is easy to administer and score, and is available in Spanish.
- *Trauma Symptom Checklist for Children (TSCC)* (Elliot & Briere, 1994; Evans, Briere, Boggiano, & Barrett, 1994; Lanktree, Briere, & Hernandez, 1995). This 54-item self-report instrument is best for use with children ages 8–16. It is quick and easy to administer and score, and appears appropriate for use with diverse client populations.

ACKNOWLEDGMENTS

We would like to thank Howard Doueck, Barbara Rittner, and Ricky Greenwald for their assistance in the preparation of this chapter.

REFERENCES

Achenbach, T. M., & Rescorla, L. A. (2001). *Manual for the ASEBA School-Age Forms and Profiles.* Burlington: University of Vermont, Research Center for Children, Youth, and Families.

American Psychiatric Association (APA). (2000). *Diagnostic and statistical manual of mental disorders* (4th ed., text rev.). Washington, DC: Author.

Berliner, L. (1997). Intervention with children who experience trauma. In D. Cicchetti & S. Toth (Eds.), *Developmental perspectives on trauma: Theory, research, and intervention* (pp. 491–514). Rochester, NY: University of Rochester Press.

Carlson, E. B., Putnam, F. W., Ross, C. A., Torem, M., Coons, P., Dill, D. L., Loewenstein, R. J., & Braun, B. G. (1993). Validity of the Dissociative Experiences Scale in screening for multiple personality disorder: A multicenter study. *American Journal of Psychiatry, 150*(7), 1030–1036.

Carrion, V. G., Weems, C. F., Ray, R. D., & Reiss, A. L. (2002). Toward an empirical definition of pediatric PTSD: The phenomenology of PTSD symptoms in youth. *Journal of the American Academy of Child and Adolescent Psychiatry, 41*(2), 166–173.

Cohen, J. (1998). Summary of the practice parameters for the assessment and treatment of children and adolescents with posttraumatic stress disorder. *Journal of the American Academy of Child and Adolescent Psychiatry, 37*(9), 997–1001.

Cook-Cottone, C. (2004). Childhood posttraumatic stress disorder: Diagnosis, treatment, and school reintegration. *School Psychology Review, 33*(1), 127–139.

Davis, L., & Siegel, L. (2000). Posttraumatic stress disorder in children and adolescents: A review and analysis. *Clinical Child and Family Psychology Review, 3*(3), 135–154.

De Bellis, M. D., Broussard, E. R., Herring, D. J., Wexler, S., Moritz, G., & Benitez, J. G. (2001) Psychiatric co-morbidity in caregivers and children involved in maltreatment: A pilot research study with policy implications. *Child Abuse and Neglect, 25*(7), 923–944.

Dyregrov, A., & Yule, W. (1995, November). *Screening measures–The development of the UNICEF screening battery.* Paper presented at the 9th Annual Meeting of the International Society of Stress Studies, Boston.

Elliot, D., & Briere, J. (1994). Forensic sexual abuse evaluations of older children: Disclosures and symptomotology. *Behavioral Sciences and the Law, 12,* 261–277.

Evans, J., Briere, J., Boggiano, A., & Barrett, M. (1994). *Reliability and validity of the Trauma Symptom Checklist for Children in a normal sample.* Paper presented at the San Diego Conference on Responding to Child Maltreatment, San Diego, CA.

Famularo, R., Kinscherff, R., & Fenton, T. (1990). Symptom differences in acute and chronic presentation of childhood posttraumatic stress disorder. *Child Abuse and Neglect, 14*(5), 439–444.

Fletcher, K. E. (n.d.). *Scales for assessing posttraumatic responses of children*. Retrieved from http://users.umassmed.edu/Kenneth.Fletcher/scales.html

Frueh, B. C., Cousins, V. C., Hiers, T. G., Cavenaugh, S. D., Cusack, K. J., & Santos, A. B. (2002). The need for trauma assessment and related clinical services in a state-funded mental health system. *Community Mental Health Journal, 38*(4), 351–356.

Garbarino, J., Dubrow, N., Kostelny, K., & Pardo, C. (1992). *Children in danger: Coping with the consequences of community violence*. San Francisco: Jossey-Bass.

Greenwald, R. (1999). *Child trauma measures for research and practice*. Retrieved from www.childtrauma.com/mezpost.html

Greenwald, R. (2000). *Lifetime Incidence of Traumatic Events–Student and Parent forms (LITE-S and LITE-P): Manual and measures*. Baltimore: Sidran.

Greenwald, R., & Rubin, A. (1999). Brief assessment of children's posttraumatic symptoms: Development and preliminary validation of parent and child scales. *Research on Social Work Practice, 9*, 61–75.

Groves, B. M., & Augustyn, M. (2004). Identification, assessment, and intervention for young traumatized children within a pediatric setting. In J. D. Osofsky (Ed.), *Young children and trauma: Intervention and treatment* (pp. 173–193). New York: Guilford Press.

Guterman, N. B., & Cameron, M. (1997). Assessing the impact of community violence on children and youths. *Social Work, 42*(5), 495–505.

Guterman, N. B., & Cameron, M. (1999). Young clients' exposure to community violence: How much do their therapists know? *American Journal of Orthopsychiatry, 69*(3), 382–391.

Guterman, N. B., Hahm, H., & Cameron, M. (2002). Adolescent victimization and subsequent use of mental health counseling services. *Journal of Adolescent Health, 30*(5), 336–345.

Hesse, A. R. (2002). Secondary trauma: How working with trauma survivors affects therapists. *Clinical Social Work Journal, 30*(3), 293–309.

Jankowski, J. (2003). Vicarious traumatization and its impact on the Pennsylvania child welfare system. *Dissertation Abstracts International, 63*(7), 2467A.

Kira, I. A. (2001). Taxonomy of trauma and trauma assessment. *Traumatology, 7*(2), 73–86.

Klapper, S. A., Plummer, N. S., & Harmon, R. J. (2004). Diagnostic and treatment issues in cases of childhood trauma. In J. D. Osofsky (Ed.), *Young children and trauma: Intervention and treatment* (pp. 139–154). New York: Guilford Press.

Lanktree, C., Briere, J., & Hernandez, P. (1995). Outcome of therapy for sexually abused children: A repeated measures study. *Child Abuse and Neglect, 19*, 1145–1155.

Lieberman, A. F., & Van Horn, P. (2004). Assessment and treatment of young children exposed to traumatic events. In J. D. Osofsky (Ed.), *Young children and trauma: Intervention and treatment* (pp. 111–138). New York: Guilford Press.

McNally, R. (1991). Assessment of posttraumatic stress disorder in children: Psychological assessment. *Journal of Consulting and Clinical Psychology, 3*, 320–325.

McNally, R. (1996). Assessment of post-traumatic stress disorder in children and adolescents. *Journal of School Psychology, 34,* 147–161.

Nader, K. O. (1997). Assessing traumatic experiences in children. In J. Wilson & T. Keane (Eds.), *Assessing psychological trauma and PTSD* (pp. 291–348). New York: Guilford Press.

Nader, K. O. (2004). Assessing traumatic experiences in children: Self-reports of DSM PTSD criteria B–D symptoms. In J. P. Wilson & T. M. Keane (Eds.), *Assessing psychological trauma and PTSD* (2nd ed., pp. 513–537). New York: Guilford Press.

Nader, K. O., & Fairbanks, L. (1994). The suppression of reexperiencing: Impulse control and somatic symptoms in children following traumatic exposure. *Anxiety, Stress and Coping: An International Journal, 7,* 229–239.

Nader, K. O., Newman, E., Weathers, F., Kaloupek, D., Kriegler, J., & Blake, D. (2004). *Clinician-Administered PTSD Scale for Children and Adolescents (CAPS-CA).* Los Angeles: Western Psychological Services. (Available at no cost at www.ncptsd.org/treatment/assessment/child_measures.html#CAPSCA)

National Center for Clinical Infant Programs. (1994). *Diagnostic classification of mental health and developmental disorders of infancy and early childhood (Diagnostic classification: 0–3).* Arlington, VA: Author.

Newman, E., & Ribbe, D. (1996). Psychometric review of the Clinician-Administered PTSD Scale for Children. In B. H. Stamm (Ed.), *Measurement of stress, trauma, and adaptation* (pp. 106–114). Lutherville, MD: Sidran Press.

Ozer, E. J., Lipsey, S. R., & Weiss, D. S. (2003). Predictors of posttraumatic stress disorder and symptoms in adults: A meta-analysis. *Psychological Bulletin, 129*(1), 52–73.

Perrin, S., Smith, P., & Yule, W. (2000). Practitioner review: The assessment and treatment of posttraumatic stress disorder in children and adolescents. *Journal of Child Psychology and Psychiatry, 41*(3), 277–289.

Peterson, K. C., Prout, M. F., & Schwartz, R. A. (1991). *Post-traumatic stress disorders.* New York: Plenum Press.

Pynoos, R. S., & Nader, D. (1993). Issues in the treatment of post-traumatic stress in children and adolescents. In J. P. Wilson & B. Raphael (Eds.), *International handbook of traumatic stress syndromes* (pp. 535–549). New York: Plenum Press.

Pynoos, R. S., Steinberg, A. M., & Goenjian, A. (1996). Traumatic stress in childhood and adolescence: Recent developments and current controversies. In B. A. van der Kolk, A. C. McFarlane, & L. Weisaeth (Eds.), *Traumatic stress: The effects of overwhelming experience on mind, body, and society* (pp. 331–358). New York: Guilford Press.

Reynolds, C. R., & Kamphaus, R. W. (1998). *Behavior Assessment System for Children Manual.* Circle Pines, MN: American Guidance Service.

Ronen, T. (2002). Difficulties in assessing traumatic reactions in children. *Journal of Loss and Trauma, 7,* 87–106.

Rutter, M. (1996). Stress research: Accomplishments and tasks ahead. In R. J. Haggerty, L. R. Sherrod, N. Garmezy, & M. Rutter (Eds.), *Stress, risk, and resilience in children and adolescents: Process, mechanisms, and interventions* (pp. 356–386). New York: Cambridge University Press.

Saigh, P. A., Yasik, A. E., Oberfield, R. A., Green, B. L., Halamandaris, P. V., Rubenstein, H., Nester, J., Resko, J., Hetz, B., & McHugh, M. (2000). The

Children's PTSD Inventory: Development and reliability. *Journal of Traumatic Stress, 13*, 369–380.

Salmon, K., & Bryant, R. (2002). Posttraumatic stress disorder in children: The influence of developmental factors. *Clinical Psychology Review, 22*, 163–188.

Saunders, B. E., Kilpatrick, D. G., Resnick, H. S., & Tidwell, R. P. (1989). Brief screening for lifetime history of criminal victimization at mental health intake: A preliminary study. *Journal of Interpersonal Violence, 4*, 267–277.

Sauter, J., & Franklin, C. (1998). Assessing post-traumatic stress disorder in children: Diagnostic and measurement strategies. *Research on Social Work Practice, 8*(3), 251–270.

Silverman, W., & Nelles, W. (1988). The Anxiety Disorder Interview Schedule for Children. *Journal of the American Academy of Child and Adolescent Psychiatry, 27*, 772–778.

Smith, P., Perrin, S., & Yule, W. (1998). Post-traumatic stress disorders. In P. Graham (Ed.), *Cognitive-behaviour therapy for children and families* (pp. 127–143). Cambridge, UK: Cambridge University Press.

Sparta, S. N. (2003). Assessment of childhood trauma. In A. M. Goldstein (Ed.), *Handbook of psychology: Vol. 11. Forensic psychology* (pp. 209–231). New York: Wiley.

Spiers, T. (2001). *Trauma: A practitioner's guide to counseling*. New York: Brunner-Routledge.

Terr, L. (1981). Forbidden games: Post-traumatic child's play. *Journal of the American Academy of Child Psychiatry, 20*, 741–760.

van der Kolk, B., Bellows, J., Cook, A., Englund, D., Silberg, J., & Waters, F. (2002). *Complex PTSD in children: I. Etiology, assessment, advocacy* [Videotape]. Nevada City, CA: Cavalcade Productions.

Webb, N. B. (Ed.). (2004). *Mass trauma and violence: Helping families and children cope*. New York: Guilford Press.

Weiss, D. S. (2004). Structured clinical interview techniques for PTSD. In J. P. Wilson & T. M. Keane (Eds.), *Assessing psychological trauma and PTSD* (2nd ed., pp. 103–121). New York: Guilford Press.

Weissman, H. N. (1991). Forensic psychological examination of the child witness in cases of alleged sexual abuse. *American Journal of Orthopsychiatry, 61*, 48–58.

Yasik, A. E., Saigh, P. A., Oberfield, R. A., Green, B., Halamandaris, P., & McHugh, M. (2001). The validity of the Children's PTSD Inventory. *Journal of Traumatic Stress, 14*, 81–94.

Yule, W., & Gold, A. (1993). *Wise before the event: Coping with crises in schools*. London: Calouste Gulbenkian Foundation.

Yule, W., & Udwin, O. (1991). Screening child survivors for post-traumatic stress disorders: Experiences from the *Jupiter* sinking. *British Journal of Clinical Psychology, 30*, 131–138.

Yule, W., & Williams, R. M. (1989). Post-traumatic stress reactions in children. *Journal of Traumatic Stress, 3*, 279–295.

CHAPTER 5

Family and Social Factors Affecting Youth in the Child Welfare System

GARY R. ANDERSON
JOHN SEITA

The purpose of this chapter is to identify and discuss the numerous family and social factors that have an impact on traumatized youth in child welfare. For children, trauma can come from multiple external sources; these sources range from witnessing some terrifying and hurtful experience through being the victims of violence. In the child welfare system, by definition, the initial source of a child's trauma is a parent. "Child maltreatment" is some form of serious, nonaccidental harm to the children that is directly attributable to actions committed or omitted by parents.

Abusive acts committed by parents include "physical abuse," in which there is some evidence of physical harm (e.g., a mark or bruise) caused by the parent's hitting the child with a hand, an implement, or some other object. Abuse can also take the form of "sexual abuse," which includes a range of actions that are sexually inappropriate, harmful, or exploitive. "Emotional abuse" is defined as acts by a parent that can cause serious behavioral, emotional, or mental disorders. Also called "psychological abuse" or "verbal abuse," this form of maltreatment is difficult to prove, because a direct link between a child's disturbance and a parent's behavior may be difficult to establish in a court of law. Emotional abuse can also be attributed to acts of omission, as well as deliberate parental assaults on the child.

Neglect can take different forms. Failure to attend to a child's clothing, food, or shelter results in "physical neglect." Failure to attend to the child's medical needs when this causes a serious health threat is central to "medical neglect". The failure to send a child to school is called "educational neglect," and failure to protect the child from harmful people or circumstances is referred to as "supervisory neglect."

In child welfare, the factors that have an impact on children relate to their parents' behavior. These parental behaviors may result in multiple traumas for a child, including physical injury or threats to the child's health, as well as emotional and psychological distress. When the powerful persons to whom a custodial child is to some degree attached and dependent prove to be inconsistent and potentially dangerous, this significantly undercuts the child's mental health and well-being. The early social worker Mary Richmond (1917) noted that no one could more powerfully hurt another person than a family member. The ability of parents to harm and traumatize their children has resulted in a series of legal provisions and in the development of a service delivery system–child protective services–whose mandate is to ensure the safety and well-being of children.

THEORIES OF CHILD MALTREATMENT

In the 1950s and early 1960s, the recognition that the actions of a child's parents could constitute a significant source of physical harm and psychological trauma to the child became more clearly understood and attended to by the medical and social service professional communities. In earlier decades, identification of child maltreatment had taken place (e.g., the case of Mary Ellen in 1873); orphanages and foster homes had also been established to care for children whose parents had died, had abandoned them, or had been deemed unfit to care for them. However, the theoretical understanding of child maltreatment and the development of a systematic response came in the second half of the 20th century. Two early conceptualizations of child trauma due to parental conduct were the "battered child syndrome" and the "world of abnormal rearing cycle."

The Battered Child Syndrome

The term "battered child syndrome" initially referred to the physical injuries sustained by a child as a result of physical abuse by a parent. Advances in medical technology made it possible to diagnose injuries and differentiate between those caused by accident and those resulting from deliberate actions or from suspicious causes. The documentation of harm through photographs, interviews, and medical examinations was viewed as an important step to provide protection for children. Training in identifying and interpreting marks on a child's body became a required procedure for child protection. Some of this recognition of injuries did not require refined medical skills; for example, it was (and is) fairly easy to tell when children presented with bruises bearing the shape of an implement that had been wielded by parents and intentionally directed at the children.

This new attentiveness to children and the trauma they could suffer became relatively widespread. The recognition that children were not the property of their parents, and that children had a right to a certain degree of health and happiness, paralleled the civil rights and women's rights movements and reduced society's tolerance of family privacy and parental privilege. It was now openly acknowledged that the maltreatment of children could result in serious physical symptoms, such as broken or fractured bones, bruises, burns, cuts, and internal injuries–indeed, even death. Moreover, it became increasingly clear that disturbing child behaviors were also correlated with parental abuse. The recognition that physical harm was accompanied by emotional harm fueled more systematic efforts to protect children from further harm and trauma. Consequently, the term "battered child syndrome" came to refer to children's experience of physical abuse resulting in both physical *and* psychological trauma (Helfer & Kempe, 1968; Kempe & Helfer, 1972).

The World of Abnormal Rearing Cycle

Concurrently, in an attempt to understand the perpetuation of child maltreatment within a family, the family and social experience of child abuse and neglect for both parents and children was analyzed. A cyclical dynamic was identified, in which deficits, losses, and traumas experienced by a person (a child and/or parent) started and reinforced a series of behavioral and emotional consequences that shaped subsequent beliefs, choices, and behaviors. This cycle was called the "world of abnormal rearing" (often abbreviated as WAR). It was theorized that the family of origin served as a training ground for interpersonal violence and/or lowered social competence (Azar & Wolfe, 1989).

According to the concept of the WAR cycle, when a child grew up in an environment of abuse and neglect, the child's views of her- or himself and others were shaped by this experience, such that future beliefs and behaviors were to some extent built upon this foundation. For example, if a little girl's parent had physically abused the child, the girl might conclude that she was "not a good person," and perhaps even that she deserved such behavior. This negative view of herself, with its accompanying belief system, would shape her success in relationships, school, and work. Disappointments in these experiences would add to a cycle of failure, further shaping the young woman's decisions about relationships and affecting her future parenting of her own child. The cycle was seen as self-perpetuating in many cases, and as having the potential to begin again. Bowlby (1988) hypothesized, "A mother who as a child suffered neglect and severe threats of being abandoned or beaten is more prone than others to abuse her child physically" (p. 37). This was not considered to be deterministic, but rather descriptive of an "appreciable minority" of abused mothers who would themselves later become abusive, with periods of prolonged anxiety punctuated by outbursts of violent anger (Bowlby, 1988, p. 84). Physical child abuse was thought to be the tip of the iceberg of parental anger and rejection, with multiple and varying effects upon the children.

The WAR cycle was seen as both beginning with and being reinforced by parental maltreatment of a child. The intervention goal would be to interrupt this cycle and encourage alternative beliefs and experiences. So, for example, having a child in a high-quality day care setting might remove that child from a negative home environment and, through consistent and skilled caregiving, promote the development of positive emotional self-concepts and behaviors. Strategies such as modulated voice control, predictable and fair rules, appropriate physical affection, courtesy, fair discipline, responsiveness from adults, and the encouragement of respectful relations among children might modify or counteract the environment experienced by the child at home (Bradley et al., 1986). Although it was a less dramatic concept than the battered child syndrome, the WAR cycle described the perpetuation of behavior resulting in multiple traumas for children and youth.

Benefits and Shortcomings of These Theories

These two viewpoints brought increasing attention to the emerging family and social issue of child maltreatment. The battered child syndrome identified child abuse as a medical emergency and reduced the sense that children were the property of parents and could be treated in any manner deemed fit by the parents. The WAR cycle described both the short- and long-term harm that resulted from child abuse and neglect, again highlighting the need for intervention to protect children and provide treatment for both children and parents. However, these concepts also supported a view of abusive parents as being different from "normal," nonabusive parents. That is, they suggested a dichotomy between people who had the potential to hurt their children and "normal" parents. More recent theorists have suggested a conceptualization of child maltreatment that is based on a continuum model of parenting. From this perspective, abuse and neglect are defined as "the degree to which a parent uses aversive or inappropriate control strategies with his or her child and/or fails to provide minimal standards of caregiving and nurturance" (Azar & Wolfe, 1989, p. 452). This focus on a broader range of parenting behaviors does not suggest that the consequences of abuse to children are not serious, however.

These two concepts, advanced by medical doctors, also implied a medical model: (1) There was a diagnosable condition called "child maltreatment"; (2) there was a victim, the child; (3) there was a perpetrator, the parent; (4) the child had the diagnosable condition, and the parent's behavior was in some way evidence of illness or other parental deficiencies; (5) typically, the child needed to be quarantined (i.e., separated from the parent); (6) both the child and the parent needed some form of treatment; and (7) hospitals and medically based interdisciplinary teams had a crucial role in the diagnosis and treatment of child abuse. Furthermore, both concepts implied a focus on child abuse rather than child neglect, even though child neglect has consistently been significantly more prevalent than physical child abuse. From both perspectives, cruel, disturbed, or sick parents were hurting unfortunate children.

The public's and the child welfare system's views of parents have often been complicated and contradictory. On the one hand, parents have been viewed as adults who are responsible for their actions and therefore should provide life's necessities and love for their children. Parents who harm their children have made bad choices, should be held responsible for their behavior, and should suffer any legal or social consequences associated with their harmful behavior. The vast majority of children in families that live in poverty are not abused or neglected by their parents. Many parents who use alcohol or other drugs, or who suffer from mental illness, do not harm their children. There is no excuse for abusing or neglecting one's children. However, the multiple stresses associated with poverty challenge consistent and positive parenting. The loss of control associated with domestic violence, mental illness, and/or the pull of addiction may also powerfully undermine parents' ability to care for children and themselves. The benefits that accrue to children raised in an attentive, loving, and resourceful home may not have been available for these parents and may not be present for their children (Seita, 1994). Also, a focus on parental failures may overlook the strengths that provide a therapeutic platform for rebuilding a struggling family. The theories of the battered child syndrome and the WAR cycle have tended to minimize both the stresses and the opportunities for support that exist in a family's environment.

These viewpoints have described and diagnosed particularly traumatic conditions for children, and have provided explanations for their views in terms of the troubles resulting from a lifelong cycle permeated by experiences of childhood trauma. Whether it was the perpetration of battering, engaging in behaviors that resulted in an abnormal world, or a range of harmful or inadequate parenting methods, the danger to children was attributed primarily to parents. But why would parents hurt their children physically and psychologically? The primary traumatization of children who are served by the child welfare system is attributable to their parents' behavior, and that behavior is affected by a range of challenges including violence, homelessness, health crises, poverty, life crises, substance abuse, impaired mental health, and other factors. The next several sections of this chapter describe a number of parental and social factors that affect the safety and well-being of children. Beyond the primary traumatization for children, the child welfare system itself can create new sources of trauma that can compound and even seem to supersede the consequences of parental harm.

PARENTAL FACTORS

The essential key to mental health is that the "infant and young child should experience a warm, intimate and continuous relationship with his mother (or permanent mother-substitute) in which both find satisfaction and enjoyment" (Bowlby, 1966, p. 11). As Bowlby indicated, this caring person (or persons) is usually the mother (or, in many cases, two parents). What if a parent is not available to be this person for some reason? For many children, there are available substitutes (e.g., grandparents, or later teachers or coaches). Their role in the children's lives may not be as timely or may not offer immediate and steady access, but such a positive relationship can have a powerful influence. But what if the person who is central to a child's early development not only lacks warmth and intimacy, but is inconsistent and negative–or, worse, harmful? The child welfare system, when it is working properly, supports families to prevent harm and separation and intervenes only when parents are judged to be a danger to their children. What factors contribute to parents' risk of harming or traumatizing their children?

Substance Abuse

In the United States, over 8 million children live with at least one parent who abuses alcohol or another drug. Substance abuse is a significant factor in both child abuse and child neglect (Young, Wingfield, & Klempner, 2001). Although the numbers vary from state to state, a high number of cases (40–80% of all families in the child welfare system) that are reported to child protective services and result in an out-of-home placement involve some form of parental substance abuse (Young et al., 2001). The abuse or neglect is attributable in these cases to the impaired cognition, as well as the lessened impulse control and self-control, that result from the use of alcohol or other substances. Prenatal abuse in the form of fetal alcohol syndrome, fetal alcohol effects, medical complications, prematurity, and/or neurological disturbances may occur in pregnant women who abuse substances (Tower, 1996).

A number of problems associated with alcohol and drug use impair parenting ability and adversely affect children. These include parental depression and the increased likelihood of mothers' being victims of violence. Moreover, alcohol and drug addiction by definition involve compulsive preoccupation with obtaining and using the substance, and this affects all aspects of the self to the point that the substance actually becomes one's primary relationship (Zuckerman, 1994). Consequently, the child maltreatment and threats to children's safety and stability that result directly or indirectly from parental substance abuse can take a number of forms. A child may be physically neglected, as a parent's resources are used to gain alcohol or drugs rather than to provide food, clothing, or appropriate shelter for the child. The child may be medically neglected, as the parent is inattentive to the child's needs or exposes the child to dangerous situations. The child may be educationally neglected, as the parent fails to send the child to school because of the parent's substance use, its aftereffects, and the parent's resulting disregard for preparing and prompting the child to attend school. The child's supervision may be neglected, resulting in exposure to potentially dangerous neighborhood environments, potentially harmful people, and domestic violence, and sometimes also in leaving young children unattended. A parent with substance abuse may not be psychologically or verbally abusive, but emotional and psychological neglect can occur due to the parent's preoccupation with substance use rather than focusing on the child's needs. In one study of children whose parents abused alcohol or opiates, all of the children were found to have suffered some form of neglect (Black & Mayer, 1980).

The use of alcohol or other substances may have a significant impact on the family's economic security and status. A parent's ability to find employment, hold employment, and acquire resources to support the family may all be seriously compromised, so that the potential cushion provided by financial resources is at risk or absent. This can jeopardize the family's housing, health, educational standing, and mental health. The substance abuse may take place in the context of the parent's poverty and/or contribute to that poverty, with resulting ill effects for the well-being of children in either case. The substance abuse may also lead to risky sexual behaviors or drug-use-related behaviors that increase exposure to HIV and heighten the risk for maternal AIDS, with its potential for devastating effects on a pregnancy, the health of a newborn, and the parent's ability to care for older children.

The implications of parental substance abuse for children are troubling. One study noted that "Children growing up in households with a substance-abusing parent demonstrate more adjustment problems, behavioral, conduct and attention deficit disorders than other children and generally function less well on many measures of behavioral and emotional functioning" (Semidei, Radel, & Nolan, 2001, p. 111). When the substance abuse causes significant parental impairment and harm to children to result in referral to child protective services and the child welfare system, children are more likely to be placed in out-of-home care. They are also likely to remain in out-of-home care longer, for the following reasons: (1) Appropriate treatment programs may be difficult to locate, particularly outpatient and inpatient programs for women with children; (2) treatment programs may require time for program implementation; (3) parents with substance abuse problems may have difficulty engaging in, remaining in, and following through with treatment programs; (4) there may be other challenging factors, such as inadequate housing or physical and mental health problems; and (5) the probability of relapse and the resulting high risk to children may complicate a plan to reunify families. The presence or absence of community resources, and the effectiveness or ineffectiveness of collaboration among child welfare agencies, substance abuse treatment programs, and other community resources, may also affect the parent's treatment success and the reunification of a family.

Federal policies introduced in the Adoption and Safe Families Act of 1997 (ASFA) have raised a number of issues regarding parents with substance abuse, their children, and child welfare system actions. AFSA requires legal permanency hearings to determine the plan and placement for children who have been under court jurisdiction for 12 months. If a child has been in an out-of-home placement for 15 out of 22 months, a petition terminating parental rights has to be introduced unless several exceptions are applicable in the case. Similar to the manner in which the advent of permanency planning developed to address foster care "drift" in the late 1970s, these tighter legal deadlines reinforce the importance of time for the healthy development of children (McAlpine, Marshall, & Doran, 2001). Children's needs for attachment and for consistent, caring parenting have underscored the urgency of making reasonable efforts to reunite children and parents in a timely manner. However, with parents who have substance abuse problems, adequate services may not be readily available (this can provide one of the exceptions for the 15-month termination deadline), or the course of treatment may not be one of steady and speedy progress.

Reducing the trauma to a child living in an impermanent out-of-home placement because of parental substance abuse may conflict with the reality of substance abuse treatment and with the time necessary for a child to gain confidence in the parent's control of the substance abuse. Some models of substance abuse describe a developmental process for recovery from alcoholism or other drug use, but this takes time, particularly for women. In addition to the need for time to move through stages of recovery, the resumption of parenting often poses a number of challenges (Hohman & Butt, 2001):

- Avoiding parentifying the child.
- Addressing poor attachment due to the parent's substance abuse, child neglect and subsequent separation from the child.
- Determining parents' expectations for themselves and for their children, working to offset the concomitant risk of disappointment and frustration.
- Dealing with parenting challenges and guilt if a child has evidence of developmental delays due to a parent's prenatal alcohol or drug use.

Child welfare workers must weigh the trauma of continued out-of-home care and separation from the parents against the potential trauma and harm if a child is returned to the home of a parent unable to maintain treatment success and avoid relapse. This is not an easy decision.

Domestic Violence

Although an understanding of the interrelationship between domestic violence and child abuse and neglect is sometimes confounded by two different service delivery systems and differing vantage points, violence in a family may have multiple expressions and multiple victims. With regard to the child welfare system, the focus is on the safety and well-being of children. Domestic violence intersects with child abuse and neglect when the abusive parent (or parental figure) is also abusive toward the child—hitting both an adult partner and a child who is present—or when the child witnesses the abuse of one parent by the other.

Child abuse is significantly more likely to occur in families where there is domestic violence; in one study, 45–70% of women in shelters reported that their children had been abused or neglected (Williams, Weil, & Mauney, 1998). When perpetrators of domestic violence either indiscriminately, accidentally, or intentionally hurt children as well as the children's mothers, the coexistence of and interrelationship between child abuse and domestic violence are quite evident. This violence poses a number of dilemmas for families and for child welfare workers. In addition to the perpetrator's role, the abused parent's ability to protect a child, seeming disregard for the child's safety, and/or exposure of the child to danger may be scrutinized. Mothers in particular may find themselves in a position of being victims of domestic violence and investigated for neglecting their children by exposing them to domestic violence. This may complicate the help-seeking process and challenge the child protective services' understanding of domestic violence. As with substance abuse, there is a need for collaboration between professionals in different systems—in this case, between child welfare and domestic violence service providers—but this cooperation is often challenged by differing perspectives and approaches.

Witnessing domestic violence may result in emotional disturbances and psychological risks for children. A child may fear for the safety of the abused parent and feel compelled to protect that parent (exposing the child to possible abuse) or may feel guilt for failing to protect the parent. Children may be confused and feel torn between the abused parent and the abusive parent. As with all child abuse and neglect, children can interpret the violence as being their own fault and something that they should have been able to prevent. The effects of witnessing domestic violence may differ with age, cognitive ability, and gender.

Whether children are covictims of or witnesses to domestic violence, the consequences for them can be deep, pervasive, and long-lasting. Many children may develop coping strategies and benefit from some social supports, but nonetheless the fear, distress, and hypervigilance about possible recurrence can be exhausting. This experience results in posttraumatic stress for many children, who may experience rage, excessive aggression, depression, numbing, panic attacks and avoidance behaviors, distrust, high-risk behaviors with other children and adults, sexualized behaviors, sleep disturbances, health problems, somatic complaints, eating disorders, and elimination disorders (Brohl, 1996).

Mental Illness

Parents with severe mental illness who abuse their children account for approximately 10% of cases (Kempe & Helfer, 1972). The number of parents with less severe mental illness, but with diagnosable cases of depression and other mood disorders, anxiety disorders, and personality disorders, is not known. Although implicated in relatively few child maltreatment cases, the severe mental illness of a parent has a profound impact on the child, as well as serious consequences for the long-term stability of the family and permanency planning for the child.

What is the harm associated with parental mental illness? Developmental theorists Mary Ainsworth and John Bowlby stated that attachment provides a child with a sense of security, a secure base (see Bowlby, 1966, 1988). This base allows the young child to make exploratory excursions and provides a measure of comfort to the child, who is increasingly aware of his or her vulnerability. Gaining confidence to explore and relate to the world and other people in that world is attainable and manageable with this sense of security. According to Bowlby (1966), this secure base develops through a dynamic equilibrium between the mother and child. If the distance between the child and parent becomes too great, this sense of security becomes threatened. The distance can be either literal physical lack of proximity or a mother's general lack of responsiveness to her infant or young child. Either type of disturbance may occur when parents suffer from severe and persistent mental illness, and this raises serious concerns about the well-being of children. A young mother with severe depression, for instance, may have a despondent mood, lack of energy, an increase in sleeping, and a persistent internal conversation characterized by self-depreciation; as a result, she may not be able to be responsive to her young child. The parent's unresponsiveness may result in neglect though failing to feed, supervise, or attend to the other needs of the child. These conditions may be compounded when the parent cares for multiple children and/or lives in social isolation. As a result, the young child may become either indiscriminately affectionate or socially unresponsive to others (Kaplan, Sadock, & Grebb, 1994).

In severe parental mental illness, neglect of the child may also result from the parent's need to attend to the illness and its symptomatology. A parent's thought processes or judgment may be impaired. The risk to the child may be heightened by the nature and intensity of parental anxieties or delusions. One standard psychiatric reference notes, "Parents who are depressed or psychotic or have severe personality disorders may view their children as bad or trying to drive them crazy" (Kaplan et al., 1994, p. 786). Such parental views may well result in neglect or abuse of a child. In other cases, high frustration and low impulse control may result in excessive physical punishment or misdirected anger, irrational beliefs about the child and the child's behavior, and agitation. Inconsistent and irrational punishment and harm to a child may influence the child's sense of self and views of the world (e.g., learned helplessness); it may also contribute to the child's future aggressiveness (Cole & Cole, 1989).

Although such views are not necessarily associated with parental mental illness, some abused children are viewed by their parents as being different from other children. Children may be considered slow in development, difficult to discipline, or excessively disobedient. Or a child's appearance or behavior may negatively remind a parent of someone else. This status as a "special child" may be a risk factor for child abuse or neglect.

A different risk factor may consist of parents' inappropriate expectations for their children. For example, a parent may expect that a child will be capable of caring for and comforting the parent. This role reversal and expectation that the child can perform a parenting role may lead to impatience and anger with the child when the child is incapable of doing so and, indeed, requires attention him- or herself. At the very least, this parentification of the child may result in neglect of the child's needs for parenting care. Bowlby (1988) hypothesized that such inverted parent–

child relationships may result in a range of anxieties and depression for children in later life.

Multiple factors should be considered with regard to these dynamics. These include (1) the influence of the child's inborn personality characteristics and genetic/temperamental makeup on his or her responsiveness to and quality of relationship with the parent; (2) the effect of two parents and/or parent substitutes, since the caregiver mother–child relationships in these cases are neither as exclusive nor as singularly powerful as the mother–child relationships Bowlby described; (3) cultural influences that shape child-raising practices and influence the nature and expression of attachment; (4) a potential array of parental strengths, coping skills, or supports, as well as the differential impacts and parental attitudes and behaviors; and (5) a range of relationships and factors in later childhood that shape and contribute to a child's experience of attachment to others and sense of security. Early deprivation in caretaking and parent–child interaction is not necessarily devastating to later development, because other relationships and factors can intervene and support a child's competency and well-being (Cole & Cole, 1989).

Traumatized Families

The separate challenges for parents noted here interact with one another, as well as with other difficulties that result from and contribute to problems for parents and risk of harm for children. It is possible to describe a "traumatized family" as well as traumatized individual family members. The connectedness of family members results in shared vulnerability, shared traumatic reactions, and varied efforts to correct or cope with problems within the family system. A traumatized family is struggling to cope with and recover from multiple injuries resulting from the extraordinary abuse or neglect of one or more family members (Figley, 1989).

This trauma to the family, and to its individual members, may have multiple features and interrelationships. For example, substance abuse and domestic violence may correlate with one another. Alcohol and other drugs may be used to self-medicate depression. Mental health challenges and substance abuse together may result in severe financial distress and homelessness. Substance abuse may result in exposure to HIV, subsequent HIV infection, and ultimately AIDS. Sometimes substance use includes illegal activity that results in criminal conviction and incarceration; this parental incarceration effectively leaves a child abandoned and dependent on the care of relatives or of unfamiliar foster patients. These problems may be compounded by still other problems, and trauma to children may result from multiple injuries, harm from several sources, and complicated and pervasive risk and danger. These problems also occur within the context of social factors that have the potential to compound the trauma further, to introduce protective elements, or both.

SOCIAL FACTORS

Parental factors are essential in understanding child abuse and neglect. However, a number of social challenges and systemic perspectives provide a crucial context for understanding parental behavior. For example, the interplay of substance abuse, domestic violence, and mental illness with parental poverty serves as an important consideration in child welfare. The negative effects of each of these difficulties are increased for a family without resources to cushion certain relationship and financial blows. The treatment opportunities (e.g., appropriate medications) that would prevent, interrupt, or ameliorate these risks may be inaccessible without financial and social resources. Poverty itself may contribute to a range of vulnerabilities and potential traumatic conditions. These vulnerabilities include unemployment or underemployment; unstable employment or multiple demanding jobs; lack of health insurance and other employment benefits, nonexistent or inferior child care options; chronic physical illness, as well as inaccessibility of medication and treatment; substandard and/or impermanent housing; poor nutrition; utility shutoffs; unreliable transportation; and difficulty in affording clothes and other resources for family members. Exposure to physical danger may be increased by the unfavorable location of housing, limited transportation options, undesirable working hours, and restricted employment options. Discrimination based on socioeconomic status may create further stress or limitations to opportunity.

Abuse may be more common among the poor, but it "occurs also in middle-class families, where it is likely to be hidden behind a façade of ultra-respectability" (Bowlby, 1988, p. 83). Although child abuse and neglect do occur in all socioeconomic groups, Leroy Pelton (1985) warned that the failure to appreciate the full effects of poverty has produced a myth of classlessness. He asserted that this diversion has reduced attentiveness to "the subculture of violence, the stresses of poverty that can provoke child abuse and neglect, and the hazardous poverty environment that heightens the dangerousness of child neglect" (p. 33). More recently, Nina Bernstein (2001) has observed that the division between child maltreatment policy and welfare policy downplays "the reality that children in foster care and at risk of entering foster care are overwhelmingly the children of the poor" (p. xiii). She asserts that policies based on a model of "deviant parents" and "unlucky children" overlook the role of socioeconomic factors and their impact on families and communities.

In considering the well-being of children and their ability to survive, cope with, or overcome certain types of harm and trauma, resiliency theory points to the interplay of three dimensions. These dimensions are (1) individual traits and capabilities, (2) family qualities and intimate protective relationships, and (3) the role of coping and protective factors in the social environment. In the child welfare system, even though there may be protective relationships within the family (e.g., a bond to siblings or an attachment to a grandparent), the parent in the family contributes to the vulnerability of the child. With this conflict in the family, the roles of social factors as sources of protective mechanisms for the child take on even greater importance than usual. Most prominently, the roles of the school and of the neighborhood/community are very significant.

Schools

The school system provides a child or young person with opportunities for relationships with caring adults, as well as an arena for potential academic, athletic, or other success (Williams, 2003, Fraser, 2004). This environment also offers a setting that is physically and emotionally safer and less conflictual than many children's homes. However, a number of pressures on schools may have the effect of compromising these positive and potentially protective qualities.

Schools are under increasing pressure from various stakeholders to meet or exceed various academic performance thresholds. This academic accountability movement may have an unintentional negative impact on students from abusive and neglectful homes. Specifically, the No Child Left Behind (NCLB) Act of 2001 has increased the pressure on schools to meet certain types of academic standards. For example, schools must meet state-mandated academic standards of performance in math, science, and literacy. This rise in accountability and performance standards, combined with sometimes severe budget cuts, has created a new set of stressors for public education. These stressors may be overlaid on a school system (particularly an urban school system) that is already underfunded, with aging buildings requiring physical and mechanical repairs, and inadequate resources for technology. Large class sizes, and an aging educational workforce that faces a classroom of students from a range of cultures, language groups, and educational levels, further heighten the educational and social challenges. The school system's ability to respond to traumatized children, and to understand and tolerate the range of behaviors that such students often initially display, may therefore be severely compromised. For example, in order to receive funds from the NCLB program, states must adopt a zero-tolerance policy for violent or persistently disruptive students. The NCLB legislation, in fact, empowers teachers to remove such students from the classroom.

The NCLB Act focuses primarily on the academic/intellectual domain of student development. Yet this narrow conception of schools' responsibility is a fairly recent one and does not fully reflect historical views of formal education. This narrow view may not be an effective way to serve youth who come to school from abusive and neglectful homes, whose developmental needs are probably not being met at home. Historically, schools were viewed as being able to meet a broader range of students' developmental needs, beyond academic performance and successful test taking. Tyler (cited in Fitzpatrick et al., 2004) listed six critical roles for schools in educating children:

- Providing information.
- Developing work habits and study skills.
- Developing effective ways of thinking.
- Helping internatize social attitudes, appreciations, and sensitivities.
- Maintaining physical health.
- Developing a philosophy of life.

With its singular academic focus, the NCLB legislation almost solely emphasizes improving student performance in math, science, and literature, and neglects the social and communal functions of public education. There is an insufficient emphasis on creating and maintaining safe schools. For students who come from homes where abuse and neglect are hampering their development in a variety of domains, the legislation is an example of an institutional force that can contribute to further alienation and marginalization of these students.

In many schools, students from troubling backgrounds behave in troubling ways. These behaviors—called "carry-in problems"—are often reflected in school settings (Long & Morse, 1996; Long & Fecser, 2001). They bring problems to school that began in the family or on the street. They display self-defeating patterns of distrust and disobedience. Assuming the worst about adults, they may replay coercive interactions learned elsewhere (Seita & Brendtro, 2004). Although many schools attempt to institute inclusive discipline strategies, too many use exclusionary punishments. Adult-wary youth see the latter as attack or rejection, and become even more aggressive or disengaged from school and teachers.

For students living on the edge, schools can become either islands of stability or arenas for battle. Research on the My Worst School Experience Scale (Hyman, 2000) showed that a surprising number of students experienced traumatic stress in school. Most commonly this was due to peer intimidation, but it also often involved humiliation from school staff.

Young people who experience abuse or neglect at home can also engage in self-isolating and withdrawn behavior. Rather than bringing attention to themselves or being combative or disruptive, these young persons are quiet, self-contained, distrustful, and aloof. With large classrooms and overoccupied educators, the abuse or neglect experienced in these students' homes is replayed in the school environment. With budget reductions shrinking or eliminating the number of adjunct personnel, such as school social workers, there are insufficient numbers of professionals available to reach out to maltreated children or youth and their families. Disruptive or withdrawn behavior may be labeled as requiring special attention. Despite relatively high rates of abused and neglected children in special education, often these children are not eligible for services.

The social environment is further shaped by educational practices that introduce or display intentional and unintentional bias with respect to race, gender, the home environment, peer group relationships, and socioeconomic status. Youth in foster care report that when their living arrangements and legal status are known, this knowledge can result in subtle and not-so-subtle prejudice (Folman & Anderson, 2004). They report that a number of teachers view foster children as troubled, disruptive, intellectually and socially limited, and as impermanent and temporary residents of their classroom. With an overrepresentation of minority children in the child welfare system, institutional forces such as racism, sexism, oppression, and denial of opportunity may also exert tremendous influence on academic success.

In positive school climates, students feel that they belong, are treated fairly, and are respected. They see the enforcement of rules as fair and beneficial. Sarcasm, ridicule, putdowns, and verbal assault from either school staff or peers are very limited or altogether absent (Seita & Brendtro, 2004). Although cliques are typical in adolescence, the school staff takes measures to minimize their impact and to support "outcasts." There is strong discouragement of any bullying or scapegoating by either students or staff. Students eagerly anticipate attendance in such schools, in spite of high academic expectations. Safe schools are a goal for children, along with positive academic and social achievements.

In summary, the school setting is a crucial environment that can provide the nurturing, sense of competency, and corrective emotional experiences that traumatized children need. However, the academic and budgetary pressures on school systems may result in conditions that work against caring relationships supporting youth resiliency. The school environment may, in fact, contribute to the challenges for maltreated children and youth by providing only negative social experiences with peers and school personnel, as well as limited opportunities for success (Sautner, 2001). The stresses introduced by such an educational setting are not mediated by caring, committed, attentive parents, and the trauma experienced in the home may not be buffered by relationships and successes at school. A child or youth ultimately loses in both settings.

Neighborhood and Community

What roles do neighborhoods play in either contributing to or ameliorating negative outcomes for children and families affected by abuse and neglect? Is the prevalence of child abuse and neglect higher in some neighborhoods than in others? What can be done within a neighborhood context to support and reclaim children who have been abused and neglected?

Although the reasons for child abuse and neglect are multifaceted, family social isolation and poverty appear to be linked to high rates of child abuse (Bethea, 1999; Gelles, 1996; Kirby & Fraser, 1997). Therefore, community risk factors that may be connected to child maltreatment include conditions that limit community involvement and foster poverty. For example, a number of inner-city communities are environmentally compromised by brownfields or other pollution. There may be an absence of employment opportunities and/or of public transportation to such opportunities. Housing may be degraded, vacant, or condemned, with high rates of nonowner occupancy. Neighborhood public schools may be nonexistent or have out-of-date facilities. There may be few houses of worship, grocery stores, recreational outlets, personal service shops, or other community amenities. The level of city services may be inadequate or inefficient. Crime rates may be higher than in other areas. In comparison to many of these features associated with urban areas, rural areas may also be physically isolated, with little access to educational, recreational, or employment outlets. This lack of services may extend to family support services such as children's clubs and organizations (Boy and Girl Scouts, 4H, Boys and Girls Clubs), tutoring or educational support, counseling, and other services. Communities interested in reducing the rates of child abuse may want to engage in strategies to reduce family isolation and economic hardships.

Historic approaches to address community risk factors that correlate with child abuse and neglect have been described as "fault fixing" (Brendtro & Ness, 1995; Seita, 1994; Burger, 1994). Fault fixing addresses specific issues and social problems, often in isolation from each other and the communities in which children and youth live, rather than focusing on the root causes of these problems. Multisystemic strategies that are community-based and family-supportive, and that aim to promote resiliency and positive youth development, may have greater promise. For example, children who have been abused are more likely to perform poorly in school, drop out of school, engage in violent behavior, join gangs, and use illegal drugs. Focusing only on these deficits may not be effective, because such a focus may overlook core causes and fail to create protective environments. Likewise, working with abusive and neglectful parents may require a more comprehensive strategy than referrals for parent education. Community partnerships between child protective services and the formal and informal resources within communities may provide opportunities for the child welfare staff to better understand both families and communities. These partnerships may identify and develop community resources, promote neighborhood-based location and provision of services (including foster care), and engage families as well as agencies in this partnership with child welfare (Waldfogel, 2000).

There are multiple avenues for reducing the isolation of parents. The first possible resource is enhancing connections with extended family members. These ties may be taxed by the parents' substance abuse, violence, or mental health challenges. But these ties can be assessed and a strengthening process begun through such approaches as family group conferencing and family-to-family intervention methods by child welfare professionals (Merkel-Holguin, 2001). Relationships with neighbors may be strained by similar challenges, and some level of community restoration may be required. The role of schools and faith communities in building these ties is crucial. Isolation can also be reduced through employment and relationships developed at work. Consequently, social policy and educational initiatives that strengthen employment may have an impact on parental isolation and functioning. The social environment of parents interacts with parental strengths and risk factors to promote positive family functioning on the one hand, or to contribute to the isolation and poverty that heighten the danger to children on the other hand.

ADDITIONAL TRAUMA CAUSED BY THE CHILD WELFARE SYSTEM

The trauma of child abuse and neglect is defined by the nature of the injury and by the person who inflicted the injury. In the case of a family entering the child welfare system, the primary person to whom the child looks for consistency, love, care, and protection has become unpredictable and potentially harmful. However, child abuse may occur in brief and relatively isolated episodes. Child neglect, although more chronic in nature, may also be accompanied by acts of attention and affection. In most cases, parents maintain some degree of caring for and attachment to their children, and children are attached to and care about their parents. Consequently, the child welfare system's response to abuse or neglect, particularly when it involves moving children to out-of-home placements, may introduce a second layer of trauma for parents and children alike.

Children may be further unintentionally traumatized by the system charged with protecting their safety and well-being. The separation from a parent, even when the parent has been abusive or neglectful, may be deeply disturbing to a child. The difficulties that arise from living with a strange new family, as well as from associated changes such as a new neighborhood and school, may also have a negative impact on children. Sometimes children are neglected and abused even in out-of-home care. They may experience multiple moves and lack of information about their futures and child welfare goals. The length of time in out-of-home care may introduce some measure of stress as well. In short, the child welfare system's commitment to preserve families, to place children in kinship care, and to prioritize goals of safety, permanency, and well-being for children may not insulate a child from further traumatization. On the other hand, the system can enhance resiliency and provide positive support for parents and children through loving foster parents, dedicated child welfare professionals, and other resources mobilized to assist the family members.

STRENGTHS

This chapter has focused on the identification of parental stresses and social conditions that heighten the risks of child abuse and neglect and of consequent trauma for children. However, parents can also employ strengths and coping mechanisms to prevent or reduce child maltreatment. For example, parents with substance abuse problems may be motivated to admit and confront their drug use or addictions in order to preserve their families. Similarly, adult victims of domestic violence may come to understand the negative impact of witnessing abuse on their children, and take steps to stop the violence or remove themselves from the abusive situation. Kinship arrangements can provide safe respite for children. Many parents with mental health challenges are still capable of responding to supportive interventions. Parents can learn strategies for managing their anger and for better parenting. Interventions such as family group conferencing can surround a traumatized family with extended family resources, and professionals can be identified and can work in partnership with the family. Even in cases of abuse and neglect, parents frequently express love for their children and a desire and willingness to at least reduce the need for child welfare involvement, if not significantly improve their functioning as parents. The informal but significant support of faith communities, and the formal support of after-school programs, Head Start, and a range of other programs, are additional resources. Foster parents, child welfare workers, other social service professionals, teachers and other school personnel, community members, and extended family members can all provide support for families and adults who take an interest in the safety, permanency and well-being of children.

IMPLICATIONS FOR PRACTICE AND POLICY

Treatment with parents needs to address the behaviors that endanger children or put them at risk. These behaviors–related to substance abuse, domestic violence, and mental health difficulties–may in turn be caused or influenced by a range of parental factors. Because of their history, emotional needs, irrational beliefs and expectations, and/or lack of knowledge, parents who hurt their children may require corrective emotional experiences and learning gained from both formal and informal personal and social supports. Resistance to treatment may be high, as parents may not view their behaviors as problematic or wrong. Engaging parents requires cultural sensitivity, outreach, and skillful intervention. Sometimes, keeping children safe dictates removal from their parents–or in a few severe cases, as allowed by ASFA, termination of parental rights.

Treatment interventions should also address the social factors that place additional demands on the parents. In particular, such interventions should target parents' isolation and their lack of resources to provide both basic and psychological needs for themselves and their children. Provision of child protective and child welfare services at the level of the neighborhood; partnerships between child welfare agencies and other service providers; and efforts to identify extended family members and engage them as partners in affirming the best interests of both parents and children all offer promising approaches.

Although treatment for parents is essential, the needs of children must not be overlooked. These children urgently need to be helped, and helpers must carefully avoid any suggestions (intentional or unintentional) of "blaming the victims." This assistance can be guided by strategies that intentionally identify, reinforce, and develop protective factors for children and youth. For example, children living in a non-nurturing or even a threatening situation may thrive in spite of those circumstances if there are teachers, coaches, clergy, neighbors, or others who connect to the children, believe in them, provide them with fair and high expectations, and support them as they seek to find a purpose in life (Benard, 1997).

These approaches can be informed by the stories of young people who have overcome horrific abuse and neglect to become what Wolin and Wolin (1993) call "individuals who have learned to love well, work well, play well." Theresa Cameron (2002), Dave Pelzer (1995), Waln Brown (1983), Edward Benzola (Benzola with Beach, 1993), Antwone Fisher (Fisher with Rivas, 2002), E. P. Jones (1990), and John Seita (Seita, Mitchell, & Tobin, 1996) have all written about their struggles to overcome child abuse and neglect, as well as the additional traumas associated with their involvement in the child welfare system. Embedded in each of these accounts are examples of resiliency and of how to promote resiliency in order to improve the lives of children suffering from abuse and neglect.

Social policies that strengthen the capacity of schools to take a holistic approach to learning and to student development; that promote employment and provide a financial safety net for families; that strengthen community development; and that provide community-based, family-supportive services will all help to address the conditions contributing to child abuse and neglect (Richmond & Bowen, 1997). The present review of the difficulties facing parents and the resulting risks to children highlights the need for multiple types of intervention, including an appreciation for extended family, close friends or "fictive kin," and faith community resources. Addressing individual, family, and community needs is essential, as the transactions between and among these systems support and complicate either harmful or supportive parenting.

SUMMARY

Within the child welfare system, understanding the traumatic effects of child abuse and neglect on children results in a focus on the behavior and the intentional harm inflicted by a parent. Child maltreatment can take place in the context of a parent's alcohol or other drug use, a violent relationship between the adults in the home, and/or the difficulties posed by a parent's mental distress or illness. These family factors frequently occur in the context of social challenges, which may include serious economic distress, unstable housing or homelessness, major health problems (e.g., HIV/AIDS), and/or parental incarceration. Schools are often unprepared to provide the safe and nurturing environments that traumatized children need, and also are unable to engage resistant or stressed parents. Because the need for attentiveness to the social and psychological needs of children is increasingly being overlooked in the current climate of curricular accountability, the school environment may introduce additional stress rather than providing a respite and resource for children. In neighborhoods and communities experiencing poverty and other stressors, internal and external conditions may promote family isolation and create difficulty in accessing appropriate resources.

Addressing child abuse and neglect requires assisting parents to reduce harm and to develop positive parenting skills. Although working to reduce substance abuse, domestic violence, and mental health difficulties is often necessary, a systemic approach to multiple factors may be most effective, given the interrelationships among various stressors. In addition, promoting the resiliency of children so that they can cope with their situation, gain a cognitive grasp of it, and experience some protection from trauma is essential. This approach recognizes that the internal strengths and positive characteristics of children can help them deal with potentially harmful experiences. Because families are linked by bonds of love, need, and proximity, there is also a role for extended family members and others who can function like family members, as well as for support from caring professionals and programs that are mobilized and accessible for maltreated children. Through the support of kin and other informal systems, as well as community and social service resources, the child welfare system should more appropriately be conceptualized as a *family* welfare system that promotes family resiliency.

REFERENCES

Azar, S., & Wolfe, D. (1989). Child abuse and neglect. In E. Mash & R. Barkley (Eds.), *Treatment of childhood disorders*. New York: Guilford Press.

Benard, B. (1993). Fostering resiliency in kids (caring and encouraging resilience in school children). *Educational Leadership, 51*(3), 44.

Benzola, E., with Beach, N. (1993). *Temporary child: A foster care survivor's story*. Fremont, CA: Real People.

Bernstein, N. (2001). *The lost children of Wilder: The epic struggle to change foster care*. New York: Pantheon Books.

Bethea, L. (1999). Primary prevention of child abuse. *American Family Physician, 59*(3), 1577–1597.

Black, R., & Mayer, J. (1980). Parents with special problems: Alcoholism and opiate addiction. *Child Abuse and Neglect, 4*, 45.

Bowlby, J. (1966). *Maternal care and mental health*. New York: Schocken Books.

Bowlby, J. (1988). *A secure base: Parent–child attachment and healthy human development*. New York: Basic Books.

Bradley, R. H., Caldwell, B. M., Fitzgerald, J. A., Morgan, A. G., & Rock, S. L. (1986). Experiences in day care and social competence among maltreated children. *Child Abuse and Neglect, 10*, 181–189.

Brendtro, L. K., & Ness, A. (1995). Fixing flaws or building strengths?: Reclaiming children and youth. *Journal of Emotional and Behavioral Problems, 4*(2), 18–24.

Brohl, K. (1996). *Working with traumatized children*. Washington, DC: Child Welfare League of America.

Brown, W. (1983). *The other side of delinquency*. Cameron, WV: William Gladden Foundation.

Burger, J. (1994). Keys to survival: Highlights in resilience research. *Journal of Emotional and Behavioral Problems, 3*(2), 6–10.

Cameron, T. (2002). *Foster care odyssey: A black girl's story*. Jackson: University of Mississippi Press.

Cole, M., & Cole, S. (1989). *The development of children*. New York: Scientific American Books.

Figley, C. (1989). *Helping traumatized families*. San Francisco: Jossey-Bass.

Fisher, A. Q., with Rivas, M. E. (2002). *Finding fish*. New York: Harper Torch.

Fitzpatrick, J., Sanders, J., & Worthen, B. (2004). *Program evaluation: Alternative approaches and practical guidelines* (3rd ed.). Boston: Allyn & Bacon.

Folman, R., & Anderson, G. (2004). *Troubled water: Foster care youth and college*. East Lansing: Michigan State University School of Social Work.

Fraser, M. (2004). *Risk and resilience in childhood: An ecological perspective* (2nd ed.). Washington, DC: NASW Press.

Gelles, R. (1996). *The book of David: How preserving families can cost children's lives*. New York: Basic Books.

Helfer, R. E., & Kempe, C. H. (Eds.). (1968). *The battered child*. Chicago: University of Chicago Press.

Hohman, M., & Butt, R. (2001). How soon is too soon?: Addiction recovery and family reunification. *Child Welfare, 80*(1), 53–70.

Hyman, I. (2000, July 13). *Dangerous schools/dangerous students: Defining and assessing student alienation syndrome*. OSEP Research Project Director's Conference, Washington, DC.

Jones, E. P. (1990). *Where is home?: Living through foster care*. New York: Four Walls Eight Windows

Kaplan, H. I., Sadock, B. J., & Grebb, J. A. (1994). *Kaplan and Sadock's synopsis of psychiatry: Behavioral sciences, clinical psychiatry* (7th ed.). Baltimore: Williams & Wilkins.

Kempe, C. H., & Helfer, R. E. (1972). *Helping the battered child and his family*. Philadelphia: Lippincott.

Kirby, L., & Fraser, M. (1997). Risk and resiliency in childhood. In M. Fraser (Ed.), *Risk and resiliency* (pp. 10–33). Washington, DC: NASW Press.

Long, N., Fecser, F., & Wood, M. (2001). *Life space crisis intervention*. Austin, TX: PRO-ED.

Long, N. J., & Morse, W. C. (1996). *Conflict in the classroom* (5th ed.). Austin, TX: PRO-ED.

McAlpine, C., Marshall, C. C., & Doran, N. H. (2001). Combining child welfare and substance abuse services: A blended model of intervention. *Child Welfare, 80*(2), 129–150.

Merkel-Holguin, L. (2001). Family group conferencing: An "extended family" process to safeguard children and strengthen family well-being. In E. Walton, P. Sandau-Beckler, & M. Mannes (Eds.), *Balancing family centered services and child well-being*. New York: Columbia University Press.

Pelton, L. (1985). *The social context of child abuse and neglect*. New York: Human Sciences Press.

Pelzer, D. (1995). *A child called It*. Deerfield Beach, FL: Health Communications.

Richmond, M. (1917). *Social diagnosis*. New York: Russell Sage Foundation.

Richmond, ., & Bowen.

Sautner, B. (2001). The safe and caring schools initiative. *Reclaiming Children and Youth, 9*(4), 197–201.

Seita, J. R. (1994). Resiliency from the other side of the desk. *Journal of Emotional and Behavioral Problems, 3*(2), 15–18.

Seita, J. R., & Brendtro, L. K. (2004). *Kids who outwit adults*. Bloomington, IN: National Educational Service.

Seita, J. R., Mitchell, M., & Tobin, C. (1996). *In whose best interest?: One child's odyssey, a nation's responsibility*. Elizabethtown, PA: Continental Press.

Semidei, J., Radel, L. F., & Nolan, C. (2001). Substance abuse and child welfare: Clear linkages and promising responses. *Child Welfare, 80*(2), 109–128.

Tower, C. (1996). *Understanding child abuse and neglect*. Boston: Allyn & Bacon.

Waldfogel, J. (2000). Reforming child protective services. *Child Welfare, 79*(1), 43–58.

Williams, B. (2003). *Closing the achievement gap: A vision for changing beliefs and practices*. Alexandria, VA: Association for Supervision and Curriculum.

Williams, E., Weil, M., & Mauney, R. (1998). Children and domestic violence: Recognizing effects and building programs. In T. Harms, A. R. Ray, & P. Rolandelli (Eds.), *Preserving childhood for children in shelters*. Washington, DC: Child Welfare League of America.

Wolin, S., & Wolin, S. (1993). *The resilient self: How survivors of troubled families rise above adversity*. New York: Villard.

Young, N. K., Wingfield, K., & Klempner, T. (2001). Serving children, youth, and families with alcohol and other drug-related problems in child welfare. *Child Welfare, 80*(2), 103–108.

Zuckerman, B. (1994). Drugs and children: Effects on parents and children. In D. Besharov (Ed.), *When drug addicts have children*. Washington, DC: Child Welfare League of America.

PART II

HELPING INTERVENTIONS

CHAPTER 6

Selected Treatment Approaches for Helping Traumatized Youth

NANCY BOYD WEBB

Trauma is not an isolated event. As the authors of the chapters in Part I clearly indicate, a multitude of interacting personal and contextual factors must be considered in the assessment of trauma in a young person (Webb, 1999, 2004). Assessment is the first critical step toward determining a treatment plan for helping. The practitioner must carefully evaluate each individual's situation and then decide how to proceed. Although many treatment choices are described in the literature (Follette, Ruzek, & Aubueg, 1998; Gil, 1991; James, 1994; Kazdin & Weisz, 2003; Malchiodi, 2003; Nader, 2001; Wilson, Friedman, & Lindy, 2001; Webb, 1999, 2004), practitioners often formulate a plan of intervention based on their own comfort, training, and experience with a specific method, and/or according to the preference and usual practice in their particular agency. Clinicians who are familiar with the research literature may prefer to use interventions that have been empirically tested, although this seriously limits the choices, as will be discussed below.

This chapter serves as an introduction to the helping interventions presented by the authors of Chapters 7–13. However, neither those seven chapters nor this one intends (or even pretends) to offer an exhaustive review of possible treatment approaches, which would be beyond the scope and purpose of this book. Rather, this chapter first deals with some issues that may influence practitioners' decisions about employing specific treatments, then presents some pertinent features of different approaches, and finally summarizes the major types of trauma treatment in work with children and adolescents. This overview provides a framework for the chapters that follow in Part II.

ISSUES IN THE TREATMENT OF TRAUMATIZED YOUTH

Practitioners who work with traumatized youth come from a variety of backgrounds, such as social work, psychology, psychiatry, nursing, and the clergy. All have different types of professional training, which tend to influence their particular perspectives on the nature of a child's problem and the best ways to help. Because this book seeks to merge the efforts of the mental health and child welfare fields in assisting traumatized young people, various helping approaches are presented. Some methods, such as eye movement desensitization and reprocessing (EMDR; see Greenwald, Chapter 13) and animal-assisted therapy (see Brooks, Chapter 11), require specialized advanced training beyond the usual preparation of master's-level clinicians. These chapters are intended to be informative rather than prescriptive, and readers who want to locate additional information or training in the use of these methods should consult the Appendix to this volume regarding specific training sites and additional resources. Other chapters in this section on helping interventions present methods that may be adapted beneficially by child welfare and other practitioners in their work in various settings. For instance, Tracy and Johnson (Chapter 7) and Ortiz Hendricks and Fong (Chapter 8) discuss ways to help youth enhance their sense of personal and cultural identity and their feelings of self-efficacy. However, before specific methods are described in detail, some overarching issues that have an impact on treatment selection are reviewed. These include the following:

- The tension between empirically supported treatment and other therapies (Ollendick, 1999; Ollendick & King, 2000).
- The polarization between supporters of psychotherapy and advocates of pharmacotherapy in the treatment of traumatized children (Oldham & Riba, 2001).
- The lack of adequate attention to the impact of racial and cultural factors in the assessment and treatment of trauma (Rosenberg, 2001; Kinzie, 2001; Nader, Dubrow, & Stamm, 1999).

The Pressure to Provide Empirically Supported Treatments

The professional literature acknowledges the tension between practitioners who subscribe to empirically based approaches and those who do not (Ollendick, 1999; Ollendick & King, 2000). Several professional groups, including the American Academy of Child and Adolescent Psychiatry, the Society of Clinical Psychology, and the Council on Social Work Education, have advocated the concept that clinical interventions should be "empirically supported" by research demonstrating that favorable client outcome is a result of specific procedures inherent in the treatment, rather than being due to chance or other factors. A typical research protocol assigns clients randomly to different treatment methods and then compares the outcomes of each method, using pre- and posttest criteria or other ways to measure success. Often the treatment approach is carefully spelled out in a manual, containing instructions and expectations that all practitioners will follow similar procedures.

Although the intent to provide service that has a proven record of efficacy is laudatory, this remains only an ideal in many settings, in which treatment decisions are based on practitioners' firmly held beliefs about the value of their respective methods. Many empirically based studies have been developed and tested by researchers in university-based settings, but some agency-based practitioners question how applicable and generalizable these methods would be in standard community practice. Addis and Krasnow (2000) concede that manuals tend to be unpopular among practicing clinicians. This may relate to the type of conformity expected in manualized approaches, which strive to ensure uniformity of intervention methods, but which possibly "stifle creativity and flexibility in the therapy process" (Ollendick & King, 2000, p. 405).

In addition to these criticisms, some professionals in the trauma field maintain that there simply have not been enough empirically supported studies completed to date to enable anyone to state emphatically that one particular method for treating traumatized children is superior to another. According to O'Donohue, Fanetti, and Elliott (1998, p. 376), "the lack of empirical treatment outcomes for children who have experienced trauma makes it difficult to recommend a specific course of action for any population other than sexually abused girls." Cognitive-behavioral treatment approaches have the strongest empirical evidence for efficacy in work with sexually abused girls, as well as with other children and adults with post-traumatic stress disorder (PTSD) (O'Donohue et al., 1998; Seedat & Stein, 2001). However, because other approaches have not been studied in controlled outcome research, we do not know "whether frequently practiced treatments from other orientations work or not" (Ollendick & King, 2000, p. 405). Finally, Nader (2001) comments that "measuring outcomes is fraught with difficulties [since] we can only know the true efficacy of our treatment methods by examining children over years into adulthood" (p. 294). Much outcome research involves follow-up investigations at 6 months or 1 year after treatment, but not over the long term.

In my opinion, the fact that a method such as play therapy has not been tested and found superior to relaxation methods in reducing symptoms does not mean that we should stop using it. It is worrisome that a comprehensive text of 25 chapters devoted to a review of evidence-based psychotherapies for children and adolescents does not even list play therapy in the index (Kazdin & Weisz, 2003). On the other hand, much "anecdotal" testimony by practitioners and clients suggests that many clinicians continue to favor and use approaches such as play therapy that have not been empirically tested. Obviously, as frequently concluded, "we need more research." However, in the meantime, traumatized clients need help, and we owe it to them to offer our best efforts—even with methods that have yet to be "scientifically" proven. Several of these are presented in Chapters 7–13, in which the authors address briefly the issue of whether the methods they espouse have been subjected to critical research review.

Psychotherapy versus Pharmacotherapy

Although many experts in the treatment of trauma recommend a "multimodal approach" that combines psychotherapy with pharmacotherapy (Oldham & Riba, 2001; Seedat & Stein, 2001), others question the use of medication with prepubertal children, because there are "too few reliable studies to generate specific recommendations" (Rosenberg, 2001, p. 51). Indeed, the use of medication with children and adolescents can be considered an ethical problem, because "the knowledge base on the safety, efficacy, and long-term impact of the majority of the commonly prescribed medications does not yet exist" (Hoagwood, 2003, p. 61).

Practitioners working with traumatized children and youth need to know that the use of medication is an unresolved issue, with differences of opinion about its efficacy and appropriateness. Physicians/psychiatrists may want to keep trying different medications in the hope that an effective one will be found, because not medicating a child means that the symptoms may continue to interfere with the youngster's development. On the other hand, parents may be reluctant to medicate their children, and practitioners must honestly report the lack of consensus about the pros and cons of doing so. Again, research will provide more definitive answers in years to come.

Racial and Cultural Factors

A child's or adolescent's cultural background can have an important influence on the response and compliance of the youth and family once they become involved in the child welfare and mental health systems. As Kinzie (2001) points out, each culture defines "normality" and "psychopathology" according to its own values and beliefs, and treatment approaches ideally should fit expected cultural norms and expectations. This is easier said than done in our increasingly multicultural society, in which approximately 25% are children of color (Ozawa, 1997), but in which culturally diverse children and adolescents are frequently misdiagnosed and improperly treated because of a lack of understanding of cultural differences (Canino & Spurlock, 2000). For example, religious and spiritual values may be very important to culturally diverse families (Boyd-Franklin, 2003), but practitioners may fail to explore these or incorporate them into the treatment plan. A case example of a 15-year-old Puerto Rican boy with an alcohol problem reported the boy's refusal to attend the various treatment programs suggested by the school counselor, such as Alcoholics Anonymous, a peer support group, and a mental health clinic (Zayas, Canino, & Suarez, 2001). However, the boy eventually agreed to speak with the Puerto Rican parish priest, because of the priest's ability to play a folk musical instrument that the boy's deceased father had played. This proved to be the beginning of a relationship that later permitted the priest to involve the boy in a number of useful church-involved activities, which led to a reduction of his alcohol consumption.

In Chapter 8 of this book, Ortiz Hendricks and Fong discuss various methods for helping culturally diverse youth in foster care explore their identity issues. Children in foster care constitute a substantial and underserved pool of child trauma cases, according to Rosenberg (2001), and more than half of these children are from minority groups (see Chapter 8; see also Maluccio, Chapter 1, and Michaels & Levine, 1992). Many culturally diverse children enter the child welfare system before the age of 5, due to their histories of physical abuse, sexual abuse, neglect, or abandonment (Benoit, 2000). Inner-city youth have been identified as at increased risk for mental health disorders, because of the high rate of poverty, gang and other violence, pregnancy, and school dropout among this population (Parson, 1997). In fact, Parson has proposed the term "urban violence traumatic stress syndrome" in referring to the detrimental effects of the environment on symptomatic inner-city youth. Treatment approaches for these young people emphasize stabilization, symptom reduction, modification of traumatic memories, and personality integration and rehabilitation (Nader, 2001).

COMPONENTS OF DIFFERENT TRAUMA TREATMENTS FOR YOUTH

The range of treatment options for traumatized youth include individual, group, and family/adjunctive approaches, with the use of more than one modality frequently recommended. These different treatments may be based on psychodynamic, cognitive-behavioral, psychoeducational, empowerment, systemic, ecological, or other theoretical orientations, and they may be offered in open-ended or time-limited formats. Despite the unique features inherent in different methods, certain commonalities exist with regard to the overall purpose and goals of helping. In particular, symptom alleviation usually constitutes a primary objective of treatment. Beyond this, different treatments vary in the extent to which they seek to help a traumatized child or youth attain an improved level of functioning. The degree to which different approaches seek to involve and make changes in the youth's family and social environment also varies.

As outlined by Nader (2001), most trauma treatments include the following procedural components:

- Review of the traumatic event(s).
- Reprocessing or redefinition of the traumatic memories.
- Restoration of a sense of safety and self-confidence.
- Promotion of an increased sense of control.

The process of this treatment can be implemented in either individual or group sessions, but the initial discussion here focuses on work with the youth on an individual basis.

INDIVIDUAL METHODS

The literature recommends that a trauma therapist helps a traumatized person to tell what happened, or to draw or play out the scene when verbalization is too frightening (Pynoos & Nader, 1998; Gil, 1991; Malchiodi, 1997, 2003). The goal in this review process is to increase the individual's understanding of the traumatic situation, with appropriate attribution of blame; it is thought that this will enable the person to put the experience in the past, and thereby will restore and promote a sense of confidence, self-control, and safety. There is a lack of unanimity about the benefits of encouraging a trauma review, however, with some reports (Litz, 2004) cautioning that this is *not* helpful, and that in some instances it may even be harmful.

The process of reviewing painful memories usually arouses anxiety, both for the client and for the clinician. It should therefore occur gradually, according to the client's ability to tolerate the accompanying stress. Children may have very low tolerance for stressful recall, and therapists using exposure methods should remind themselves of the principle "Respect the trauma membrane, and above all do no harm" (Lindy & Wilson, 2001). The term "trauma membrane" refers to the ego defenses people develop to protect themselves from anxiety and stress. With this in mind, prior to beginning the traumatic review, clinicians should spend some time teaching traumatized individuals various methods of stress management (e.g., deep breathing and positive imagery) as a way to help them manage their stressful feelings (Bevin, 1999; Doyle & Stoop, 1999; see discussion below). Nader (2001) emphasizes that practitioners using exposure methods with young clients should have a thorough knowledge of general psychotherapeutic principles, a knowledge of trauma in particular, and an understanding of children/adolescents and how to work with them. Furthermore, they should have access to supervision and consultation to assist them in their work.

Age Considerations

All treatment methods should be age-appropriate, and with younger children whose verbal abilities are limited, the trauma review process typically involves play therapy (James, 1994; Gil, 1991; Webb, 1999). In a detailed case example involving a 9-year-old refugee boy with selective mutism, the clinician used a toy bathtub and a rag doll to encourage the youngster to recount his own near-drowning as he crossed the Rio Grande River with his family, and then the subsequent witnessing of his mother's rape (Bevin, 1999). At several points during the child's play reenactments, the therapist made encouraging comments, such as "You made it," and "You had to be very strong to endure that" (p. 175). These are examples of cognitive restructuring, which helped to transform the boy's anxiety associated with his frightening memories into a sense of pride that he had survived. The therapist concluded that "the play reenactment helped [the boy] turn passivity into activity and provided an outlet for his frustration and anger" (p. 181).

Type I versus Type II Trauma

The case described by Bevin (1999) involved a child who endured a *single* traumatic experience, referred to by Terr (1991) as Type I trauma (referring to *one* sudden shock). This differs from Type II trauma, which is more typical of children in the child welfare system—many of whom have experienced "a *series* of external blows" (p. 19, emphasis added) such as ongoing physical or sexual abuse. These situations qualify as Type II traumas, for which treatment usually requires several different forms of interventions, often over many years.

Doyle and Stoop (1999) presented the case of a 10-year-old boy who had suffered multiple abuses since early childhood. The abuse included being sold into prostitution as a preschooler, and later being kidnapped and tortured by a satanic cult. When the youngster at age 10 set a fire that killed several relatives, he was placed in a residential treatment center, where numerous treatment methods were provided. These included individual and group therapy, as well as specialized programs such as music therapy, garden therapy, and woods therapy. The published description of the boy's individual treatment demonstrated his creation of a cartoon lifeline and the use of puppets to enable the youngster to identify painful elements of his life history that led up to the fire. Each session began and ended with some guided imagery exercises, to help the boy learn how to relax at the beginning of the session, and to restore a sense of calm at the end after he had confronted numerous anxiety-producing traumatic memories. The boy's treatment lasted for several years. Unfortunately, when he returned to live in the community when he was in late adolescence, he became involved in petty crime and was incarcerated. The case illustrates the serious impact of severe early abuse on later development and the challenge of rehabilitation, even when extensive and intensive treatment is provided.

The cases described by Bevin (1999) and by Doyle and Stoop (1999) demonstrate the process of trauma review with children as an essential component of their individual treatment.

GROUP METHODS

With seriously traumatized youngsters, individual treatment is preferred over group methods, because of the extensive support and encouragement these youngsters need in the process of dealing with painful memories. Furthermore, individual therapy for a severely traumatized youth avoids the possible negative impact on other group members of exposure to the details of the extremely traumatic experiences.

In less extreme circumstances, when children share similar traumatic histories, group modalities can be an effective treatment choice. For example, a 12-session school-based group was formed with children ages 9–11 years, all of whom had witnessed various forms of violence (Nisivoccia & Lynn, 1999). The group helped the members express and deal with their feelings of anger, ongoing fears, and sense of vulnerability, as they engaged in activities structured to promote the sharing of their experiences.

Group approaches have also been reported as helpful with sexually abused girls. The content of these groups often includes a component of education and social learning, in addition to trauma exposure and anxiety reduction training (Deblinger, McLeer, & Henry, 1990; Pelcovitz, 1999). Bereavement groups following the World Trade Center tragedy of September 11, 2001 have helped many children and adolescents share their feelings associated with their traumatic grief experiences (Cohen et al., 2001; Hartley, 2004; Malekoff, 2004). Some agencies and programs, such as hospices, refer to such bereavement groups as "supportive" rather than "therapy" groups (Burrough & Mize, 2004). The implication is that the groups are not intended to provide therapy to people who have preexisting or coexisting psychological problems, but for those whose "normal" process of grief can be facilitated in a group. With traumatized adolescents, group therapy is often the treatment of choice, because they usually are more comfortable with peers than they would be in individual treatment with an adult therapist. Group participation allows adolescents to express their feelings therapeutically through a variety of methods, such as music, dance, poetry, and journal writing (Malekoff, 2004). Whatever the treatment approach, the methods must be age-appropriate, and must respect developmental abilities and preferences regarding activities designed to foster communication and promote healing.

FAMILY WORK

Adjunctive work with biological or foster family members of traumatized youth may occur in either individual, conjoint, or group formats. Whenever possible, strong efforts must be made to help caretakers understand the reasons for the youth's continuing symptomatic behavior, such as jumpiness or withdrawal, so that they will respond with patience rather than criticism. A model treatment program for the nonoffending parents of sexually abused girls included parent education, parent–child communication, and instruction in therapeutic behavior management (Deblinger et al., 1990). Because traumatized youth often continue to show high levels of reactivity in situations when they feel threatened or stressed, those living with these youngsters need to receive education about predictable effects of trauma, as well as about methods for helping the youngsters learn how to manage their feelings of stress. When a youth has a history of family violence, the nonoffending parent, as well as siblings, can benefit from individual and group treatment. Trauma occurs in a context, and the appropriate treatment should include all the witnesses (Groves, 2002).

Many children and adolescents in the child welfare system may never have known or had any contact with their biological families, due to long-term separations related to the effects of substance abuse, poverty, incarceration, mental illness, or other serious problems. In other cases, youngsters have suffered neglect or abuse at the hands of their only known parent; this experience generates feelings of profound loss, grief, and rage. In Chapter 10, Crenshaw and Hardy describe the long-term individual treatment of such a child, who was placed in a residential treatment program as a result of his mother's neglect/abuse and subsequent incarceration. In cases such as this, in which multiple abuses and abandonment have led to feelings of despair and loss of trust, youth will require long-term treatment. Furthermore, when these children are placed in foster homes, the foster parents should receive regular guidance and emotional support in individual and/or group sessions designed to educate and sensitize them regarding the impact of trauma and the management of its aftereffects.

Ongoing or sequential/intermittent treatment of a youngster may be essential to maintain stability throughout his or her developmental course when predictable life stresses threaten to upset the status quo. The very nature of adolescent development may cause the youth to ponder previous abuses from a more mature perspective that questions the injustice of his or her experience. This can lead to anger and acting-out behavior when memories of earlier traumas become triggered by the adolescent's own physical development and growing interest in the opposite sex. Intermittent therapy at such critical periods may help the youth understand and deal with the resurgence of feelings related to past traumas (Holmbeck, Greenley, & Franks, 2003).

TIME CONSIDERATIONS AND SPECIFIC TYPES OF TREATMENT

Impact of Assessment on Choice of Treatment Method

The selection of a treatment method or methods for trauma is not an easy, "one size fits all" prescription. Because people respond differently to the same type of traumatic event, some treatments will be more effective with some and other options will work better with others, depending on their backgrounds and other factors. Ultimately, the choice of treatment method must take into account an assessment of multiple factors, including the nature of the trauma itself, each person's unique personal history, and the type of support available. Among factors to be evaluated in an individual's history are the youth's age/developmental stage, his or her typical method of responding to stress, and the specific meaning being attributed to this particular traumatic situation. Some young people have suffered numerous painful losses and assaults on their psyches, in contrast to others who have managed to live lives relatively unscathed by trauma. These *individual factors* interact with the *specifics of the trauma event/circumstances*, and with the *response of the network of community, family, and friends surrounding the traumatized individual.* This intermingling of factors serves as the basis for the "tripartite assessment" that informs the understanding of each person's particular response to a traumatic situation (Webb, 1999, 2002, 2003, 2004). Once clinicians have completed this assessment, they are in a better position to select the appropriate treatment method. For example, knowing about a 10-year-old's history of repeated sexual and physical abuse will help a practitioner determine that this child clearly requires more intensive and extensive treatment than six sessions in a support group. Conversely, a 5-year-old with no past trauma/loss history who witnessed a car accident will probably not require long-term treatment.

Determining the Length of Treatment

Nader (2001, 2004), Goenjian et al. (1997), and March, Amaya-Jackson, Foa, and Treadwell (1999) suggest the following general guidelines regarding long versus short-term treatment:

- Mildly to moderately traumatized children/adolescents: 2–16 sessions.
- Moderately to severely traumatized youth (especially those exposed to life threat and/or multiple bloody deaths or injuries): 1–3 years or more.

These guidelines appear to refer to Type I traumas. Practitioners who employ EMDR will generally plan for fewer sessions, as discussed below. Youth who have been chronically abused/neglected (Type II traumas) may require ongoing treatment for 2–3 years, with subsequent follow-up sessions periodically, as future developmental stresses threaten the capacity of the growing youth to maintain stability.

Traumatized youth may periodically avoid any focus on their experiences and memories of abuse. Nader (2004) points out that periods of numbing and avoidance may be interspersed with their attempts to recall and deal with aspects of their traumatic experiences. Therefore, it is acceptable for treatment to occur in a segmented, discontinuous format. In addition, differences in the ability of various family members to work on issues related to their traumatic past must be honored: "Individual children and family members will have different recovery rates, trauma issues, and readiness to focus on or resolve specific issues" (Nader, 2004, p. 60). Again, practitioners must adapt to the emotional readiness of each of their clients.

Debriefing and Psychological First Aid

Many practitioners believe that time considerations play a critical role in the treatment of trauma. The provision of intervention 2–14 days after a traumatic event in the form of debriefing has been recommended following Type I traumas, in order to "defuse" the experience and reduce later symptom formation (Mitchell & Everly, 1993; Williams, 2004). As previously mentioned, however, other authors (Litz, 2004) discredit the use of such groups. Proponents of debriefings describe them as occurring in a single-session format that aims to help individuals examine and review their personal experiences in dealing with the critical incident (traumatic event), and then provides education and information about possible future responses, such as jumpiness and sleeping problems. Debriefings are *not* considered to be therapy sessions, and people who do not wish to participate should not be pressured to do so (Mitchell & Everly, 1993; Williams, 2004). The length of a debriefing session varies according to the age of the participants; it can range from 15 minutes for preschoolers to 1–2 hours or more for high school students and adults. School crisis teams typically use debriefings when traumatic events have been experienced together by a number of students.

There has been considerable acceptance of the value of debriefings following a shared traumatic experience, despite studies that have reported negative or mixed results. According to an article in the *Psychotherapy Networker*, "research up to this point indicates that [debriefing] has little positive impact, or at least much less impact than most treatments" (Lebow, 2003, p. 79). This suggests that schools and other community programs need to reassess whether they want to continue using this method with pupils and others, in view of these questions about its efficacy.

The term "psychological first aid" has been used to refer to group screenings and interventions in school settings following a traumatic event (Nader, 1997; Pynoos & Nader, 1998). These interventions include drawing and narrative (storytelling) exercises that provide diagnostic information that can help identify children at risk of PTSD reactions related to their traumatic experiences. Another benefit comes from the group discussion that follows the drawing and storytelling exercises; this provides cathartic relief and the opportunity for the children to normalize some of their responses and obtain accurate information about the trauma they experienced. This particular aspect of psychological first aid is similar to what happens in a debriefing group (Chemtob, Thomas, Law, & Cremniter, 1997; Williams, 2004; Mitchell & Everly, 1993). However, the components of risk assessment (diagnosis) and therapeutic treatment of children's traumatic responses in the psychological first aid model go far beyond debriefing. In addition to the drawing and storytelling exercises, the first aid assessment also includes the administration of a semi-structured individual screening inventory (the Childhood Post-Traumatic Stress Response Index, CPTS-RI; Frederick, Pynoos, & Nader, 1992) that permits the triage and screening of children in need of further mental health services. Informal reports from children who have received these directive and interactive psychological first-aid interventions have been very positive.

Cognitive-Behavioral Approaches

The rationale of cognitive-behavioral therapy is that thoughts determine feelings, which in turn influence behaviors. This is the opposite of psychodynamic theory, which maintains that feelings determine both thoughts and behaviors. When a youngster has been traumatized, he or she may respond with various symptoms of depression and anxiety, as well as PTSD symptoms (such as reexperiencing, avoidance, and arousal). Cognitive-behavioral practitioners assume that a person's thoughts and attributions about the trauma create the resulting stress, rather than elements of the event itself. Therefore, cognitive-behavioral methods focus on alleviating and managing the distressing thoughts through the use of such techniques as thought stopping, cognitive restructuring, guided imagery, controlled breathing, and behavior management. An essential component of the cognitive-behavioral approach is exposure through encouraging the individual to tell (draw or play out) his or her story about the event, including the worst moment. The expectation is that the emotions attached to the event will become less intense with repeated exposure. During this recall, the therapist alters any distortions or misinformation the person may report. Some researchers using this method with children have renamed the exposure component as the process of "creating a trauma narrative," because of the possible negative connotations of deliberately requiring a child to revisit his or her painful traumatic experiences (Cohen et al., 2001).

Cohen et al. (2001) have published a manual for cognitive-behavioral treatment of traumatic grief in children, following the terrorist attacks of September 11, 2001. The manual distinguishes traumatic grief from other types of bereavement and includes a protocol for 16-session parallel groups of children and parents, with some conjoint sessions. An excerpt from a cognitive-behavioral group session appears in Malekoff (2004), in which the group members shared their wishes that they could have protected their respective parents from the World Trade Center collapse. An example of cognitive reprocessing occurred when the group worker engaged the group members in challenging the ability of anyone to have known in advance about this tragedy. To summarize, the cognitive-behavioral interventions emphasized in Cohen et al.'s (2001) manual include the following:

- Stress inoculation methods, such as relaxation, thought stopping, cognitive coping, and increasing a sense of safety.
- Gradual exposure that increases the ability of participants to discuss the traumatic death without accompanying negative emotions of terror and rage.
- Cognitive processing of thoughts about the death, including the correction of inaccurate cognitions (as illustrated above).

As mentioned previously, there has been considerable empirical support for cognitive-behavioral therapy, which can be used in individual, family, or group modalities.

Eye Movement Desensitization and Reprocessing

Using bilateral activation of the brain through back-and-forth movements or sounds, EMDR incorporates a number of interventions typical of cognitive-behavioral treatment, such as exposure and the encouragement of more adaptive cognitions regarding the traumatic situation. There is a growing body of empirical evidence that EMDR is effective in the treatment of trauma, and it tends to achieve reduction of symptoms in fewer sessions than other therapies (Lebow, 2003; Greenwald, 1998; see also Greenwald, Chapter 13).

EMDR has been used with children of all ages and for various kinds of loss and trauma (Greenwald, 1998). The younger the child, the more likely it is that a parent or caretaker will be included as part of the child's treatment. For example, the child may sit on the parent's lap as the therapist moves a magic wand or puppets in front of the child's face to encourage bilateral eye movements, while telling a story that has themes similar to the child's traumatic experience.

Chapter 13 of this book, and other writings by Greenwald (1998, 2005), provide details of how EMDR may be incorporated into trauma treatment that also utilizes cognitive, play, art, and other methods to bring about symptom alleviation. Unlike the cognitive-behavioral therapy approach described above, which deals primarily with the *current* trauma, EMDR focuses on *past* memories related to trauma/loss experiences that may be influencing the present distress. After completing a series of 8–12 back-and-forth eye movements or sound "sets" the therapist asks the client to make an assessment of his or her level of discomfort when thinking about the distressing feeling associated with the trauma. This assessment is referred to as the "subjective unit of disturbance" (SUDS) rating. Children can be asked to respond with their hands to the question "How big is the worry now?" Sometimes older children and adolescents consider the process of participating in the eye movements to be "weird," and practitioners can give them the option of using electrical "tappers" that emit low-frequency vibrations. These may be held in the hands or attached to the ankles during the process of first thinking about a worry, and then thinking, about how they will feel when the worry is no longer present (two separate steps). Obviously, this latter concept incorporates the cognitive method of thought substitution.

Practitioners of EMDR openly admit that they do not understand the reasons for the method's effectiveness. Despite the lack of a valid biological explanation, however, EMDR is becoming increasingly accepted as one of the preferred treatments for PTSD, and it can be included as part of the therapy process with traumatized children and adolescents.

EMDR requires specialized training beyond the typical clinical master's degree in social work or psychology. The details about this training are summarized in the Appendix to this volume.

Play/Art and Other Expressive Therapies

For the purpose of this discussion, the term "play therapy" is used to include all forms of expressive and creative therapies, such as art, music, sandplay, and various other play methods. As previously mentioned, therapists who treat children must use symbolic ways to communicate with young clients who are incapable of and/or unwilling to spend 45 minutes talking to an adult about the terrible thing or things that happened to them. In fact, because of the avoidance reactions that are typical of PTSD, even adults shirk from the detailed recounting of a traumatic experience.

Play therapists have unlimited resources in the form of toys, art materials, board games, and stories to assist them in communicating with traumatized children. Initially, the therapist should acknowledge that he or she knows about the trauma the child has experienced, and should suggest that during their time together they can sometimes talk and sometimes play (Webb, 2001). Many children, hearing that play is an option, will choose an activity that deals symbolically with the trauma, without consciously realizing the connection. The play therapist notices the child's selection and the manner in which the child proceeds. Some children create a displaced version of their experience—for example, by playing with human-eating dinosaurs, by tipping over a dollhouse, or by having toy cars crash in numerous and massive pile-up accidents. Under these circumstances, the play therapist may comment about the frightening things that are happening and how scary it must be for the people who are being eaten by a dinosaur, are in the house, or are in the cars. It is not advisable for the therapist to make any direct acknowledgment about the connection to events in the child's life, especially early in treatment, because this would make the child more anxious and disrupt the ongoing play.

Some play therapy approaches are directive, and others are nondirective. Directive approaches are more appropriate for traumatized children, who usually are reluctant and need a lot of encouragement and support to deal with their painful experiences. The degrees of direction can range from asking a child to show with the dolls what happened to him or her, to simply asking, "What else happened?" in the middle of a child's spontaneous reenactment of an aggressive scene. A child may be uncomfortable or reluctant to recreate the traumatic scene, especially in the early stages of treatment, when the child has not yet established a trusting relationship with the therapist. Children with histories of physical or sexual abuse have often been sworn to secrecy, and practitioners must always make certain that the children's safety is assured. When court proceedings related to abuse are anticipated, it is contraindicated for a therapist to give any kind of direction to a child during the court investigation period. Once the court proceedings are completed and the child has been referred for therapy, it will take some time for the child to develop some comfort with the therapist. Prior to initiating any trauma reenactment, the therapist should teach the child some relaxation techniques.

Play methods may be used individually, in groups, and with family members to assist in dealing with the feelings associated with difficult and painful past events. Many parents are unfamiliar with the concept of play therapy and will require an explanation of how children "play out" their feelings, just as adults talk about them. Members of some cultures may not understand this and may not agree regarding the child's use of play as communication. Again, the play therapist must be prepared to offer explanations regarding the rationale and usefulness of the method.

There is a lack of empirical studies to support the use of play therapy with traumatized children. However, the literature recounts numerous examples of successful treatment outcomes using art therapy (Malchiodi, 1997; Roje, 1996), music therapy (Loewy & Stewart, 2004), sandplay (Carey, 1999, 2004), play with puppets/dolls (Webb, 1999, 2001), and storytelling (O'Toole, 2002). Even when dealing with stressful feelings, children enjoy the process of play therapy, and they benefit greatly from the understanding and validation they experience through the helping relationship. This is especially true for children with abusive backgrounds whose self-esteem has suffered because of their negative experiences. Many chapters in this book attest to the potential for healing and growth through joining with a child or adolescent on his or her own developmental level.

Combined Methods

Many practitioners employ a blend of helping methods; they find that an eclectic approach allows them to fit treatment to each client, rather than treating all clients in the same manner. Most methods build on the helping relationship between the therapist and the child or adolescent. When the practitioner conveys respect for the young client and a genuine desire to help, the choice of method builds on this foundation. Flexibility and knowledge of different treatment methods will ultimately benefit both the practitioner and the clients. The chapters that follow offer some rich examples of effective therapeutic interventions with children and adolescents who have suffered numerous traumas, but who, as a result of creative therapy approaches, now face the future with enhanced skills and ability to meet new developmental challenges.

REFERENCES

Addis, M. E., & Krasnow, A.D. (2000). A national survey of practicing psychologists' attitudes toward psychotherapy treatment manuals. *Journal of Consulting and Clinical Psychology, 68*, 331–339.

Benoit, M. B. (2000). Foster care. In B. J. Sadock & V. A. Sadock (Eds.), *Kaplan and Sadock's comprehensive textbook of psychiatry* (7th ed., pp. 2873–2877). Philadelphia: Lippincott Williams & Wilkins.

Bevin, T. (1999). Multiple traumas of refugees—near drowning and witnessing of maternal rape: Case of Sergio, age 9, and follow-up at age 16. In N. B. Webb (Ed.), *Play therapy with children in crisis: Individual, group, and family treatment* (2nd ed., pp. 164–182). New York: Guilford Press.

Boyd-Franklin, N. (2003). *Black families in therapy: Understanding the African American experience* (2nd ed.). New York: Guilford Press.

Burrough, C., & Mize, D. (2004). Ongoing, long-term grief support groups for traumatized families. In N. B. Webb (Ed.), *Mass trauma and violence* (pp. 142–160). New York: Guilford Press.

Canino, I., & Spurlock, J. (2000). *Culturally diverse children and adolescents. Assessment, diagnosis, and treatment* (2nd ed.). New York: Guilford Press.

Carey, L. (1999). *Sandplay therapy with children and families*. Northvale, NJ: Aronson.

Carey, L. (2004). Sandplay, art, and play therapy to promote anxiety reduction. In N. B. Webb (Ed.), *Mass violence and trauma* (pp. 216–233). New York: Guilford Press.

Chemtob, C. M., Tomas, S., Law, W., & Cremniter, D. (1997). Postdisaster psychosocial intervention: A field study of the impact of debriefing on psychological distress. *American Journal of Psychiatry, 154*(3), 415–417.

Cohen, J. A., Greenberg, T., Padlo, S., Shipley, C., Mannarino, A., Deblinger, E., & Stubenbort, K. (2001, September). *Cognitive-behavioral therapy for traumatic grief in children: Treatment manual* (rev. ed.). Pittsburgh, PA: Center for Traumatic Stress in Children and Adolescents, Department of Psychiatry, Allegheny General Hospital.

Deblinger, E., McLeer, S. V., & Henry, D. (1990). Cognitive behavioral treatment for sexually abused children suffering from post-traumatic stress: Preliminary findings. *Journal of the American Academy of Child and Adolescent Psychiatry, 29*, 747–752.

Doyle, J. S., & Stoop, D. (1999). Witness and victim of multiple abuses: Case of Randy, age 10, in a residential treatment center, and follow up at age 19 in prison. In N. B. Webb (Ed.), *Play therapy with children in crisis: Individual, group, and family treatment* (2nd ed., pp. 131–163). New York: Guilford Press.

Follette, V. M., Ruzek, J. I., & Abueg, F. R. (Eds.). (1998). *Cognitive-behavioral therapies for trauma*. New York: Guilford Press.

Frederick, C., Pynoos, R., & Nader, K. (1992). *The Childhood Post-Traumatic Stress Reaction Index (CPTS-RI), a copyrighted inventory*. Available from measures@twosuns.org.

Gil, E. (1991). *The healing power of play: Working with abused children*. New York: Guilford Press.

Goenjian, A. K., Karayan, I., Pynoos, R. S., Minassian, D., Najarian, L. M.,

Steinberg, A. M., & Fairbanks, L. A. (1997). Outcome of psychotherapy among early adolescents after trauma. *American Journal of Psychiatry, 154*, 536–542.

Greenwald, R. (1998). EMDR: New hope for children suffering from trauma and loss. *Clinical Child Psychology and Psychiatry, 3*(2), 279–287.

Greenwald, R. (2005). *Child trauma handbook: A guide for helping trauma-exposed children and adolescents.* New York: Haworth Press.

Groves, B. M. (2002). *Children who see too much: Lessons from the Child Witness to Violence Project.* Boston: Beacon Press.

Hartley, B. (2004). Bereavement groups soon after traumatic death. In N. B. Webb (Ed.), *Mass violence and trauma* (pp. 167–190). New York: Guilford Press.

Hoagwood, K. (2003). Ethical issues in child and adolescent psychosocial treatment research. In A. E. Kazdin & J. R. Weisz (Eds.), *Evidence-based psychotherapies for children and adolescents* (pp. 60–75). New York: Guilford Press.

Holmbeck, G. N., Greenley, R. N., & Franks, E. A. (2003). Developmental issues and considerations in research and practice. In A. E. Kazdin & J. R. Weisz (Eds.), *Evidence-based psychotherapies for children and adolescents* (pp. 21–41). New York: Guilford Press.

James, B. (1994). *Handbook for treatment of attachment-trauma problems in children.* New York: Free Press.

Kazdin, A. E., & Weisz, J. R. (Eds.). (2003). *Evidence-based psychotherapies for children and adolescents.* New York: Guilford Press.

Kinzie, J. D. (2001). Cross-cultural treatment of PTSD. In J. P. Wilson, M. J. Friedman, & J. D. Lindy (Eds.), *Treating psychological trauma and PTSD* (pp. 255–277). New York: Guilford Press.

Lebow, J. (2003, September–October). War of the worlds: Researchers and practitioners collide on EMDR and CISD. *Psychotherapy Networker,* 79–83.

Lindy, J. D., & Wilson, J. P. (2001). Respecting the trauma membrane: Above all, do no harm. In J. P. Wilson, M. J. Friedman, & J. D. Lindy (Eds.), *Treating psychological trauma and PTSD* (pp. 432–445). New York: Guilford Press.

Litz, B. (Ed.). (2004). *Early intervention for trauma and traumatic loss.* New York: Guilford Press.

Loewy, J., & Stewart, K. (2004). Music therapy to help traumatized children. In N. B. Webb (Ed.), *Mass violence and trauma* (pp. 191–215). New York: Guilford Press.

Malchiodi, C. (1997). *Breaking the silence: Art therapy with children from violent homes.* Belmont, CA: Brooks/Cole.

Malchiodi, C. A. (Ed.). (2003). *Handbook of art therapy.* New York: Guilford Press.

Malekoff, A. (2004). *Group work with adolescents: Principles and practice* (2nd ed.). New York: Guilford Press.

March, J., Amaya-Jackson, L., Foa, E., & Treadwell, K. (1999). *Trauma focused coping treatment of pediatric post-traumatic stress disorder after single-incident trauma* (Version 1.0). Unpublished protocol.

Michaels, D. T., & Levine, C. (1992). Estimates of the number of motherless youth orphaned by AIDS in the United States. *Journal of the American Medical Association, 268*(24), 3456–3460.

Mitchell, J. T., & Everly, G. S., Jr. (1993). *Critical incident stress debriefing: An opera-*

tions manual for the prevention of trauma among emergency services and disaster workers. Ellicott City, MD: Chevron.

Nader, K. (2001). Treatment methods for childhood trauma. In J. P. Wilson, M. J. Friedman, & J. D. Lindy (Eds.), *Treating psychological trauma and PTSD* (pp. 432–445). New York: Guilford Press.

Nader, K. (2004). Treating traumatized children and adolescents. Treatment issues, modalities, timing, and methods. In N. B. Webb (Ed.), *Mass trauma and violence: Helping families and children cope* (pp. 50–74). New York: Guilford Press.

Nader, K., Dubrow, N., & Stamm, B. H. (Eds.). (1999). *Honoring differences: Cultural issues in the treatment of trauma and loss.* Philadelphia: Taylor & Francis.

Nader, K. O. (1997). Treating traumatic grief in systems. In C. R. Figley, B. E. Mazza, & B. N. Mazza (Eds.), *Death and trauma: The traumatology of grieving* (pp. 159–192). Washington, DC: Taylor & Francis.

Nisivoccia, D., & Lynn, M. (1999). Helping forgotten victims: Using activity groups with children who witness violence. In N. B. Webb (Ed.), *Play therapy with children in crisis: Individual, family, and group treatment* (2nd ed., pp. 74–103). New York: Guilford Press.

O'Donohue, W., Fanetti, M., & Elliott, A. (1998). Trauma in children. In V. M. Folette, J. I. Ruzek, & F. R. Abueg (Eds.), *Cognitive-behavioral therapies for trauma* (pp. 355–382). New York: Guilford Press.

Oldham, J. M., & Riba, M. B. (2001). Introduction to the Review of Psychiatry Series. In S. Eth (Ed.), *PTSD in children and adolescents* (pp. xiii–xvi). Washington, DC: American Psychiatric Press.

Ollendick, T. H. (1999). Empirically supported treatments: Promises and pitfalls. *The Clinical Psychologist, 52,* 1–3.

Ollendick, T. H., & King, N. J. (2000). Empirically supported treatments for children and adolescents. In P. C. Kendall (Ed.), *Child and adolescent therapy: Cognitive-behavioral procedures* (2nd ed., pp. 386–425). New York: Guilford Press.

O'Toole, D. (2002). Storytelling with bereaved children. In N. B. Webb (Ed.), *Helping bereaved children: A handbook for practitioners* (2nd ed., pp. 323–345). New York: Guilford Press.

Ozawa, M. (1997). Demographic changes and their implications. In M. Reisch & E. Gambrill (Eds.), *Social work in the twenty-first century* (pp. 8–27). Thousand Oaks, CA: Pine Forge Press.

Parson, E. R. (1997). Posttraumatic child therapy (P-TCT): Assessment and treatment factors in clinic work with inner-city children exposed to catastrophic community violence. *Journal of Interpersonal Violence, 12,* 172–194.

Pelcovitz, D. (1999). Betrayed by a trusted adult: Structured time-limited group therapy with elementary school children abused by a school employee. In N. B. Webb (Ed.), *Play therapy with children in crisis: Individual, group, and family treatment* (2nd ed., pp. 183–199). New York: Guilford Press.

Pynoos, R. S., & Nader, K. (1998). Psychological first aid treatment approach to children exposed to community violence: Research implications. *Journal of Traumatic Stress, 1*(4), 127–155

Roje, J. (1996). LA '94 earthquake in the eyes of children: Art therapy with elementary school children who were victims of disaster. *Art Therapy, 12,* 1263–1284.

Rosenberg, J. E. (2001). Forensic aspects of PTSD in children and adolescents. In S. E. Eth (Ed.), *PTSD in children and adolescents* (pp. 33–58). Washington, DC: American Psychiatric Press.

Seedat, S., & Stein, D. J. (2001). Biological treatment of PTSD in children and adolescents. In S. Eth (Ed.), *PTSD in children and adolescents* (pp. 87–116). Washington, DC: American Psychiatric Press.

Terr, L. C. (1991). Childhood traumas: An outline and overview. *American Journal of Psychiatry, 20,* 741–759.

Webb, N. B. (Ed.). (1999). *Play therapy with children in crisis: Individual, group, and family treatment* (2nd ed.). New York: Guilford Press.

Webb, N. B. (Ed.). (2002). *Helping bereaved children: A handbook for practitioners* (2nd ed.). New York: Guilford Press.

Webb, N. B. (2003). *Social work practice with children* (2nd ed.). New York: Guilford Press.

Webb, N. B. (Ed.). (2004). *Mass violence and trauma.* New York: Guilford Press.

Williams, M. B. (2004). How schools respond to traumatic events: Debriefing interventions and beyond. In N. B. Webb (Ed.), *Mass violence and trauma* (pp. 120–141). New York: Guilford Press.

Wilson, J. P., Friedman, M. J., & Lindy, J. D. (Eds.). (2001). *Treating psychological trauma and PTSD.* New York: Guilford Press.

Zayas, L. H., Canino, I., & Suarez, Z. E. (2001). Parenting in mainland Puerto Rican families. In N. B. Webb (Ed.), *Culturally diverse parent–child and family relationships* (pp. 133–156). New York: Columbia University Press.

CHAPTER 7

The Intergenerational Transmission of Family Violence

ELIZABETH M. TRACY
PAMELA J. JOHNSON

Ellie Brown is a 31-year-old European American woman living in a rural Midwestern town. She and her husband of 10 years have been separated for the past 8 months. Both have a history of severe alcohol and drug abuse, as well as of depression. The two oldest of their children (Billy, 9, and Candace, 11) have been placed in the temporary custody of the paternal grandparents. The youngest (Jamie, 4) is living with foster parents who have experience in dealing with emotionally disturbed youngsters, because his grandparents were unable to cope with his explosive temper tantrums and escalating aggression.

Ellie grew up in a very poor family in the same rural community where she now lives. Her early family life was chaotic: Chronic and palpable conflict was always present between her parents, and this ongoing tension often erupted into physical fights between them, especially when they had been drinking. As a child, Ellie experienced episodes of harsh and physically abusive discipline "for her own good," as her parents put it.

Ellie began to smoke tobacco and experiment with alcohol at the age of 12. In recent years her main drug of choice has been crack cocaine, though she has often resorted to methamphetamine ("crank") when nothing else was available. She has a history of manic–depressive episodes that began when she was 19, though her more usual emotional state over the years has been a persistent and severe depression.

Her husband is actively using alcohol and cocaine, and disappears for weeks at a time. He has not worked in months. Even as recently as 2 years ago, Ellie and Johnnie were relatively sober, owned their own home, and Johnnie's contractor business was taking hold. However, once Ellie and Johnnie started to use cocaine on a regular basis (and then crack cocaine), the losses were rapid and catastrophic. They lost their house and the business; there were frequent problems with the law; and child protective services (CPS) became involved when concerned relatives reported that the children were frequently unsupervised. Further investigation by CPS revealed that Ellie was often verbally and emotionally abusive with the children. As she became unable to deal with her anger during Jamie's temper tantrums, she locked him in a closet on a regular basis while the two older children were at school.

As she tries to comply with a case management plan designed to enable her to regain her children, it is a confusing and frightening time for Ellie. She has no money, no job, and no marketable skills with which to earn a living wage. She misses her children and feels tremendous guilt and shame for their loss. These feelings sometimes trigger her substance use, which then makes her feel even more remorseful, especially as a relapse "resets the clock" in terms of how soon—or even whether—she can get her children back. Even more confusing, memories of sexual abuse in her family of origin are just beginning to surface, and she has begun to experience the signs and symptoms of posttraumatic stress disorder (PTSD).

The case example presented above illustrates the connections mental health and child welfare practitioners frequently see between clients' histories of trauma, substance abuse, and mental disorders in their families of origin, and the consequent effects on the clients' current parenting. Practitioners often recognize that exposure to violence in one generation tends to be replicated in similar patterns of behavior and attitudes in the next. In particular, emerging evidence suggests that trauma is a risk factor for the development of both substance use and mental disorders, and that often these take the form of co-occurring ("dual") disorders (Ouimette & Brown, 2003). This combination of childhood exposure to violence, parental substance abuse, and subsequent impaired or compromised parenting in one generation appears to be strongly implicated in creating a traumatic developmental context for the children in the next.

This chapter helps students and practitioners to clarify elements in the "intergenerational transmission of violence," which is often related to experiences of exposure to violence, to subsequent substance abuse and/or dependence, and to mental disorder. The chapter begins by broadly outlining the scope of the interrelated problems and their potential for serious emotional, behavioral, and neuropsychological sequelae in such mothers and their children. This is followed by a discussion of the interrelated effects of trauma, substance abuse, and mental illness on parenting roles and capacities. Finally, implications are presented for trauma-informed assessment and intervention with mothers, children, and families, especially with respect to parental roles and competencies.

This chapter focuses on women and their children. Although we recognize that men too are victims of violence, women represent a high proportion of those who have experienced lifetime trauma, and historically their needs as a group for treatment of substance use and mental disorders have gone largely unaddressed and underserved. Women with histories of exposure to violence, substance use disorders, and mental health problems also tend to have stressful life conditions–limited resources, unsupportive families, poor job skills, few social network supports, and serious health problems–which contribute to and exacerbate their difficulties in sustaining themselves and their children (Cash & Wilke, 2003). Furthermore, these realities may seriously impair their ability to fulfill their roles as mothers. Consequently, treatment providers often must respond to the multiple needs of such women.

SCOPE OF THE PROBLEM: IMPACT OF VIOLENCE ON WOMEN AND THEIR CHILDREN

The cumulative impact of ongoing domestic violence, child maltreatment, and related substance abuse exacts an enormous toll in terms of physical injury, emotional pain, and social dysfunction at the individual, family, and community levels across the United States. The Centers for Disease Control and Prevention (CDC) report that about 1.5 million women and 834,700 men are physically and/or sexually assaulted by an intimate partner each year (CDC, 2004a). Domestic violence victimization in women is highly correlated with depression; long-term gynecological, neurological, and stress-related health problems; and substance abuse (American Medical Association, 2001; Substance Abuse and Mental Health Services Administration [SAMSHA], 2000). Between 51% and 97% of women with serious mental illnesses have experienced some form of physical or sexual abuse in their lifetime (SAMHSA, 2000). Among women in treatment for a drug or alcohol use disorder, 41–71% report being sexually abused, either as children or as adults (Alexander, 1996). Women who have experienced any form of abuse as children are more likely to report drug dependence as adults, while women who have experienced both physical and sexual abuse double their risk for substance abuse, compared with women who have experienced only one type of abuse (Najavits, Weiss, & Shaw, 1997). Furthermore, there is consistent research evidence that for women, mental disorders, particularly depression and posttraumatic stress disorder, frequently co-occur with substance abuse (Kelley, 2003).

The negative impact of mothers' exposure to violence extends to their children as well. The Child Welfare League of America (CWLA, 2003) reports that between 1.5 and 3.3 million children witness violence at home annually. Moreover, in at least 30% of cases of domestic violence (and some estimates run as high as 60%), child abuse is occurring as well: Of those men who abuse their female partners, it has been found that as many as 50–70% also abuse the partners' children (CWLA, 2003). Women involved in domestic violence—whether as victims or as perpetrators—are also more likely to abuse and/or neglect their children (Jones, Gross, & Becker, 2002). In general, the overlap between child maltreatment and domestic violence is thought to range from 30% to 60% of all cases that involve either (National Clearinghouse on Child Abuse and Neglect Information, 2002).

Both intimate partner violence perpetration and child maltreatment are in turn highly correlated with substance abuse and addiction (Sedlak & Broadhurst, 1996; CDC, 2000). Rates of co-occurring domestic violence perpetration and substance abuse are thought to range from 23% to as high as 100% (Corvo & Carpenter, 2000). According to the CWLA (2003), 70% of child maltreatment cases involve substance abuse, and a child whose parents have problems with alcohol or other drugs are three to four times more likely to be abused and/or neglected than those children whose parents do not. Cash and Wilke (2003) found that having been sexually abused prior to the age of 15, having an alcoholic parent, and having an extended family history of substance abuse significantly predicted the odds of a mother's neglecting her children later in life.

Childhood exposure to violence, whether as victim and/or as witness, is common to all of the foregoing phenomena, and is highly correlated with subsequent emotional dysregulation and a propensity to aggress against others (e.g., Lewis, 1992; Perry, 1997; Karr-Morse & Wiley, 1997; Dutton, 1999; Sappington, 2000; Teicher, 2002; CWLA, 2003). Furthermore, childhood exposure to violence is associated with psychological, interpersonal, and sexual difficulties that persist into adulthood (e.g., Harris, 1996; van der Kolk & McFarlane, 1996; Davis & Petretic-Jackson, 2000; Ouimette & Brown, 2003), and with significant neurocognitive deficits that undermine information-processing and problem-solving capabilities throughout the life course (e.g., Dodge, Bates, & Pettit, 1990; Warnken, Rosenbaum, Fletcher, Hage, & Adelman, 1994; CDC, 2004b). Figure 7.1 illustrates the possible causal relationships between and among childhood trauma, PTSD, substance abuse, and propensity for violence.

Such patterns often seem to "run in families" across generations. Although there is controversy about the precise rates of transmission of violence from one generation to the next, it has been fairly consistently found across studies that about one-third of those victimized as children go on to perpetrate violence against others as adults (Cerezo, 1997; Buchanan, 1998; Simons & Johnson, 1998; Pears & Capaldi, 2001).

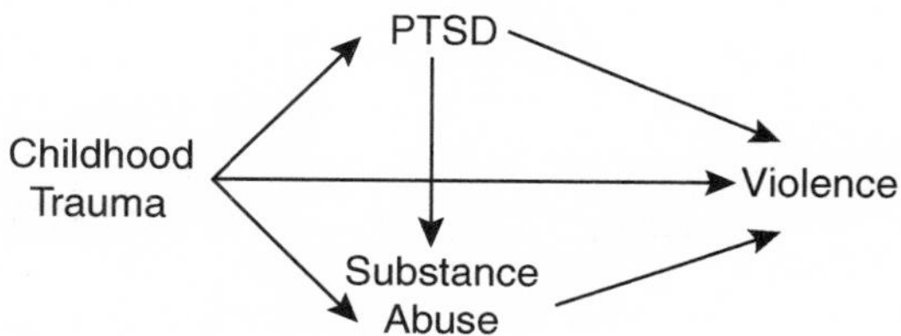

FIGURE 7.1. Childhood trauma, PTSD, substance abuse, and violence. From Lisak and Miller (2003). Copyright 2003 by the American Psychological Association. Reprinted by permission.

EFFECTS OF TRAUMA, SUBSTANCE ABUSE, AND MENTAL DISORDERS ON PARENTING ROLES AND CAPACITIES

It is beyond the scope of this chapter to discuss the neurophysiological effects of trauma, substance abuse, and mental illness in detail. (See Perry, Chapter 3, this volume, for a more in-depth discussion.) It is crucial for practitioners to recognize and understand that there is often a strong neurophysiological component underlying particular behavioral and emotional patterns and responses. This understanding helps to determine appropriate modes of assessment and intervention, and to sustain an empathic and trusting working relationship. It is not that such notions as "will" and "intent" are beside the point, or that a client is incapable of marshaling directed energy, but rather that in the earlier stages of healing and recovery the client's emotional reactivity may override the ability to function, including the ability to parent, and this is in part a function of neurobiological processes. For example, a woman just learning to manage her flashbacks may not yet be ready to benefit from formal (didactic, cognitively based) parent education training, because her emerging memories may be at an emotional, preverbal level that are not consonant with higher language functions.

Neurobiological and psychological functions and capabilities reinforce one another over time, evolving from an individual context of familial, sociocultural, and environmental experience; these functions and capabilities are then encoded (incorporated) into the structure and function of the brain at the level of cells, tissues, and structures (Perry, 1997; Karr-Morse & Wiley, 1997; Siegel, 1999; van der Kolk, 2001; van der Kolk & McFarlane, 1996; Teicher, 2002). It is thought that these neurological changes in turn lead to increased risk of developmental lags and distortions, aggressive behavior, susceptibility to PTSD, and substance abuse and dependence. In children, exposure to traumatogenic processes during critical developmental windows is thought to undermine their capacity for healthy attachment, for the development of self-soothing and self-monitoring behavior, and for emotional resilience; again, one result is increased susceptibility to substance abuse and dependence (Dutton, 1999, 2002; De Bellis, 2002; Anderson, Teicher, Polcari, & Renshaw, 2002; Vasquez, 1998; Gunnar & Donzella, 2002). Although some effects are amenable to intervention after the fact, others may not be fully reversible. Therefore, timely intervention with parents and their children is important (Weinstein & Weinstein, 2000).

During assessment, the clinician may observe the neurophysiological effects of trauma manifested in several domains (see Table 7.1). For example, in terms of affect, a mother may exhibit irritability, depression, and emotional numbing. Cognitively, she may experience intrusive thoughts and dissociation. Her behavior may include aggression, high tolerance for inappropriate behavior, and avoidance of trauma-related situations. Each of these in turn may affect the mother's ability to parent.

For example, a possible effect of dissociation on parenting sometimes involves withdrawal or lack of focused attention on the child. A mother's irritability may be associated with low tolerance for the child's typical behaviors. The child's range of activity may be restricted, because the mother's inability to feel safe and her own patterns of avoidance of perceived threats cause her to be overly protective. A mother's intense mood states and emotional instability may alienate or frighten the child, which in itself can be traumatogenic, and therefore may undermine typical development (Schuengel, Bakermans-Kranenburg, & van IJzendoorn, 1999). It should also be noted that in this population, many women have never received nurturing parenting themselves, which further compromises their ability to parent.

In addition, maternal substance use, abuse, and dependence have been associated with parenting deficits, such as parentification of the child (role reversals), difficulties with organizing and completing caretaking activities (preparing meals, supervision, etc.), and exposing and/or introducing the child to alcohol and drugs (Tracy, 1994). By the same token, parental mental illness has its own set of impacts on parenting; for example, the observed effects of depression on the parent–child interaction, such as the mother's lack of responsiveness to the child's cues, are associated with subsequent language delays (Schuengel et al., 1999).

IMPLICATIONS FOR ASSESSMENT

Given the accumulation of risks and stressors facing women with histories of exposure to violence and subsequent substance use and mental disorders, assessment should include proper screening for a history of trauma, so as to distinguish the signs, symptoms, and sequelae of current sub-

TABLE 7.1. Trauma Symptoms and Potential Effects on Parenting

Domain	Typically observed responses to trauma	Potential effects on parenting
Cognitive	• Intrusive thoughts • Intrusive images • Amnesia • Derealization/ depersonalization • Dissociation	• Preoccupation, withdrawal, lack of presence, and lack of focused attention while attempting to parent • Difficulty in providing stability, adhering to routines, and keeping track of scheduled activities involving the child
Affective	• Anger/irritability • Anxiety/nervousness • Depression • Shame • Hopelessness • Sense of isolation, loneliness • Emotional numbing • Feeling different from others	• Difficulty in feeling close or connected to child, withdrawal • Low tolerance for child's age-appropriate "acting out" • Pervasive fear of hurting child, feeling unable to keep child safe • Inadvertent communication of negative emotions regarding physical contact, bodily functions of child (e.g., changing diapers, bathing)
Behavioral	• Increased activity • Aggression • High tolerance for inappropriate behavior • Low tolerance for chaotic, busy, or complex environments/situations • Avoidance (often unconscious) of triggering and/or trauma-related situations	• Increased risk of child maltreatment • Difficulty setting appropriate boundaries and limits • Easily overwhelmed with everyday demands of parenting • Restriction of child's range of activities and experiences due to the mother's avoidance of perceived threats
Physiological	• Arousal due to autonomic hyperreactivity to trauma triggers • Sensory numbing • Absence of "normal" reaction to events	• Child must often cope with mother's erratic and unpredictable behavioral reactions and mood states, which do not always correspond in easily understandable ways with situations and events
Multiple domains	• Flashbacks • Age regression • Nightmares • Rigid and/or limited notion of range of acceptable behaviors • Unsure as to what constitutes "normal" family life and parenting behaviors	• Mother's intense mood states, levels of fear, and emotional instability may frighten child • Chronic fatigue due to sleep problems may undermine coping skills • Difficulty assuming authority, making decisions, advocating for self and/or child • Difficulty distinguishing between discipline and punishment • Difficulty establishing safe environment for child

Note. Based on information from SAMHSA (2000) and Harris and the Parenting Workgroup (2001).

stance abuse from those of trauma-related disorders. Such screening must take place in a supportive atmosphere that minimizes attendant shame and humiliation. At a minimum, the clinician and/or team should assess for the following, both at baseline and on an ongoing basis:

- *Screen for exposure to significant traumatic events.* The emotional pain of abuse may deter people from seeking help, and often people in treatment do not talk about their traumatic experiences or become aware of them until well into treatment (Goodman, Dutton, & Harris, 1997). Adult survivors of childhood trauma commonly suppress memories as a means of coping, or minimize the impact of those traumatic events they do remember, sometimes to the point of idealizing what was in fact an abusive situation (see, e.g., Courtois, 1999). Consequently, the level of violence a woman actually experiences may never be accurately assessed or dealt with in treatment. Table 7.2 lists examples of interview questions to screen for childhood maltreatment.

TABLE 7.2. Direct Questions to Screen for a History of Childhood Abuse or Neglect

Questions about trauma events

- Were there any significant traumatic events in your family while you were growing up? For example, did any of the following events occur in your family: death of a parent or sibling, hospitalization of a parent or sibling, incarceration of a parent or sibling, divorce, or chronic disease?
- Were you treated harshly as a child?
- Did you ever experience physical, sexual, or emotional abuse as a child?
- Did you experience inappropriate physical or sexual contact with an adult or person at least 5 years older than you while you were growing up?
- When you were a child, was there violence in your household, such as battering of family members, involving siblings or a parent and his or her partner?
- Do you feel that your parents neglected you while you were growing up? For example, were there ever periods during which you did not have adequate food, clothing, shelter, or protection by your parents?
- Did your parents use alcohol or drugs frequently when you were growing up? Did you ever use alcohol or drugs with them?

Questions about circumstances that may suggest traumatic events

- Have you or has anyone in your family ever been involved with the child protective system?
- Did you ever live away from your parents? Were you ever in foster care? Were any of your siblings ever in foster care?
- When you were a child, were there any periods when you felt unsafe or in danger?
- When you were growing up, did anyone in your family use alcohol or drugs? How did their alcohol or drug use affect you as a child?
- Have you ever felt that abuse or neglect was justified based on your misbehavior or shortcomings? (In other words, did you feel that the abuse was your fault and that you deserved it?)

Note. Data from Substance Abuse and Mental Health Services Administration (SAMHSA) (2000).

• *Assess the mother's current mental health symptoms, especially posttraumatic stress, depressive, and dissociative symptoms.* Such an assessment should include screening for ongoing physical violence, emotional abuse, and/or verbal abuse in significant relationships. It should also include screening for alcohol and drug abuse/dependence (for an overview of assessment of substance use disorders, see King & Bordnick, 2002; see also American Psychiatric Association, 2000). Table 7.3 lists examples of instruments that assess trauma and mental health status.

• *Assess the child's safety, which is influenced by the stresses facing the mother and the support available to her.* It is important to know the child's and family's daily schedule, involvement with other agencies (particularly CPS), and the role of significant others and extended family members in the care of the child (SAMHSA, 2000).

• *Assess aspects of the parenting role, such as knowledge of child development, parenting skills, and discipline styles.* For example, Table 7.1, discussed earlier, lists possible effects of trauma specific to parenting.

• *Be familiar with and assess child symptoms that may be related to witnessing or experiencing violence.* These may include sleep difficulties, somatic complaints, hypervigilance, regression, withdrawal, numbing, difficulty concentrating, and increased separation anxiety (Child Witness to Violence Project, 2004).

IMPLICATIONS FOR PRACTICE

The premise underlying the following practice guidelines is that helping professionals should approach issues of trauma, family violence, and substance use in an integrated fashion. Because the focus of this chapter is on direct practice skills, service delivery issues required for such an approach are not fully addressed (for such a discussion, see, e.g., Institute for the Advancement of Social Work Research, 2003) although we recognize that services need to be adapted within the context of different treatment settings and philosophies (e.g., child welfare, mental health, and/or substance abuse). This section provides a brief overview of what is known about empirically based trauma interventions, particularly those that address PTSD symptoms, and some common features of integrated approaches. A number of program exemplars are highlighted, and resources for additional information on practice approaches are included, in Appendices 7.1 and 7.2 to this chapter, respectively.

Much clinical research is still needed to develop precise practice guidelines for trauma interventions. The International Society for Traumatic Stress Studies (Foa, Keane, & Friedman, 2000) concludes that although research shows the effectiveness of cognitive-behavioral therapy and pharmacotherapy, relatively little is known about other treatments

TABLE 7.3. Standardized Screening Instruments for Trauma, Substance Abuse, and Mental Health Symptoms

- *Addiction Severity Index (ASI)*. The fifth edition of ASI is a 161-item multidimensional structured clinical interview designed to collect information about substance abuse and client functioning in various life areas for adults seeking treatment for substance abuse.
- *Beck Depression Inventory (BDI)*. The BDI is a 21-item scale designed to measure the severity of depression by assessing the presence and severity of affective, cognitive, motivational, vegetative, and psychomotor components of depression. The BDI is one of the most widely used measures of depression in clinical practice.
- *Brief Symptom Inventory (BSI)*. The BSI is designed to reflect the psychological symptom patterns of psychiatric and medical clients. The BSI takes approximately 10 minutes to administer and has 53 items.
- *Child Maltreatment Interview Schedule (CMIS)*. The CMIS is a 46-item tool based on behavioral descriptions; it assesses emotional, physical, and sexual abuse.
- *Childhood Maltreatment Questionnaire (CMQ)*. The CMQ elicits information about the frequency of maltreatment on or before the age of 17.
- *Childhood Trauma Questionnaire (CTQ)*. The CTQ is a 10- to 15-minute questionnaire that provides a brief and relatively noninvasive screening of childhood trauma experiences.
- *Diagnostic Interview Schedule (DIS)*. The most recent version of DIS (Version 4), is designed to elicit data relating to most *Diagnostic and Statistical Manual of Mental Disorders*, fourth edition (DSM-IV) adult diagnoses on both a lifetime and current basis.
- *Mini International Neuropsychiatric Interview (MINI)*. The MINI was designed as a brief structured interview to screen for the major psychiatric disorders in DSM-IV. It contains 120 questions covering 17 Axis I disorders from DSM-IV.
- *Parent–Child Relationship Inventory (PCRI)*. The PCRI is a 78-item self-report questionnaire designed for clinical use. The PCRI assesses six areas of parenting, including parental satisfaction, support, involvement, communication, limit setting, and autonomy.
- *Posttraumatic Stress Diagnostic Scale (PDS)*. The PDS is a 49-item tool that assesses all DSM-IV criteria for PTSD.
- *Screen for Posttraumatic Stress Symptoms (SPTSS)*. The SPTSS is a brief, 17-item self-report tool used to screen for PTSD symptoms; it is especially useful for clients with histories of multiple traumatic events or whose trauma history is unknown.
- *Structured Clinical Interview for DSM-IV Axis I Disorders (SCID-I)*. The SCID-I is an extremely detailed interview tool that comprehensively reviews all DSM-IV Axis I disorders.
- *Symptom Checklist 90–Revised (SCL-90-R)*. This is a brief, multidimensional inventory designed to screen for a broad range of psychological problems and symptoms of psychopathology.
- *Trauma Symptom Checklist–40 (TSC-40)*. The TCS-40 is a 40-item self-report tool that evaluates symptomatology in adults resulting from childhood or adult traumatic experiences.
- *Trauma Symptom Inventory (TSI)*. The TSI is a 100-item test designed to evaluate posttraumatic stress and other psychological consequences of traumatic events.
- *Traumatic Events Scale (TES)*. The TES evaluates a wide range of both childhood and adult traumas.

Note. For more information about and citations for these tools, see Substance Abuse and Mental Health Services Administration (SAMHSA) (2000).

either specific to PTSD alone or in combination with other treatments. Some other empirically based treatments to explore past trauma, such as exposure therapy (Foa, Dancu, & Hembree, 1999), do not address the substance abuse and case management issues so often seen in a treatment population of women. The society does recommend that PTSD be treated simultaneously with comorbid chemical abuse/dependence.

Intervention with families with a history of intergenerational violence must take a systems perspective; it must also take into consideration the developmental needs of both the adults and the children involved. Many children exposed to trauma neither are assessed for, nor receive, treatment. This is partly due to the fact that while trauma is often related to the nature of the caregiving received, the child's access to treatment is paradoxically dependent on the neglectful and/or abusive caregiver's making the necessary arrangements. Likewise, as stated earlier, the extent to which the mother has been exposed to violence can be underestimated for a variety of reasons, and so she may have received little mental health treatment specific to trauma, in spite of multiple contacts across a wide spectrum of service providers.

It is important, then, that trauma and abuse be addressed in conjunction with other services the family receives, such as substance abuse treatment or parenting skills training. In addition to the mother's needs, the needs of the children must be addressed. Therefore, parenting programs should consider the impact of lifetime exposure to violence on *all* family members, and must necessarily incorporate program elements such as an emphasis on safety for both the mother and child, as well as case management to address multiple service needs.

Adults with histories of childhood trauma tend to share a number of clinical characteristics. These include having severe substance use disorders; starting substance use at a very young age; using substances in order to manage signs and symptoms of PTSD (i.e., "self-medication"); making suicide attempts; and having relationship problems that make it hard for them to trust and to accept help, thus rendering them more vulnerable to relapse (SAMHSA, 2000). The presence of PTSD has been associated with higher rates of relapse after substance abuse treatment, and there is some evidence that addressing PTSD along with substance abuse treatment reduces relapse rates over substance abuse treatment alone (Brown, 2000). Because of this, practitioners should be knowledgeable about interventions to address PTSD.

Cohen, Mannarino, Zhitova, and Capone (2003), in a review of empirically based treatment for child-abuse-related posttraumatic stress and substance abuse in adolescents, conclude that the available evidence suggests an integrated treatment approach that includes both cognitive behavioral interventions (particularly trauma-focused ones) and family treatment strategies. Trauma-focused cognitive-behavioral treatment includes the following components: stress management training, psychoeducation, "gradual exposure" to constructing a trauma narrative, recognizing and coping with triggers and reminders of past abuse, cognitive processing, and problem-solving and safety skills. Some specific treatment components common to empirically supported interventions include (1) developing a trusting therapeutic relationship; (2) enhancing stress management; (3) developing mood management, social, and problem-solving skills; (4) challenging and correcting inaccurate cognitions that contribute to negative mood states or self-destructive behaviors; (5) enhancing parenting skills; and (6) decreasing family violence. Use of psychopharmacological treatments to target PTSD symptoms is also recommended.

Similarly, treatment for trauma in dually diagnosed women typically consists of several components: (1) supportive group therapy so that these women can learn that they are not alone, and can share coping strategies; (2) cognitive reframing to replace self-damaging assumptions (such as the assumption of personal blame) with more self-affirming thought patterns; and (3) social and emotional skills training in managing the neuropsychological sequelae of sexual and physical abuse, such as learning to establish a healthy female identity, healing the sexual self, maintaining physical and emotional safety, developing self-soothing abilities, and honing parenting skills (Harris, 1996). Seeking Safety, for example, is an evidence-based, integrated treatment model for PTSD and substance abuse in women, and is based on the following central treatment themes (Najavits, 2002; Najavits et al., 1997; Najavits, Weiss, Shaw, & Muenz, 1998):

1. Safety as the first and most urgent clinical goal–for example, discontinuing substance use, reducing suicidality, letting go of dangerous relationships, stopping self-harm behaviors such as cutting, and learning about and gaining control of symptoms such as dissociation.
2. Integrated treatment of PTSD and substance use by the same clinician; this provides opportunities for women to see the connections between the trauma they have experienced and their use of substances.
3. Focus on ideals that have been lost due to trauma and substance use, such as respect, commitment, and honesty.
4. Cognitive-behavioral interventions to teach such skills as self-control, relapse prevention, and coping skills, and to strengthen healthy decision making and thought patterns.
5. A focus on interpersonal relationships, mobilizing supportive rela-

tionships, and setting boundaries with respect to destructive relationships.
6. Case management services to provide for other service needs.
7. Therapeutic processes such as highlighting the positive, giving clients as much control as possible, and avoiding harsh confrontation and power struggles.

Appendix 7.1 describes several other types of trauma-informed interventions that address the needs of women and their children. These selected program exemplars represent strategies for addressing trauma issues at multiple levels. In addition, these projects are also examining ways to incorporate trauma-informed parenting skills education and training into treatment services.

MANAGING CHALLENGING CLINICAL PRACTICE ISSUES

A number of sensitive clinical issues are inevitably present in work with women and children who have been exposed to violence.

Balancing Therapeutic Tasks

Workers should avoid an exhaustive focus on past trauma and recovery of memories, to the exclusion of time for emotional rest and healing, practicing new skills, and formulating steps toward a healthy future. In any given session, a worker should be mindful of balancing the time spent exploring the past with the time needed to focus on skill building, regaining emotional equilibrium, and preparing to function in the present. The worker should also focus on validating the woman's emotions associated with her lived experiences rather than on verifying the factual details of the trauma, which may not be a realistic goal, depending on the setting and the situation.

Nurturing Mom, While Monitoring Mothering

A tension exists for the worker between the reparenting process integral to therapeutic work with the mother (through modeling, teaching, and giving instructive feedback) and monitoring the safety of her children. The worker needs to develop a trusting, open relationship with the mother, but must also be vigilant to dangers that may be present due to the mother's limited parenting skills. It is not uncommon for chaos, disorganization, and crisis to interrupt needed work with these clients, and also to distract workers from real dangers in the environment.

Transference and Countertransference Issues

The following transference issues are to be expected in working with women who have histories of trauma: playing one social service worker against the other (e.g., "splitting," secret keeping); minimizing or denying facts to avoid disclosure of embarrassing or shameful details (e.g., extent of violence in the home, or severity of substance abuse); reactivity to the worker as an authority figure, due to victimization by past authority figures; and difficulty in developing trusting relationships with service providers.

Countertransference issues the worker must consider include these: the sympathy evoked by the client's circumstances, which may in turn lead to enabling; the worker's reactivity to the dependency and control needs of the client; vacillating between "rescuing" and feeling victimized by the client with multiple needs; maintaining integrity of professional boundaries and relationships when advocating for the client across service systems; and the possibility that a *worker's* prior trauma may trigger certain unhelpful reactions to the client and her family (e.g., engaging in blame of an aggressive adolescent boy without recognition that he may have been victimized as well).

Avoidance of Retraumatization

It is important that intervention strategies address PTSD arousal symptoms while avoiding techniques that might retraumatize a woman (Harris, 1996). Therefore, a worker should limit the use of confrontation and treatment modes that may trigger or reinforce feelings of shame and self-blame, such as direct didactic teaching, which may be experienced as intimidating. Also, the worker should permit the client to limit the degree of exposure to terrifying memories, to avoid being overwhelmed. Treatment staff members should also review their program's policies in such areas as use of restraints and time outs, and in programmatic responses to difficult situations such as relapse or noncompliance, to ensure that institutional remedies are trauma-informed and do not reproduce patterns of oppression.

SUMMARY AND CASE APPLICATION

This chapter has discussed the often interrelated problems of exposure to violence, substance abuse, and mental health symptoms present in many women's lives, and has provided an overview of trauma-informed assessment and intervention with mothers and children. As practitioners, we are just beginning to explore effective approaches in working with mothers and children exposed to violence, and integrated service models are still being developed. However, as this book attests, women and children served in child welfare and mental health settings often present with multiple problems rooted in the experience of trauma. Therefore, practitioners need to be mindful of the potential impact of possible trauma on mothers, as well as its effects on their sons and daughters, and thus to formulate their intervention approaches accordingly.

We now return to the case scenario at the beginning of this chapter. What follows is a brief description of possible services for Ellie Brown and her children. The service plan assumes that a complete assessment has been completed for all involved adults and children, as well as of the overall family system; that integrated delivery of required services is available in Ellie's community; that staff members are trained in the impact of trauma and will employ trauma-informed interventions, that they have the time and resources to carry out a high-quality treatment plan; and finally, to the extent possible, that the interventions used will have an empirical base.

With this context in mind, and with the overriding goal of safely reuniting Ellie and her children, we suggest the following as immediate objectives:

1. Ensure that Ellie's basic needs (housing, food, etc.) are being met.
2. Help Ellie to establish and maintain sobriety.
3. Conduct a complete psychiatric assessment and initiate treatment for Ellie, so as to decrease her depressive episodes and stabilize her mood.
4. Facilitate Ellie's understanding of the relationship between her substance abuse and PTSD symptomatology.
5. Facilitate her safe exploration of trauma issues and concurrent development of related coping skills.
6. Help Ellie to develop and build positive child management techniques.
7. Support the paternal grandparents in their current caregiving role.
8. Ensure that Jamie (the 4-year-old, currently living with foster parents) is provided with an assessment and intervention as indicated.
9. Establish clear, well-maintained lines of communication with CPS, such that Ellie and all related professionals (including the social services caseworker) are clear about what is required to achieve family unification, and in what time frame(s).

Interventions that might be employed to meet these objectives include case management through the local social welfare department, so as to ensure a basic standard of living for Ellie while she completes treatment; substance abuse treatment (individual, group); and mental health treatment (individual, group), which includes psychopharmacological management, cognitive-behavioral treatment for depression, psychoeducation, and targeted interventions to address PTSD history and symptomatology (e.g., exposure therapy, eye movement desensitization and reprocessing, and/or a Seeking Safety group). Intensive home-based services that include a case management component and behavioral training in parenting skills and behavior management might be an effective service delivery strategy; the home-based worker, using a multisystemic perspective, could also mobilize and coordinate school-based resources, such as a family resource center or supportive school social work services. In addition to these clinical services, the family members will need support and advocacy in negotiating and meeting the requirements of CPS as they move toward reunification.

APPENDIX 7.1. SELECTED PROGRAM EXEMPLARS

• *Trauma Recovery and Empowerment Model (TREM; www.communityconnectionsdc.org).* TREM is a comprehensive group intervention for women who have suffered sexual, physical, or emotional abuse. Core assumptions of TREM are that (1) some current dysfunctional behavior may have originated as a coping response to trauma; (2) repeated trauma deprives women of the opportunity to develop certain coping skills; (3) trauma severs connections to family, community and self; and (4) women who have been abused feel powerless. The TREM intervention occurs in 33 sessions over a 9-month period. Themes addressed in the sessions include empowerment; trauma recovery; trauma recovery issues of blame, responsibility, and forgiveness; and closing rituals (Harris & the Community Connections Trauma Work Group, 1998; Copeland & Harris, 2000) Supplemental material is included for special populations of women, such as incarcerated women, parenting women, adolescent girls, and women who abuse.

• *Seeking Safety (www.seekingsafety.org).* Seeking Safety is a primarily cognitive-behavior intervention providing integrated treatment for women with PTSD and substance dependence. The program's 25 topic areas deal with cognitive, behavioral, and interpersonal domains, and each topic emphasizes a coping skill to promote safety. The model can be adapted for group or individual use, and includes a case management component. The treatment has been found to improve PTSD symptoms, problem solving, and depression, and to decrease substance abuse and suicidality. A therapist's manual containing all handouts and materials is available to implement this model (Najavits, 2002).

• *Violence Intervention Program for Children and Families (VIP; www.medschool.lsuhsc.edu/vip).* VIP utilizes a multidisciplinary systemic treatment approach and operates through the Department of Psychiatry, Louisiana State University

Health Sciences Center in New Orleans (Appleyard & Osofsky, 2003). Services are tailored to each family's needs and include individual treatment for the parent and/or child (through cognitive-behavioral therapy, play therapy, narrative therapy), infant–parent therapy, parental counseling, and guidance. Parent education on the impact of violence on children and how to keep children safe is provided. Referrals to sources of support in the community are utilized as well (e.g., Big Brothers/Big Sisters, after-school programs, school-based intervention).

• *San Francisco Child Trauma Research (www.nccp.org/initiative_20.html).* Under the direction of Dr. Alice Lieberman, this program of the San Francisco General Hospital and the University of California at San Francisco's Department of Psychiatry targets preschool-age children and their mothers who have been involved with domestic violence (Lieberman, Van Horn, Grandison, & Pekarsky, 1997). The treatment model consists of weekly home-based psychotherapy sessions and places equal emphasis on the child and mother, both of whom may be experiencing traumatic reactions. The sessions focus on developing appropriate and nonpunitive parenting skills, encouraging symbolic play, putting feelings into words, and expressing negative feelings in nondestructive ways. Wraparound case management services are provided to meet basic needs. The intervention can last for up to 1 year, although there is a less intense 16-week model. Several outcome studies of the intervention are currently underway. The program also engages in training, consultation, and advocacy.

• *Child Witness to Violence Project (CWVP; www.bmc.org/pediatrics/special/cwtv/overview.html).* The CWVP of the Department of Developmental and Behavioral Pediatrics, Boston Medical Center, is a counseling, advocacy, and outreach project focusing on children exposed to community and domestic violence. In addition to counseling services provided to children and families, the project offers national and state training on issues of violence for social service professionals. Project goals are to identify children who have witnessed violence, to provide developmentally appropriate counseling to help children and families heal, and to train caregivers of young children to identify and help children exposed to violence. The project website contains useful information about common symptoms of exposure to violence, and lists helping resources for parents and caregivers.

APPENDIX 7.2. PERTINENT CURRICULA, TRAINING PROGRAMS, AND RESOURCES

Websites

• *National Consumer Supporter Technical Assistance Center (www.ncstac.org).* The Women and Trauma Project provides resources, educational materials, and links to a network of organizations to help empower women who have survived trauma.

• *Invisible Children's Project, the National Mental Health Association (www.nmha.org).* This project seeks to address the unmet needs of the children of parents who have mental illness or co-occurring disorders. These children are often "invisible" to many mental health service providers, who tend to view adults in service systems in isolation from their children.

- *Substance Abuse and Mental Health Services Administration (SAMSHA; www.samhsa.gov).* See especially the following Programs in Brief: Women, Co-Occurring Disorders and Violence; Homeless Families: Women with Mental and/or Addictive Disorders and Their Children; Residential Women and Children/Pregnant and Postpartum Women; and Children of Substance-Abusing Parents. A Web-based course for professionals is available–Silence Hurts: Alcohol Abuse and Violence Against Women (http://pathwayscourses.samsha.gov/vawp/vawp_intro_pg1.htm).
- *Center for Substance Abuse Treatment (www.health.org).* The following publications, among others, can be obtained from this clearinghouse:

Substance abuse treatment and domestic violence (DHHS Publication No. SMA 97-3163).

Substance abuse treatment for persons with child abuse and neglect issues (Treatment Improvement Protocol [TIP] Series 36, DHHS Publication No. SMA 00-3357).

- *Minnesota Center against Violence and Abuse (www.mincava.umn.edu).* This is a searchable website with access to research, training, and multimedia resources. A training curriculum (Collaborating for Women and Child Safety) for multidisciplinary teams to enhance practice when domestic violence and child maltreatment occur can be accessed through the Minnesota Rural Project for Women and Child Safety (www.mincava.umn.edu/rural/).

Videos

- *Women Speak Out.* A 40-minute video about trauma issues to use as a staff training tool. Available from Community Connections (www.communityconnectionsdc.org).
- Trauma and substance abuse I: Therapeutic approaches (46-minute video); Trauma and substance abuse II: Special treatment issues (40-minute video). The second of these describes special issues of trauma and substance abuse; the first describes new integrated treatment models. Available from Cavalcade Productions (www.cavalcadeproductions.com).

Clinical Resources

Christophersen, E. R., & Mortweet, S. L. (2001). *Treatments that work with children: Empirically supported strategies for managing childhood problems.* Washington, DC: American Psychological Association.

Evans, P. (1996). *The verbally abusive relationship: How to recognize it and how to respond* (2nd ed). Center City, MN: Hazelden Foundation.

Harris, M., & the Community Connections Trauma Work Group. (1998). *Trauma recovery and empowerment: A clinician's guide for working with women in groups*. New York: Free Press.

Harris, M., & the Parenting Workgroup. (2001). *Non-traditional parenting interventions: The impact of early trauma on parenting roles.* Washington, DC: Community Connections. (Available from Community Connections at www.communityconnections-dc.org)

Najavits, L. M. (2002). *Seeking safety: A treatment manual for PTSD and substance abuse.* New York: Guilford Press.

REFERENCES

Alexander, M. J. (1996). Women with co-occurring addictive and mental disorders: An emerging profile of vulnerability. *American Journal of Orthopsychiatry, 66*, 61–69.

American Medical Association (2001, October). *October is domestic violence awareness month.* Retrieved from www.ama-assn.org/ama/pub/category/6451.html

American Psychiatric Association. (2000). *Diagnostic and statistical manual of mental disorders* (4th ed., text rev.). Washington, DC: Author.

Anderson, C. M., Teicher, M. H., Polcari, A., & Renshaw, P. F. (2002). Abnormal T2 relaxation time in the cerebellar vermis of adults sexually abused in childhood: Potential role of the vermis in stress-enhanced risk for drug abuse. *Psychoneuroendocrinology, 27*(1–2), 231–244.

Appleyard, K., & Osofsky, J. D. (2003). Parenting after trauma: Supporting parents and caregivers in the treatment of children impacted by violence. *Infant Mental Health Journal, 24*(2), 111–125.

Brown, P. J. (2000). Outcome in female patients with both substance use and posttraumatic stress disorders. *Alcoholism Treatment Quarterly, 18*(3), 127–135.

Buchanan, A. (1998). Intergenerational child maltreatment. In Y. Danieli (Ed.), *Intergenerational handbook of multigenerational legacies of trauma* (pp. 535–552). New York: Plenum Press.

Cash, S. J., & Wilke, D. J. (2003). An ecological model of maternal substance abuse and child neglect: Issues, analyses, and recommendations. *American Journal of Orthopsychiatry, 73*(4), 392–404.

Centers for Disease Control and Prevention (CDC). (2000). *Male batterers: Fact sheet.* Retrieved from www.cdc.gov/ncipc/factsheets/malebat.htm

Centers for Disease Control and Prevention (CDC). (2004a). *Intimate partner violence: Fact sheet.* Retrieved from www.cdc.gov/ncipc/factsheets/ipvfacts.htm

Centers for Disease Control and Prevention (CDC). (2004b). *Child maltreatment: Fact sheet.* Retrieved from www.cdc.gov/ncipc/factsheets/cmfacts.htm

Cerezo, M. A. (1997). Abusive family interaction: A review. *Aggression and Violent Behavior, 2*(3), 215–240.

Child Welfare League of America (CWLA). (2003). *National fact sheet 2003: Making children a national priority.* Retrieved from www.cwla. org/advocacy/nationalfactsheet03.htm

Child Witness to Violence Project. (2004). *Symptoms of witnessing violence.* Retrieved from www. bmc.org/pediatrics/special/CWTV/recognize/recognize_symptons.html

Cohen, J. S., Mannarino, A. P., Zhitova, A. C., & Capone, M. E. (2003). Treating child abuse-related posttraumatic stress and comorbid substance abuse in adolescents. *Child Abuse & Neglect, 27,* 1345–1365.

Copeland, M. E., & Harris, M. (2000). *Healing the trauma of abuse: A women's handbook.* Oakland, CA: New Harbinger.

Corvo, K., & Carpenter, E. H. (2000). Effects of parental substance abuse on current levels of domestic violence: A possible elaboration of intergenerational transmission processes. *Journal of Family Violence, 15*(2), 123–135.

Courtois, C. A. (1999). *Recollections of sexual abuse: Treatment principles and guidelines.* New York: Norton.

Davis, J. L., & Petretic-Jackson, P. A. (2000). The impact of child sexual abuse on adult interpersonal functioning: A review and synthesis of the empirical literature. *Aggression and Violent Behavior, 5*(3), 291–328.

De Bellis, M. D. (2002). Developmental traumatology: A contributory mechanism for alcohol and substance use disorders. *Psychoneuroendocrinology, 27,* 155–170.

Dodge, K. A., Bates, J. E., & Pettit, G. S. (1990). Mechanisms in the cycle of violence. *Science, 250,* 1678–1683.

Dutton, D. G. (1999). Traumatic origins of intimate rage. *Aggression and Violent Behavior, 4*(4), 431–447.

Dutton, D. G. (2002). The neurobiology of abandonment homicide. *Aggression and Violent Behavior, 7,* 407–421.

Foa, E. B., Dancu, C. V., & Hembree, E. A. (1999). A comparison of exposure therapy, stress inoculation training and their combination for reducing posttraumatic stress disorder in female assault victims. *Journal of Consulting and Clinical Psychology, 67*(2), 194–200.

Foa, E. B., Keane, T. M., & Friedman, M. J. (Eds.). (2000). *Effective treatments for PTSD: Practice guidelines from the International Society for Traumatic Stress Studies.* New York: Guilford Press.

Goodman, L. A., Dutton, M. A., & Harris, M. (1997). The relationship between violence dimensions and symptom severity among homeless, mentally ill women. *Journal of Traumatic Stress, 10*(1), 51–70.

Gunnar, M. R., & Donzella, B. (2002). Social regulation of the cortisol levels in early human development. *Psychoneuroendocrinology, 27*(1–2), 199–220.

Harris, M. (1996). Treating sexual abuse trauma with dually diagnosed women. *Community Mental Health Journal, 32*(4), 371–385.

Harris, M., & the Community Connections Trauma Work Group. (1998). *Trauma recovery and empowerment: A clinician's guide for working with women in groups.* New York: Free Press.

Harris, M., & the Parenting Workgroup. (2001). *Non-traditional parenting interventions: The impact of early trauma on parenting roles.* Washington, DC: Community Connections at www.communityconnectionsdc.org.

Institute for the Advancement of Social Work Research. (2003, October). *Social work contributions to public health: Bridging research and practice. Lessons from child maltreatment and domestic violence.* Washington, DC: Author.

Jones, L. P., Gross, E., & Becker, I. (2002). The characteristics of domestic violence victims in a child protective service caseload. *Families in Society: The Journal of Contemporary Human Services, 83*(4), 405–415.

Karr-Morse, R., & Wiley, M. S. (1997). *Ghosts from the nursery: Tracing the roots of violence*. New York: Atlantic Monthly Press.

Kelley, S. J. (2003). Cumulative environmental risk in substance abusing women: Early intervention, parenting stress, child abuse potential and child development. *Child Abuse and Neglect, 27*, 993–995.

King, M. E., & Bordnick, P. S. (2002). Alcohol use disorders: A social worker's guide to clinical assessment. *Journal of Social Work Practice in the Addictions, 2*(1), 3–31.

Lewis, D. O. (1992). From abuse to violence: Psychophysiological consequences of maltreatment. *Journal of the American Academy of Child and Adolescent Psychiatry, 31*(3), 383–391.

Lieberman, A. F., Van Horn, P., Grandison, C. M., & Pekarsky, J. H. (1997). Mental health assessment of infants, toddlers, and preschoolers in a service program and a treatment outcome research program. *Infant Mental Health Journal, 18*(2), 158–170.

Lisak, D., & Miller, P. M. (2003). Childhood trauma, posttraumatic stress disorder, substance abuse and violence. In P. Ouimette & P. J. Brown (Eds.), *Trauma and substance abuse: Causes, consequences and treatment of comorbid disorders* (pp. 73–88). Washington, DC: American Psychological Association.

Najavits, L. M. (2002). *Seeking safety: A treatment manual for PTSD and substance abuse*. New York: Guilford Press.

Najavits, L. M., Weiss, R. D., & Shaw, S. R. (1997). The link between substance abuse and posttraumatic stress disorder in women: A research review. *American Journal on Addictions, 6*, 273–283.

Najavits, L. M., Weiss, R. D., Shaw, S. R., & Muenz, L. R. (1998). "Seeking safety": Outcome of a new cognitive behavioral psychotherapy for women with PTSD and substance dependence. *Journal of Traumatic Stress, 11*, 437–456.

National Clearinghouse on Child Abuse and Neglect Information. (2002). *In harm's way: Domestic violence and child maltreatment*. Retrieved from www.calib.com/nccanch/pubs/otherpubs/harmsway.cfm

Ouimette, P., & Brown, P. J. (Eds.). (2003). *Trauma and substance abuse: Causes, consequences, and treatment of comorbid disorders*. Washington, DC: American Psychological Association.

Pears, K. C., & Capaldi, D. M. (2001). Intergenerational transmission of abuse: A two-generational prospective study of an at-risk sample. *Child Abuse and Neglect, 25*, 1439–1461.

Perry, B. D. (1997). Incubated in terror: Neurodevelopmental factors in the "cycle of violence." In J. D. Osofsky (Ed.), *Children in a violent society* (pp. 124–149). New York: Guilford Press.

Sappington, A. A. (2000). Childhood abuse as a possible locus for early intervention into problems of violence and psychopathology. *Aggression and Violent Behavior, 5*(3), 255–266.

Schuengel, C., Bakermans-Kranenburg, M. J., & van IJzendoorn, M. H. (1999). Frightening maternal behavior linking unresolved loss and disorganized infant attachment. *Journal of Consulting and Clinical Psychology, 67*(1), 54–63.

Siegel, D. J. (1999). *The developing mind: Toward a neurobiology of interpersonal experience*. New York: Guilford Press.

Sedlak, A. J., & Broadhurst, D. D. (1996). *Executive summary of the third national incidence study of child abuse and neglect*. Retrieved from www.calib.com/nccanch/pubs/statinfo/nis3.cfm

Simons, R. L., & Johnson, C. (1998). An examination of competing explanations for the intergenerational transmission of domestic violence. In Y. Danieli (Ed.), *International handbook of multigenerational legacies of trauma* (pp. 553–570). New York: Plenum Press.

Substance Abuse and Mental Health Services Administration (SAMHSA). (2000). *Substance abuse treatment for persons with child abuse and neglect issues* (Treatment Improvement Protocol [TIP] Series 36, DHHS Publication No. SMA 00-3357). Washington, DC: U.S. Department of Health and Human Services.

Teicher, M. H. (2002). Scars that won't heal: The neurobiology of child abuse. *Scientific American, 286*(3), 68–75.

Tracy, E. M. (1994). Maternal substance abuse: Protecting the child, preserving the family. *Social Work, 39*(5), 534–540.

van der Kolk, B. A. (2001). The psychobiology and psychopharmacology of PTSD. *Human Psychopharmacology: Clinical Experience, 16*, S49–S64.

van der Kolk, B. A., & McFarlane, A. C. (1996). The black hole of trauma. In B. A. van der Kolk, A. C. McFarlane, & L. Weisaeth (Eds.), *Traumatic stress: The effects of overwhelming experience on mind, body, and society* (pp. 3–23). New York: Guilford Press.

Vasquez, D. M. (1998). Stress and the developing limbic-hypothalamic-pituitary-adrenal axis. *Psychoneuroendocrinology, 23*(7), 663–700.

Warnken, W. J., Rosenbaum, A., Fletcher, K. E., Hoge, S. K., & Adelman, S. A. (1994). Head-injured males: A population at risk for relationship aggression? *Violence and Victims, 9*(2), 153–166.

Weinstein, J., & Weinstein, R. (2000). Before it's too late: Neuropsychological consequences of child neglect and their implications for law and social policy. *University of Michigan Journal of Law Reform, 33*(4), 561–613.

CHAPTER 8

Ethnically Sensitive Practice with Children and Families

CARMEN ORTIZ HENDRICKS
ROWENA FONG

Child abuse and neglect are never easy topics to discuss or deal with, and when cultural diversity exists between foster parents and children or between workers and families, the complexity intensifies. Cultural competence is necessary for providing services to diverse clients, especially children and families traumatized by poverty, discrimination, exploitation, family or community violence, incarceration, and substance abuse (Fong, McRoy, & Ortiz Hendricks, 2005). Child welfare workers may recognize trauma in the lives of the diverse children and families brought to their attention, but they need help to incorporate this knowledge into their practice and interventions. Biological families, child welfare workers, and foster parents need to work with each other in culturally sensitive and competent ways in the best interests of children, who deserve protection, a resolution of their foster care placements, and permanency planning.

Everyone has a culture, but special attention needs to be directed toward particular cultural groups in U.S. society that are likely to need a range of human services because of differences in the following factors:

- Understanding of health, mental health, illness, and disability.
- Family customs, social patterns, child-rearing practices, and religious values.
- Language skills and literacy (language assistance for people with limited English proficiency is required by federal law).
- Experiences of colonialism or exploitation due to ethnic, racial, social, or class-related discrimination.

Included among these populations are four major racial/ethnic "minority" groups in the United States: African Americans; Hispanic or

Latino/Latina Americans; Asian Americans and Pacific Islanders; and Native Americans/First Nations Peoples. The term "minority" has historically referred to people who have been subjected to differential treatment and oppression in the United States. However, when "minority" may soon become inaccurate or obsolete in a numerical sense, "the former minorities gradually increase to become the majority" (Webb, 2001, p. 5). Some persons in these groups have been U.S. residents for hundreds of years, whereas others are recent immigrants or refugees; still, members of both groups are faced with prejudice, racism, and discrimination on a daily basis. The unique needs of these groups require skilled and knowledgeable responses that are culturally competent, and so this chapter begins by defining the concept of "cultural competence."

The chapter then examines the disparities and disproportionate representation of certain racial/ethnic populations within the child welfare system, the institutional arrangements that contribute to this overrepresentation, and the kinds of responses needed to reduce it. The chapter also explores ways to enhance culturally competent child welfare practice with traumatized children and families by making the following more readily available:

- *Culturally competent personnel*–service providers, paraprofessionals, and administrators with appropriate skills, knowledge, and attitudes.
- *Culturally competent services*–interventions and treatments proven effective with individuals from the diverse communities likely to be served.
- *Culturally competent organizations*–policies, administrative procedures, and management practices designed to ensure access to culturally appropriate services and competent personnel.

CULTURAL COMPETENCE

Cultural competence requires hard work, commitment, and experience. It entails more than speaking a client's language or gaining specialized knowledge about a particular cultural group. "Cultural competence" means understanding the value of culture as perceived by clients, and appreciating how culture guides behavior and gives meaning to life (Fong, 2004; Lum, 1999; Webb, 2001). It also involves, when appropriate, taking indigenous interventions and giving them high priority within the treatment plan, because they reflect cultural values that are strengths and should be used as resources (Fong, Boyd, & Browne, 1999).

Culture both determines and influences individual health and mental health beliefs, family practices, human behavior, and even the outcomes of interventions. Culture "affects everything we think and do from how we treat our aging relatives, to when and how we recognize a child's transition into adulthood, to what we do when we feel sick" (Center for Cross-Cultural Health, 1997, p. x). "Cultural competence . . . implies a heightened consciousness of how clients experience their uniqueness and deal with their differences and similarities within a larger social context" (National Association of Social Workers [NASW], 2001, p. 8).

The NASW, in its *Standards for Cultural Competence in Social Work Practice*, defines cultural competence as "the process by which individuals and systems respond respectfully and effectively to people of all cultures, languages, classes, races, ethnic backgrounds, religions, and other diversity factors in a manner that recognizes, affirms, and values the worth of individuals, families, and communities and protects and preserves the dignity of each" (NASW, 2001, p. 11). Fundamentally, cultural competence is the ability and the will to respond sensitively to the needs of clients, based on an understanding of both their culture and the worker's own culture; it also includes respect for clients' abilities to use their culture as a resource, strength, or tool to meet common human needs. Culturally competent child welfare practice "involves a range of professional knowledge, skills and values that addresses the complex cultures emerging in a society from the interplay of power and privilege associated with race and ethnicity, gender and sexual orientation, religion and spirituality, social class and status, age and abilities" (Ortiz Hendricks, 2004a). The emphasis in this definition is on the fact that some groups are granted power and privilege while others are oppressed, in large part because of characteristics they cannot control.

Social agencies have tended to put the burden of responsibility on workers to become culturally competent. According to Lum (1999), "the worker achieves cultural competence after developing cultural awareness, mastering knowledge and skills, and implementing an inductive learning methodology" (p. 175). But cultural competence is both a personal and an organizational quest. It requires more than individual awareness and sensitivity, the hallmarks of culturally competent practice. Agencies have spent thousands of dollars yearly training workers to become more culturally aware and sensitive; providing them with knowledge of different client groups; educating them about the impact of cultural differences on help-seeking behaviors; and encouraging them to adapt intervention strategies for different populations and needs. However, attention to workers' individual growth in knowledge and skills is insufficient without simultaneously paying attention to the agency context within which the workers serve clients (Fong & Gibbs, 1995; Ortiz Hendricks & Fong, 2005; Nybell & Gray, 2004).

According to the Minnesota Department of Human Services (2004, executive summary) it is not a choice but a necessity for child welfare organizations to become more culturally competent, for these reasons:

- The demographics of the U.S. and individual states are rapidly becoming more diverse.
- Disparities in health and service outcomes exist between mainstream and diverse populations.
- Access barriers mean clients' needs are not identified and effective service is not provided.
- Culture influences assessment accuracy and service effectiveness so quality may suffer.
- Law and accreditation standards increasingly demand cultural competence.
- Liability exposure increases and costs rise when services are not effective.
- Competition in funding and business markets favor the culturally competent organization."

OVERREPRESENTATION OF CHILDREN AND FAMILIES OF COLOR IN THE CHILD WELFARE SYSTEM

The most challenging and controversial issue facing the child welfare system today is the disproportionate representation of racial/ethnic minority children and families in the system, particularly Hispanic Americans and African Americans (Freeman, 2005; McRoy & Vick, 2005; Suleiman, 2003). "Over-representation of adolescents of color in the juvenile justice system result from decisions made very early on regarding the need to remove children from their homes; decisions that are based in some large part on the family's color or race" (Walker, 2000, p. 6). A few examples should help demonstrate this point.

> Mr. and Mrs. G speak English only minimally. They are from Honduras, and when the child welfare investigator came to their home there was no Spanish interpreter. The G children were removed from the home at 3:00 one morning based on a neighbor's allegation of child abuse and child endangerment. The parents were not informed where the children were being taken; nor were they ever asked whether the family had relatives who could care for the children. The investigator also did not take the son's asthma medication. In a panic, the parents tried to find out where the children were in order to deliver the medication. Ultimately, the family physician delivered a new prescription to the police. In order to attend the court hearing, Mr. G had to pay a coworker 2 days' wages to cover for him for 1 day at the restaurant where he worked. At the courthouse, the appointed attorney was not present, so Mr. G simply lost 2 days' wages. In the end, the children spent 10 days in foster care whereupon the neighbor recanted the allegation. The family was left confused and wondering why the children were removed so abruptly and traumatically, and why they were returned to the family so quickly.

The Coalition for Asian American Children and Families (CAACF, 2001, p. 12) described the case of Mr. S, an immigrant from Bangladesh, who was worried because his 13-year-old daughter was failing in school. He found her diary; though he could not read her English well, he could understand that some entries were about boys and maybe about sex too. Mr. S, in fury, told his daughter that he was going to have a talk with her teacher. The daughter panicked and told a friend, who suggested she should claim that her father was abusing her. The friend told a teacher, and all three of the S children were immediately taken from the family home and placed in a non-Muslim, non-Bangladeshi foster home. The youngest child, a 3-year-old girl who could not speak English, refused to wash or eat in the foster home. The father was advised by his court-appointed lawyer to plead guilty in order to end the case quickly, although the father did not understand the admission of guilt or its ramifications.

Mrs. R, a recent immigrant from Haiti, arrived at a hospital at 11:45 A.M. with her 6-year-old son (who was running a fever) and her 4-year-old daughter in tow. She spent the next 12 hours waiting for someone to treat her son, or at least to talk to her. When midnight arrived and the nurses had done little more than take her son's temperature, she decided to leave and go home. As she walked out, however, she was apprehended by security guards and escorted back into the emergency room. The nurse explained to Mrs. R that the hospital suspected child abuse and was taking her son away. This worried mother was trying to do the best for her child, and someone who did not know her and would not even talk to her was accusing her of abusing her child.

These three examples all demonstrate the immediate trauma to these families caused by the loss of control and the blatant disempowerment. They also highlight the unwarranted lingering problems because of the traumatization suffered by the parents and children together and separately. "Trauma" is defined in the *Diagnostic and Statistical Manual of Mental Disorders*, fourth edition, text revision (DSM-IV-TR; American Psychiatric Association, 2000) as experiencing or witnessing an event that involves threatened or actual death, serious injury, or danger to the physical integrity of oneself or others, especially loved ones or close associates. In addition, the individual's response to the traumatic event involves intense helplessness, fear, or horror. In children, this may be expressed instead by disorganized or agitated behavior. Family members in each of the case examples described above could be said to meet at least partial criteria for the DSM-IV-TR diagnostic category of posttraumatic stress disorder (assuming that the children and even the parents believed that the physical integrity of loved ones was at risk), although more details about each case would need to be known for a formal diagnosis to be made. Much miscommunication and misinformation transpire in cases such as these, causing unnecessary additional burdens to overly stressed immigrants or refugees and to non-English-speaking families. Many of these families are traumatized by the communities they live in and the situations they find themselves in; they may also suffer from other stressors, such as mental or physical problems, substance abuse, or family violence. Even the act of immigrating from one country to another can be considered a highly traumatic event. These families are then further traumatized by the child welfare system, which can suddenly remove children from their homes, fail to inform parents or children about where the children are going, and proceed to put the children and families through multiple placements and court procedures.

These examples also demonstrate the range of ethnic diversity that child welfare workers are faced with today all over the United States, and they exemplify the dilemmas that confront families and workers alike. Although the United States is now a multilingual nation, the political context of the English language makes access to social services difficult for language-minority client populations. In addition to language barriers, the stress of immigration, sociocultural dislocation, and discriminatory U.S. policies toward immigrants contribute to the likelihood that immigrant families are more vulnerable and therefore more likely to enter the child welfare system. Child abuse and neglect may be the result of failed systems of care that further traumatize parents and children of color, who are at greatest risk (Smith & Fong, 2004). When parents cannot find adequate help for their own or their children's problems, they often do not know where they can turn to for help or lack understanding of the kind of help they may receive.

HISPANIC OR LATINO[1] DEMOGRAPHICS AND CHILD WELFARE STATISTICS

The 2000 U.S. census clearly demonstrated how diverse the country is and how immigration patterns continue to change the demographic landscape

[1]The question of how to name this multiethnic population is often debated. The label "Hispanic" was coined in the mid-1970s by federal bureaucrats in response to a concern that the government was misidentifying segments of the population by classifying those with ancestral ties to the Spanish culture as either Chicano/Chicana, Cuban, or Puerto Rican (Schmidt, 2003). "Hispanic" is used by those interested in advancing social and cultural goals, and this term generally refers to persons of Spanish origin who are Spanish speaking and often have Spanish surnames. "Latino/Latina" is a term used by those primarily concerned with equality and activism. It generally refers to persons who are of Caribbean, Central American, or South American ancestry, and includes indigenous peoples who lived in these countries before the European and African peoples settled there. Many people use the terms interchangeably. Most Hispanics prefer to be identified by terms indicating their national origin, but these may have several variations. For example, a man from Mexico may call himself, Mexican, Mexican American, or Chicano (an indigenous and activist name), or a Puerto Rican woman may refer to herself as Borinqueña, after the island's original name, Boriqua.

of the population. In 2000, the Hispanic population comprised 12.5% of the U.S. population, or 35,305,818 million people (U.S. Bureau of the Census, 2000–2001). This represented an increase of 57.9% from 1990, or from 22.4 million to 35.3 million in 10 years. This made the U.S. the second largest Hispanic country in the world, and this population is expected to increase to 97 million by 2050 (Logan, 2001). Hispanics live in every state of the union, but are concentrated in nine states: California, Texas, and New York have the largest populations, followed by Florida, Illinois, New Jersey, New Mexico, Arizona, and Colorado. Two-thirds of Hispanics of Mexican origin reside in either California or Texas; Puerto Ricans are concentrated in the northeastern states of New York, New Jersey, and Pennsylvania; and two-thirds of Cuban Americans live in Florida. In the past decade, there has also been more than a 100% increase in the Hispanic populations of Washington, Oregon, Idaho, West Virginia, Virginia, Pennsylvania, South Carolina, and most of New England.

Child welfare workers need to keep in mind other distinguishing characteristics of the Hispanic population as reported by the U.S. Bureau of the Census (2000, 2000–2001, 2001):

- The extraordinary growth of the Hispanic/Latino population can be primarily attributed to immigration rather than to increasing birthrates.
- Hispanics are an urban population to a greater extent than most other Americans; they tend to concentrate in large metropolitan centers such as Los Angeles, New York City, and Chicago.
- Hispanics are considered a young population, with a median age of 25.8 years. Thirty-six percent of Hispanics are under 18 years old, in comparison to 24% for non-Hispanic whites.
- Fifty-seven percent of Hispanics have graduated from high school, compared to 88% of non-Hispanic whites.
- Hispanic family households are larger than their non-Hispanic white counterparts, with 31% of Hispanic families consisting of five or more persons, compared to 12% of non-Hispanic white households.
- Hispanics are a population particularly at risk for poverty; they are three times more likely (22.8%) than non-Hispanic whites (7.7%) to be poor.
- Hispanics are more likely than non-Hispanic whites to work in service occupations, almost twice as likely to be employed as operators and laborers (22% vs. 12%), and less likely than non-Hispanic whites to have earnings of $35,000 or more (23% vs. 49%).

Many of these factors significantly increase the likelihood for Hispanics to be a population at risk. Consider the fact that the Latino/Latina child foster care population almost doubled from 8% in 1990 to 15% in

September 2002 (Suleiman, 2003), and that even the latter figure is considered an underestimate of the number of Hispanic children in the child welfare system. Suleiman's report for the Committee for Hispanic Children and Families notes that Latino/Latina children constituted at least 20% of the foster care population in Colorado and Massachusetts; more than 30% in Arizona, California, Connecticut, and Texas; and over 50% of the foster care population in New Mexico.

There is a tremendous dearth of research, policy, and programs concerning the fact that Hispanics are overrepresented in criminal justice, juvenile delinquency services, and public welfare programs, but they are underutilizing health and mental health care services (Ortiz Hendricks, 2004b). Poverty may be the principal underlying reason for the disproportionate number of maltreatment reports among Hispanics, and it can be attributed to a number of factors that child welfare workers should keep in mind: brevity of stay in the United States, size of the family, undocumented status, minimum-wage jobs, financial support of family members in countries of origin, youth of the population, single-parent households, lack of marketable skills, residence in inner-city neighborhoods, substandard housing, inadequate schools, and limited English-speaking proficiency. Racism and discrimination further oppress Hispanics in the U.S., and put all Hispanic groups at risk.

AFRICAN AMERICAN DEMOGRAPHICS AND CHILD WELFARE STATISTICS

The percentage of African American children who enter the system and remain in out-of-home care is greater than their proportion of the country's population (Anderson, 1997). African Americans account for 15% of all children under 18 in the United States, but they account for 25% of substantiated maltreatment reports and 38% of the children in foster care. European American children constitute 66% of the child population, but only 36% of all substantiated maltreatment reports (McRoy & Vick, 2005). Racial disparities are even more pronounced in out-of-home care. African American children account for 45% of the total number of children in foster care (U.S. Department of Health and Human Services [DHHS], 2001). African American and Native American children are five times more likely to be in out-of-home placement than their European American counterparts; they are more likely to experience multiple placements; and they stay in placement longer and are less likely to be reunified with their parents (U.S. DHHS, 2001). Several studies have confirmed that African American children tend to have longer lengths of stay in foster care than European American and Hispanic children (Wulczyn, Onerleke, & Haigth, 2002; Schmidt-Tieszen & McDonald, 1998). In addition, African American children are more likely to be placed with kin, which makes reunification less likely; thus African American children may remain in the child welfare system longer than children of other races (Ards, Chung, & Myers, 1999; Terling, 1998). Both African American and Hispanic children are less likely than European American children to be adopted, and African American children from urban areas have the lowest rates of adoption (Wulczyn et al., 2002).

ASIAN AMERICAN MYTHS AND UNDERREPRESENTATION

Less information is available about Asian and Pacific Islander children, who comprise 4% of the U.S. population and are frequently described as underrepresented among child maltreatment cases, with only 1% of the substantiated child maltreatment reports. Asian American children may indeed be underrepresented in the child welfare system. Ferrari (2002) states, "Cross cultural literature suggests that child maltreatment is less likely in cultures where children are valued for [their] economic utility, for perpetuating family lines and cultural heritage, and for sources of emotional pleasure and satisfaction" (p. 795). Another perspective on this, however, is that since the traditional Asian cultural value is to dote on children in their younger years so that the children will take care of the parents as they age, child maltreatment that may be occurring may not be reported because of shame and disapproval within the larger Asian community.

Although it is true that children are highly valued in most Asian groups—especially boys, because the males continue the family line—there may be still elements of neglect and emotional abuse that do not get reported because of the shame this would bring upon the nuclear and extended family members. In addition, Kuramoto and Nakashima (2000) report risk factors for alcohol and other drug use among Asians and Pacific Islanders to include shame and denial, discrimination and racism, immigration and acculturation issues, and pressures to succeed. Lie (2005) states that child welfare issues among Southeast Asian refugee and immigrant populations are not well documented. The few publications available tend to focus on child abuse and its psychoemotional effects, unaccompanied minors, school dropouts, and gangs. Segal (2000) concludes from her research on child abuse among Vietnamese refugees, "Common methods of identifying the occurrence of child abuse may not be valid in its assessment among populations that fear repercussions of admitting to the use of corporal punishment to discipline their children" (p. 159).

The myth that Asian Americans are a model minority group without problems is as problematic as the stereotypes and persistent derogatory characterizations of Asian Americans. The CAACF (2001) reported that data on Asian children in foster care are misleading at best, and it looked to different types of measurements for the prevalence of Asian Americans in the child welfare system. For example, according to the New York State Department of Social Services, 162 "Oriental" children were in foster care in 2000. The Coalition pointed out that "oriental" is an offensive term to most Asian Americans, but that the subcategories listed under this term were Vietnamese, Cambodian, and Laotian. Missing were the four largest Asian groups in New York State–Chinese, Korean, Filipino/Filipina, and South Asian Indian. Thus New York was clearly undercounting Asian American child maltreatment reports in the state. The CAACF pursued other avenues to determine the statistics on Asian American children in child welfare. They contrasted the small number of Asian children referred to the Division of Child Protection with the 581 requests for Asian-language interpreters; the latter figure indicated that 27% of all referrals to child protective services were Asian American children and families.

NATIVE AMERICANS AND COLONIALISTIC PRACTICES

American Indians, Alaska Natives, and other First Nations Peoples of North America have endured a succession of traumatic and systematic assaults by foreign governments on their Nations, communities, and families (Evans-Campbell & Walters, 2005). The American colonialization of the Native American tribes and the pressure to send their children to off-reservation boarding schools, established in the late 1800s, has had enduring traumatic consequences for many parent–child relationships among the various Native tribal groups (Brave Heart, 2001; Yellow Bird, 2005; Weaver, 2001).

The boarding schools, which were a form of forced out-of-home placement, devalued traditional Native language practices, customs, and beliefs. As a result, they created tremendous tensions between parents and children and between young adults and reservation communities. Poverty, discrimination, and racist attitudes and practices also contributed to major stressors for Native families, resulting in alcohol consumption and the use of other substances among some tribal members, young and old (Earle & Cross, 2005; Ledesma & Starr, 2000; Smith & Fong, 2004). In addition to the boarding school experiences, another negative practice disrupting Native American families was the Indian Adoption Project supported by the Child Welfare League of America from 1958 to 1968. This practice was thought to be "in the best interest" of the "forgotten child" on the reservations (Glover, 2001, p. 208).

Although these events may be perceived as historical contexts of discriminatory practices, the current status of Native peoples continues to include discriminatory stereotypes. The most blatant of these are the assumptions that alcohol consumption is a problem for all Native Americans and that all children raised on reservations are neglected. Ledesma and Starr (2000), in protest, state:

> Unfortunately the one area of American-Indian life that has received attention from the dominant society in the popular press and media is the high rate of alcohol abuse and the impact of [fetal alcohol syndrome/fetal alcohol effects]. While attention is needed to remediate substance abuse problems, substance abuse throughout the life course in Indian country must be examined in context. Not every Indian child is exposed to alcohol or drugs; not every child experiments [with] or family has been assaulted by alcohol; there are many caregivers of children who have not had or no longer have problems with substance abuse. (p. 136)

In summary, Native Americans have been falsely stereotyped; Asian Americans have been incorrectly labeled with myths; and African Americans and Latinos/Latinas have been overrepresented in the child welfare system. Clearly this system is in dire need of improvements to make it a more culturally competent service organization. To achieve such improvements, an understanding of the factors that contribute to the overrepresentation of minorities within the system is warranted.

FACTORS CONTRIBUTING TO OVERREPRESENTATION

There are several key factors in the overrepresentation of minority children, especially African Americans and Hispanics, in the child welfare system. Perhaps the primary factor, again, is the disproportionate poverty found among minority families (U.S. DHHS, 2003). There is a strong correlation between poverty and minority status in the United States, and children of color are more than twice as likely to live in poverty as non-Hispanic whites (U.S. Bureau of the Census, 2001). Almost one-third of African American (30%) and Hispanic (27%) children live in poverty, while only 10% of European American children live in poverty (U.S. Bureau of the Census, 2001). As for the relationship between income and child maltreatment, the Third National Incidence Study of Child Abuse and Neglect (NIS-3) found that abuse was 14 times more common and neglect was 44 times more common in poor families (Sedlak & Broadhurst, 1996). The NIS-3 also revealed that the incidence of child maltreatment in families with annual incomes under $15,000 was 47 per 1,000, whereas the incidence fell to 2 per 1,000 in families with annual incomes above $30,000. "The greater incidence of maltreatment among low-income families combined with the over-representation of families of color living in poverty suggests a plausible explanation for the disproportional representation of minority children in the child welfare system" (U.S. DHHS, 2003, p. 4).

Others argue that the disproportionate representation of minority children in the child welfare system is a result of differential treatment by race or racial bias in decision making by human service professionals (Morton, 1999). One study (Chasnoff, Kandress, & Barrett, 1990) found that although white and black pregnant women were equally likely to test positive for drugs, black women were 10 times more likely to be reported to child protective services after delivery. This finding has tremendous importance for African Americans and other racial/ethnic groups overrepresented in the child welfare system, given that drug abuse is currently seen as the major reason for child welfare involvement with families (U.S. General Accounting Office, 1994). It also indicates that health and human service professionals may make decisions about cases that are influenced by race.

Reported rates of substance use/abuse and treatment utilization also vary according to ethnicity. The 1999 National Household Survey on Drug Abuse (Substance Abuse and Mental Health Services Administration, 2000) indicates that Native Americans are the ethnic group reporting the highest rate of illicit substance use (10.6%), followed by African Americans (7.7%), Hispanics (6.8%), and European Americans (6.6%). The group with the lowest rate of illicit substance use is Asians. Respondents who reported multiethnic backgrounds actually reported a higher level of illicit substance use than any single ethnic group (11.2%). Studies also show that as many as two-thirds of parents whose children were placed in alternative care by the state were involved in substance abuse (Famularo, Kinscherff, & Fenton, 1992). Attending to the needs of addicted parents and providing preventive services should thus go a long way in reducing child welfare caseloads, particularly cases involving families and children of color.

A 2003 exploratory study by the U.S. DHHS's Children's Bureau that interviewed child welfare administrators, supervisors, and direct service workers listed a range of other factors in the overrepresentation of children of color in the child welfare. In addition to the factors just noted (i.e., poverty, bias on the part of professionals, and substance abuse), possible reasons for the overrepresentation include, but are not limited to, the following:

- Poor families are more likely to live in resource-poor communities and are isolated from other communities that might offer support and services.
- Impoverished families have more need to contact public service

systems such as public hospitals or welfare agencies, due to the problems they are experiencing, and frequent contact with these systems makes them more visible at times of greatest risk.
- Families of color frequently lack important information about how the child welfare system works, the financial resources to negotiate the system, and the confidence to advocate for themselves.
- Families of color generally live in vulnerable communities where they experience oppression firsthand. These communities have limited opportunities and greater vulnerability to such social ills as drugs and violence.
- Disproportionality is often a direct result of discriminatory policies and practices within the larger society against particular minority groups and leads to the overreporting of parents of color for child abuse and neglect.
- Increased media attention to extreme cases of child abuse and neglect has put supervisors and workers under increased scrutiny and pressure to substantiate more cases and bring more children into care.
- The reason why some child welfare workers bring preconceived biases against minority groups into their work is that they lack exposure to cultures other than their own, and have no context for understanding the cultural norms and practices of minority populations.
- There exist biases and differences in perception regarding what constitutes abuse and discipline across cultures.

The child welfare workers interviewed in the U.S. DHHS (2003) study also indicated confusion with carrying out federal policies regarding the Multi-Ethnic Placement Act and the Adoption and Safe Families Act (ASFA); concerns regarding transracial placements and adoptions; shortened timelines under ASFA; limited resources; and limited permanency options for children as making their jobs more complex and difficult.

REDUCING THE OVERREPRESENTATION

As we have shown, families and children of color are traumatized by multiple factors in the environment that stress and deplete their health and mental health in the United States. Social arrangements and social policies maintain violent families and violent communities in the inner cities and on the fringes of suburbs. The only way to change these social arrangements is to examine the child welfare, social welfare, health, and mental health care systems, while simultaneously working to remedy the problems that bring children into the system in the first place. The well-being of children is inevitably interwoven with the well-being of their parents (Sun, 2000). Poverty, violence, substance abuse, and mental health problems are among the factors fueling the growth of child maltreatment, and as a result, protecting children and reducing the level of trauma that they are exposed to will require more than mere child protective services or foster care placements (McRoy & Vick, 2005). Dramatic social changes and broad responses are needed in many areas, including education, public welfare, child welfare, juvenile justice, criminal justice, substance abuse, health, and mental health programs—which often interact with the very same families, but do not collaborate in their care or treatment. Creating safe environments, including adequate housing, nutrition, and health care, is a prerequisite to achieving a notable downward trend in all forms of maltreatment.

Given the diversity of child welfare populations, culturally competent services that acknowledge the cultural experiences and backgrounds of families and the circumstances surrounding their situations are essential to effective prevention of maltreatment and protection of traumatized children. Linguistic and cultural barriers often prevent certain ethnic groups from receiving adequate services, once they are identified as having serious family problems.

The U.S. DHHS (2003) report described in the preceding section makes the following recommendations to reduce overrepresentation of children of color in the child welfare system: (1) Emphasize prevention and preventive services; (2) build public and private agency partnerships; (3) find additional resources to support families to stay together; (4) recruit minority foster care and adoptive families; (5) recruit culturally diverse and competent staffers; (6) hire more workers to work with smaller caseloads; (7) build in administrative supports; (8) locate external resources to serve families; (9) enhance agency resources to serve families; (10) provide outreach to communities and establish connections; and (11) establish coalitions, councils, or other collaborative boards to examine the issue of overrepresentation and problem-solve ways to reduce it. This report and many other studies indicate that human service professionals know what is needed to reduce disparities in child welfare. What are needed is the power and resources to implement these well-established and well-thought-out recommendations.

CULTURALLY COMPETENT CHILD WELFARE ORGANIZATIONS

Child welfare staff members need to feel competent and effective in carrying out very complex roles and functions. In order to do this, they require the support and guidance of culturally competent organizations. These organizations need to enact a two-pronged strategy: (1) continued recruitment and retention of diverse workers who can understand the language and culture of diverse clients; and (2) ongoing preparation of all staff members to be culturally and linguistically effective practitioners. Cultural competence begins with administrative supports and encouragement, high-quality supervision and oversight, strong peer relationships, and manageable caseloads. It also requires well-educated, well-trained, and experienced child welfare workers, who can effectively deal with increasingly troubled and diverse families. Child welfare workers need to understand the changing demographics and the increases in undocumented immigrant families, unaccompanied refugee minors, and human trafficking victims (most of whom are women and children).

Child welfare agencies need to help workers keep abreast of new policies and procedures, as well as changing state and federal laws. Agencies need to train staff members to adopt new strategies for dealing with such client-specific issues as mental illness, addiction, AIDS, and incarceration. Workers need to be prepared to identify and intervene in these problems and make proper referrals for treatment when indicated, and they have to do this in culturally competent ways that strengthen families and children of color. Furthermore, child welfare workers need to be trained to identify the interrelationship among substance abuse, family violence, and mental health problems within child maltreatment, since they may be the only constant and stable resources in the lives of maltreating parents with substance abuse and/or mental illness. They are also in a unique position for helping traumatized parents move toward treatment, due to the legal sanctions attached to child protective investigations.

Child welfare workers need to collaborate with other service systems that have an impact on the families and children they serve. For example, they may have to work with the staff in a correctional facility to decide how to best address the family-related and treatment needs of incarcerated mothers. Child welfare workers will also need to collaborate with substance abuse treatment programs to help them address parenting skills and child maltreatment issues. Indeed, in many ways, child welfare workers, supervisors, foster parents, and other stakeholders in child well-being will have to become generalists rather than specialists to be more successful in meeting the needs of African American, Hispanic American, Asian American, and Native American clients.

Ongoing, agency-sponsored, and well-crafted training opportunities for all levels of the child welfare staff need to remain a priority for culturally competent organizations. Child welfare workers report needing more training in cultural awareness and sensitivity, especially in light of observed incidents of staff bias toward children and families of color. As stated earlier, sometimes child welfare workers make decisions based on race or the socioeconomic backgrounds of families, rather than on the specific merits of a case. Specifically, differential decision making often results in African American or impoverished families' being more likely to have children removed from the home or to have parental rights terminated. More extensive training that focuses on cultural, sociological, and psychological factors in decision making among child welfare staff is necessary to address such difficult and complex issues as racial or socioeconomic bias.

Cultural competence requires a holistic approach that combines biological, psychological, social, and spiritual elements in services. Such an approach gives clients the opportunity to address other major problems they may have, such as depression, low self-esteem, and family problems. Culturally competent practice includes, but is not limited to, knowledge of a range of cultures, histories, world views, values, and beliefs; understanding of communication patterns and appropriate interviewing techniques; strengths and differences among and within diverse racial/ethnic groups; cultural expectations and help-seeking behaviors; and the integration of traditional, indigenous practices that attend to the spiritual needs of families and children of color.

Culturally competent child welfare organizations do not just attend to the micro level or genesis of individual problems; they emphasize the importance of structural problems that require structural changes. Culturally competent organizations work at securing both the internal and external resources needed to strengthen families. Internal resources, such as kinship care and family group decision making, might include support services to diverse foster and adoptive families that will enable them to take on new challenges (e.g., caring for a traumatized child from a different culture or religion). External resources, such as One Child One Church, might include relationships with churches or other agencies that can provide such necessities as food, housing, employment opportunities, and child care options. They may also include expanded mental health and substance abuse treatment programs to meet the needs of families of color.

A recent study by the New York City Department of Health and Mental Hygiene (Engstrom et al., 2003) uncovered the startling fact that 57% of referrals for outpatient mental health clinic services for children in the Bronx do not lead to treatment. The study findings highlighted the severity and complexity of the mental health problems presented by children compared to the extended average wait for services, as well as the high attrition rate for children prior to receiving any treatment or services. This study depicts "a system that is not meeting the needs of children who are presenting for outpatient mental health clinic services in the Bronx" (Engstrom et al., 2003, p. 2). The clinic capacity, was at maximum suggesting the need for expanded mental health services in the Bronx, and the clinical staff did not have the linguistic ability to serve Spanish-speaking parents and guardians adequately. These children and families might be referred to a child welfare agency, due to the lack of mental health services in the Bronx. Collaboration between the child welfare and mental health system could result in some creative solutions to the mental health needs of Bronx children and forestall referrals to child protective services.

Furthermore, not enough is known about successful interventions for parents with substance abuse or mental illness who abuse or neglect their children. Research is needed to enhance treatment options for recovery from substance misuse while ensuring child safety and family stability. Research is needed on practice interventions and outcomes to determine which approaches are more successful with which clients, particularly within racial/ethnic groups and with women in particular. In addition, research is needed on resiliency to determine the factors that keep families intact and healthy. And most importantly, there is a need for research on racial disproportionality that moves beyond the bare statistics. Qualitative studies in combination with exploratory quantitative studies could provide an increased understanding of the complex issue of disproportionality, along with effective strategies that a child welfare system could undertake to reduce this. Empirical studies of disproportionality need to be inclusive of the range of diversity found in child welfare caseloads. Research also needs to "unpack" large ethnic groupings and to analyze subgroup or intergroup relationships. For example, there are few studies that examine the disproportionate numbers of Central American or Southeast Asian immigrants in child maltreatment reports or their relationship to other groups.

It is not hard to imagine the possibility of depression and health problems among young parents (particularly single mothers) of color—who often are struggling financially with little education and job skills; with little social support and often enormous social isolation; and with extensive lifelong histories of trauma due to personal violence, substance abuse, and discrimination. It is ethically unacceptable to be involved in improving the efficacy of a system that takes children away from their families without simultaneously being involved in advocating to remedy the problems that bring these children, especially children of color, into the system in the first place. Everything is connected, and this is the spirit in which culturally competent child welfare workers and organizations should approach traumatized families and their children.

REFERENCES

American Psychiatric Association. (2000). *Diagnostic and statistical manual of mental disorders* (4th ed., text rev.). Washington, DC: Author.

Anderson, G. R. (1997). Introduction: Achieving permanency for all children in the child welfare system. In G. R. Anderson, A. Ryan, & B. Leashore (Eds.), *The challenge of permanency planning in a multicultural society*. New York: Haworth Press.

Ards, S., Chung, C., & Myers, S. (1998). The effects of sample selection bias on racial differences in child abuse reporting. *Child Abuse and Neglect, 22*(2), 103–115.

Brave Heart, M. (2001). Culturally and historically congruent clinical social work assessment with Native clients. In R. Fong & S. Furuto (Eds.), *Culturally competent practice: Skills, interventions, and evaluations.* Boston: Allyn & Bacon.

Center for Cross-Cultural Health. (1997). *Caring across cultures: The providers' guide to cross-cultural health care.* St. Paul, MN: Author.

Chasnoff, I. J., Kandress, H. J., & Barrett, M. E. (1990). The prevalence of illicit-drug and alcohol use during pregnancy and discrepancies in mandatory reporting in Pine County, Florida. *New England Journal of Medicine, 322*, 1202–1206.

Coalition for Asian American Children and Families (CAACF). (2001). *Crossing the divide: Asian American families and the child welfare system.* New York: Author. (Available at www.cacf.org)

Earle, K., & Cross, T. (2005). Cumulative effects of federal policy on American Indian families. In R. Fong, R. McRoy, & C. Ortiz Hendricks (Eds.), *Intersecting child welfare, substance abuse and family violence: Culturally competent approaches.* Alexandria, VA: Council on Social Work Education.

Engstrom, M., et al. (2003, August). *Children's mental health needs assessment in the Bronx.* New York: New York City Department of Health and Mental Hygiene, Division of Mental Hygiene, Bureau of Planning Evaluation and Quality Improvement.

Evans-Campbell, T., & Walters, K. (2005). Catching our breath: A decolonialization framework for healing indigenous families. In R. Fong, R. McRoy, & C. Ortiz Hendricks (Eds.), *Intersecting child welfare, substance abuse and family violence: Culturally competent approaches.* Washington, DC: Council on Social Work Education.

Famularo, R., Kinscherff, R., & Fenton, T. (1992). Parental substance abuse and the nature of child maltreatment. *Child Abuse and Neglect, 16*(4), 476–484.

Ferrari, A. (2002). The impact of culture upon childrearing practices and definitions of maltreatment. *Child Abuse and Neglect, 26*, 793–813.

Fong, L. G. W., & Gibbs, J. T. (1995). Facilitating service to multicultural communities in a dominant culture setting: An organizational perspective. *Administration in Social Work, 19*(2), 1–24.

Fong, R. (Ed.). (2004). *Culturally competent practice with immigrant and refugee children and families.* New York: Guilford Press.

Fong, R., Boyd, C., & Browne, C. (1999). The Gandhi technique: A biculturalization approach for empowering Asian and Pacific Islander families. *Journal of Multicultural Social Work, 7*, 95–110.

Fong, R., McRoy, R., & Ortiz Hendricks, C. (Eds.). (2005). *Intersecting child welfare, substance abuse and family violence: Culturally competent approaches.* Alexandria, VA: Council on Social Work Education.

Freeman, E. (2005). A systems perspective. In R. Fong, R. McRoy, & C. Ortiz Hendricks (Eds.), *Intersecting child welfare, substance abuse and family violence: Culturally competent approaches.* Alexandria, VA: Council on Social Work Education.

Glover, G. (2001). Parenting in Native American families. In N. B. Webb (Ed.),

Culturally diverse parent–child and family relationships. New York: Columbia University Press.

Kuramoto, F., & Nakashima, J. (2000). Developing an ATOD prevention campaign for Asian and Pacific Islanders: Some considerations. *Journal of Public Health Management Practice, 6*(3), 57–64.

Ledesma, R., & Starr, P. (2000). Child welfare and the American Indian community. In N. Cohen & Contributors, *Child welfare: A multicultural focus* (2nd ed., pp. 117–142). Boston: Allyn & Bacon.

Lie, G. (2005). Family violence, child welfare, and substance abuse in Southeast Asian refugee populations. In R. Fong, R. McRoy, & C. Ortiz Hendricks (Eds.), *Intersecting child welfare, substance abuse and family violence: Culturally competent approaches.* Alexandria, VA: Council on Social Work Education.

Logan, J. R. (2001). *The new Latinos: Who they are, where they are.* Retrieved from http://mumford1.dyndns.org/cen2000/report.html

Lum, D. (1999). *Culturally competent practice: A framework for growth and action.* Pacific Grove, CA: Brooks/Cole.

McRoy, R., & Vick, J. (2005). Intersecting child welfare, substance abuse and domestic violence. In R. Fong, R. McRoy, & C. Ortiz Hendricks (Eds.), *Intersecting child welfare, substance abuse and family violence: Culturally competent approaches.* Alexandria, VA: Council on Social Work Education.

Minnesota Department of Human Services. (2004, May). *Guidelines for culturally competent organizations* (2nd ed.). St. Paul: Author.

Morton, T. D. (1999). The increasing colorization of America's child welfare system: The overrepresentation of African American children. *Policy and Practice, 57*(4), 23–30.

National Association of Social Workers (NASW). (2001). *Standards for culturally competent social work practice.* Washington, DC: Author.

Nybell, L. M., & Gray, S. S. (2004). Race, place, space: Meanings of cultural competence in three child welfare agencies. *Social Work, 49*(1), 17–26.

Ortiz Hendricks, C. (2004a, October). *The national health status of racial and ethnic minority children.* Paper presented at Closing the Disparity Gap for Racial and Ethnic Minority Children: An Investment in Our Future, First National Child Health and Child Welfare Conference, U.S. Department of Health and Human Services, Washington, DC.

Ortiz Hendricks, C. (2004b, January). *A strategic plan for the development of the Latina/o social work workforce.* Report for the Latino Social Work Task Force, National Association of Social Workers, New York City Chapter.

Ortiz Hendricks, C., & Fong, R. (2005). Cultural competency and intersectionality: Bridging practices and redirecting research. In R. Fong, R. McRoy, & C. Ortiz Hendricks (Eds.), *Intersecting child welfare, substance abuse and family violence: Culturally competent approaches.* Alexandria, VA: Council on Social Work Education.

Schmidt, P. (2003, November 28). Academe's Hispanic future: The nation's largest minority group faces big obstacles in higher education, and colleges struggle to find the right ways to help. *Chronicle of Higher Education,* p. A8.

Schmidt-Tieszen, A., & McDonald, T. P. (1998). Children who wait: Long term foster care or adoption? *Children and Youth Services Review, 20*(1–2), 13–28.

Sedlak, A. J., & Broadhurst, D. D. (1996). *Third National Incidence Study of Child*

Abuse and Neglect: Final report. Washington, DC: U.S. Department of Health and Human Services, Administration on Children, Youth and Families, National Center on Child Abuse and Neglect.

Segal, U. (2000). Exploring child abuse among Vietnamese refugees. In D. de Anda & R. Becerra (Eds.), *Violence: Diverse populations and communities.* New York: Haworth Press.

Smith, M., & Fong, R. (2004). *The children of neglect: When no one cares.* New York: Brunner-Routledge.

Substance Abuse and Mental Health Services Administration. (2000). *National household survey on drug abuse.* Washington, DC: U.S. Department of Health and Human Services.

Suleiman, L. P. (2003). *Creating a Latino child welfare agenda: A strategic framework for change.* New York: Committee for Hispanic Children and Families.

Sun, A.-P. (2000). Helping substance-abusing mothers in the child welfare system: Turning crisis into opportunity. *Families in Society, 81*(2), 142–151.

Terling, T. (1999). The efficacy of family reunification practices: Reentry rates and correlates of reentry for abused and neglected children reunited with their families. *Child Abuse and Neglect, 23*(12), 1359–1370.

U.S. Bureau of the Census. (2000). *Presence of children under 18 years old: Households by total money income in 1999.* Washington, DC: Author.

U.S. Bureau of the Census. (2000–2001). *Series of updates on Hispanic demographics.* Washington, DC: Author.

U.S. Bureau of the Census. (2001). *Poverty statistics.* Washington, DC: Author.

U.S. Department of Health and Human Services (DHHS), Children's Bureau, Administration for Children and Families. (2003, December). *Children of color in the child welfare system: Perspectives from the child welfare community.* Washington, DC: Author.

U.S. Department of Health and Human Services (DHHS), Children's Bureau, Administration for Children and Families. (2001). *Adoption and foster care analysis and reporting system.* Washington, DC: Author.

U.S. General Accounting Office. (1994). *Foster care: Parental drug abuse has alarming impact on young children* (HEHS-94–89). Washington, DC: Author.

Walker, J. S. (2000). *Caregivers speak about the cultural appropriateness of services for children with emotional and behavioral disabilities.* Portland, OR: Research and Training Center on Family Support and Children's Mental Health, Portland State University.

Weaver, H. (2001). Native Americans and substance abuse. In S. L. A. Straussner (Ed.). *Ethnocultural factors in substance abuse treatment.* New York: Guilford Press.

Webb, N. B. (Ed.). (2001). *Culturally diverse parent–child and family relationships.* New York: Columbia University Press.

Wulczyn, F., Oberleke, B., & Haigth, J. (2002). *Placement outcome, 1990–1999: A report from the Multistate Foster Care Data Archive.* Unpublished report, Chaplin Hall Center for Children, Chicago.

Yellow Bird, M. (2005). The continuing effects of American colonialism. In R. Fong, R. McRoy, & C. Ortiz Hendricks (Eds.), *Intersecting child welfare, substance abuse and family violence: Culturally competent approaches.* Alexandria, VA: Council on Social Work Education.

The road to literacy is lined with limericks and Leprechaun Lattes.

jumpstart
CONNECT EARLY

JUMPSTART NEW ENGLAND
jstart.org

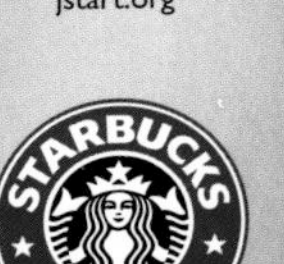

CHAPTER 9

Children with Disabilities in Child Welfare

Empowering the Disenfranchised

PATRICK SHANNON

Individuals with disabilities experience oppression and domination in all aspects of their lives. Approximately 17% of children ages 0–17 experience some form of disability (Decouflé, Boyle, Paulozzi, & Lary, 2001). It has been estimated that 1 in 6 children ages 0–17 experience at least one developmental disability, and that approximately 3 million Americans have developmental disabilities (Newman, Christopher, & Berry, 2000). Children with disabilities are particularly vulnerable to domination by others. A disturbing manifestation of this oppression is the increased incidence of maltreatment of such children. Children with disabilities appear to be more susceptible to maltreatment than children without disabilities (Sobsey, 1994). Research estimates suggest that children with disabilities are 1.7 to 10 times more likely to be maltreated than children who do not have disabilities (Ammerman & Balderian, 1993; Crosse, Kay, & Ratnofsky, n.d.; Sobsey & Varnhagen, 1988; and Sullivan & Knutson, 2000). Sullivan and Knutson (2000) reported that children with disabilities were also more likely than children without disabilities to be maltreated more frequently and in multiple ways. In addition, these authors reported that children with disabilities are 3.8 times more likely to be victims of neglect, 3.1 times more likely to be victims of sexual abuse, 3.8 times more likely to be victims of physical abuse, and 3.9 times more likely to be victims of emotional maltreatment than children without disabilities.

Crosse et al. (n.d.) and Sullivan and Knutson (2000) explored the relationship between type of disability and risk of maltreatment, and found that children with behavioral disorders were at highest risk of maltreatment followed by children with speech/language disorders, mental retardation, and health impairments. These researchers also found that children with disabilities who were maltreated were more likely to be male than maltreated children without disabilities. The majority of perpetrators in cases of nonsexual maltreatment are family members, particularly mothers. However, sexual abuse of children with disabilities is committed more frequently by males who are not members of the children's families, such as teachers, health care providers, residential care providers, transportation providers, babysitters, and peers (Ammerman & Balderian, 1993; Sobsey, 1994).

Not surprisingly, children with disabilities are disproportionately represented in state child protection programs (Sullivan & Knutson, 2000). Child protection programs, however, often consider disabilities to be a secondary concern, and thus have yet to integrate specific services for children with disabilities into their programs (Hughes & Rycus, 1998). State child protection systems have historically lacked not only procedures for identifying and documenting the presence of disabilities among children receiving child protection services, but the expertise to serve such children effectively (Ammerman & Balderian, 1993; Bonner, Crow, & Hensley, 1997; Camblin, 1982). Before any further exploration of the intersection between disabilities and abuse and neglect, it is essential to define what is meant by "disability." This chapter focuses on developmental disabilities—that is, delays in or concerns about cognitive, emotional/behavioral, gross and fine motor, learning, physical, and speech/language development. In addition, the chapter focuses on the intersection between the developmental disability and child welfare systems, and on practices that empower children with disabilities, families, child welfare staff, and other professionals.

DEVELOPMENTAL DISABILITY

Definition of the Concept

The definition of a "developmental disability" has evolved from a classification based on a specific diagnosis such as cerebral palsy, epilepsy, or mental retardation to a broader definition based on functional impairment. The federal government's Administration on Developmental Disabilities (ADD, 2001) defines a developmental disability as a physical or mental impairment that begins before age 22 and alters or substantially inhibits a person's capacity to do at least three of the following:

1. Take care of oneself (dress, bathe, eat, and perform other daily tasks).
2. Speak and understand clearly.
3. Learn.

4. Walk/move around.
5. Make decisions.
6. Live independently.
7. Earn and manage an income.

Examples of developmental disabilities include attention-deficit/hyperactivity disorder, autism and other pervasive developmental disorders, fetal alcohol syndrome, learning disabilities, mental retardation, epilepsy, cerebral palsy, genetic disorders such as Down's syndrome or fragile X syndrome, and speech/language disorders. The vagueness of the definition has made it easier to identify individuals experiencing developmental limitations who are eligible for needed services. However, the broadness of the definition also presents problems for child protection workers, related to determining appropriate services to meet these children's unique needs. There are a myriad of programs and resources available to support children with developmental disabilities and their families through federal and state developmental disability systems. However, stronger ties are needed between the child protective system (CPS) and the developmental disability system, in order to better meet the needs of children with developmental disabilities.

The Developmental Disability System

The federal agency responsible for overseeing the federal developmental disability system is the U.S. Department of Health and Human Services, Administration on Children and Families, ADD. ADD requires each state to have three separate functional systems to provide supports and services to individuals with disabilities, their families, and organizations that provide direct services. First, each state must have a protection and advocacy (P&A) system to protect and promote the rights of individuals with disabilities. The P&A and client assistance programs constitute a nationwide network of congressionally mandated, legally based, disability rights agencies. Information about each state's P&A system can be retrieved from the website of the National Association of Protection and Advocacy Systems (NAPAS; see www.napas.org). Each state's P&A system is responsible for providing referral, information, and legal representation and advocacy to individuals with disabilities on the following disability-related issues: special education; employment; housing; assistive technology; access to mental health and/or developmental disability services; medical services; financial assistance; vocational rehabilitation; elimination of physical barriers in public places; and freedom from abuse, neglect, and unwarranted restraint and seclusion (see the NAPAS website).

Second, each state must have an agency that provides direct services and supports to individuals with disabilities. ADD's State Councils on

Developmental Disabilities program provides financial support to each state to promote activities for a developmental disabilities council in that state. Each council is mandated to develop and implement a statewide plan to increase independence, productivity, inclusion, and integration into the community of people with developmental disabilities, through systems change efforts, capacity building, and advocacy. A list of state councils may be found at www.acf.dhhs.gov/programs/add/states/ddcs.htm. Finally, the Association of University Centers on Disabilities promotes policy, practice, research, and training for and about individuals with developmental and other related disabilities through a national network of university centers on disabilities (UCD). A complete list of each state's university centers may be found at www.aucd.org.

Children and their families are entitled to a host of services through the Individuals with Disabilities Education Act (IDEA). IDEA requires states to provide comprehensive programs for infants, toddlers, and school-age children and their families. The legislation promotes family-centered service delivery for all children with disabilities. Another important piece of federal legislation affecting children with disabilities is the Rehabilitation Act of 1973 (Public Law 93-112). The act focuses on providing training and placement of people with disabilities in full-time, part-time, or supportive employment in competitive jobs. In addition, training provided under the auspices of the act emphasizes skills needed by individuals with disabilities to live independently in their communities. Section 504 of the Rehabilitation Act protects rights of people with disabilities in schools and other educational programs that are federally funded by ensuring access to educational facilities and programs, including colleges and universities (Capper, 1996).

CHILD PROTECTION AND DEVELOPMENTAL DISABILITIES

CPS workers have regular and frequent contact with a population of children at high risk for developmental disabilities. Many environmental factors commonly associated with risk of maltreatment are also risk factors for developmental disabilities, such as poor nutrition, inadequate medical care, poor prenatal care, unsanitary living environments, exposure to toxic substances such as lead, high rates of substance abuse, poor supervision of children, and lack of nurturing and stimulation (Hughes & Rycus, 1998). Children who enter the CPS often have not received adequate medical care or services that may result in early identification and intervention. Many factors associated with risk of developmental disability are preventable, or at least their developmental impact can be limited. Child welfare workers are therefore in a unique position to identify children with developmental disabilities and to provide supportive services that may mitigate the impact on the children's developmental outcomes and on the families. Understanding the potential environmental and social factors that make children with disabilities more vulnerable to abuse and neglect is an essential first step in designing intervention programs to meet their needs.

Why Are Children with Developmental Disabilities at Higher Risk of Maltreatment?

Prevention of maltreatment of children with disabilities, and effective intervention in such maltreatment, are dependent upon an adequate understanding of the reasons for these children's increased risk of maltreatment. There are many possible explanations why these children experience higher rates of maltreatment. Factors related to parents and families, children, service systems, and societal attitudes have all been suggested as reasons that place children with disabilities at higher risk of maltreatment (Ammerman & Balderian, 1993; Mitchell & Buchele-Ash, 2000). Family stress and the ability of family members to cope with stress may be associated with maltreatment of children with disabilities. Examples of stress include change in lifestyle experienced by caregivers, a child's temperament and responsiveness, the degree of specialized care required, parental disability, emotional or psychological problems of another family member, family social isolation, severity of a child's disability, and other stressors unrelated to a child's disability (Hughes & Rycus, 1998; Pearson, 1996; Sullivan & Knutson, 2000). Hughes and Rycus (1998) speculated that other family members sometimes view a child with a disability as a threat, because the needs of the child disrupt family routines and family relationships. Also, parents are frequently forced to leave their place of employment to care for their child, which can affect the family's socioeconomic status. Child factors such as impaired communication, poor self-defense abilities, and the potential for exhibiting problem behaviors have also been suggested as reasons for the higher rates of maltreatment for these children (Ammerman & Balderian, 1993; Sobsey, 1994; White, Benedict, Wulff, & Kelley, 1987).

Maltreatment itself can be the cause of disability for some children. There is evidence that children who are maltreated are at greater risk of experiencing emotional difficulties, language impairment, cognitive impairments, and/or physical disabilities (Cohen & Warren, 1990). Ammerman and Balderian (1993) reported that nearly 25% of children who were victims of abuse and 50% of children who suffered from neglect were permanently disabled as a result of their maltreatment. In 1993, the National Center on Child Abuse and Neglect estimated that 36.6% of substantiated cases of maltreatment were the primary cause of disabilities

(U.S. Department of Health and Human Services, 1995). Environmental deprivation, often experienced in cases of neglect, has been associated with higher rates of developmental delays in infants and toddlers as well (Ammerman & Balderian, 1993). Finally, Sobsey (1994) has speculated that North American society devalues persons with disabilities, and Goldson (1997) has suggested that children with disabilities are sometimes dehumanized and treated as property by their caretakers, making it easier for the caretakers to justify maltreatment.

Identification of and Intervention for Children with Developmental Disabilities

Few state child welfare agencies note the presence of children with disabilities in their records (Sullivan & Knutson, 2000). Bonner et al. (1997) reported that only seven states reported the presence of any disability in their abuse records in 1994, and that even fewer recorded the specific disabilities. The few states reporting numbers of children with disabilities contrasts with the reports of maltreatment; for example, in 1982, nearly half of all states recorded disability status of maltreated children (Camblin, 1982). In addition, few states have provided disability-related training to CPS workers, despite the fact that programs and services for children with disabilities and for children who are victims of maltreatment have improved in the last decade.

Identification of children with developmental disabilities by the CPS does not necessarily translate into effective services to assist with coping with the trauma they may have experienced. CPS workers have difficulty meeting the needs of children with developmental disabilities who have been maltreated, due to the complexity of their behavioral, cognitive, physical, social, and special health needs (Hanley, 2002). Sobsey (1994) has speculated that inadequate services are the result of inadequate training of child welfare professionals regarding screening and assessment procedures and strategies for preventing maltreatment of children with disabilities. CPS workers are knowledgeable about abuse and neglect, but they are not necessarily equipped to identify and respond to the unique needs of children with disabilities and their families.

Orelove, Hollahan, and Myles (2000) conducted a study in Virginia regarding the training needs for child welfare and other professionals working with children with disabilities who have been maltreated. Parents, educators, and CPS investigators were asked about their knowledge level, experience, and training interests regarding maltreatment of children with developmental disabilities. All three groups indicated limitations in knowledge on how to recognize children with disabilities (9%) and strategies to respond to maltreatment of such children (14%). Ammerman and Balderian (1993) cited training of child welfare professionals as an essential element in preventing maltreatment of children with disabilities. Poor coordination of services between different providers and across all professions reduces the effectiveness of efforts to prevent and respond to maltreatment of these children (National Symposium on Abuse and Neglect of Children with Disabilities, 1995). However, Mitchell, Turbiville, and Turnbull (1999) have noted that early intervention and developmental disability professionals also need training regarding definitions of abuse and neglect, and that they specifically need training to distinguish between characteristics of a disability and indicators of abuse or neglect. For example, if a child with a feeding tube is undernourished, is the issue a caretaker's lack of knowledge about how to use and maintain the feeding tube, or is it medical neglect?

> Linda placed a call to her local child protection agency asking for help with her 5-year-old son, Jimmy, who had cerebral palsy and moderate mental retardation. Jimmy was diagnosed at age 18 months with spastic quadriplegia, which affects all four limbs and the trunk, as well as the muscles that control the mouth, tongue, and pharynx. As a result, Jimmy was unable to eat, drink, use the toilet, or complete basic hygiene functions independently. Linda was responsible for round-the-clock care for Jimmy's self-care needs. Linda sought services from the local developmental disability agency, but was able to receive only basic case management services, and was not able to access an aide to help with in-home self-care or respite services so that she could have a break from Jimmy's round-the-clock care. Linda reported that she was unable to provide an adequate level of care for him.
>
> Linda was a single mother with two other children. Two years prior, Linda had an open case with the same child protection office regarding a substantiated case of neglect for her two older children. Both children remained at home, and the case was closed 6 months later. The CPS worker knew Linda well. He reported that she was a committed parent who sometimes lacked good judgment, but had few resources to draw upon for support. After verifying that Linda was correct about not being eligible for in-home aide services and the absence of respite care in her community, the CPS worker and his supervisor discussed with Linda the only potential option they could generate. They suggested that Linda agree to opening a new case, whereby she admitted to unintentional neglect of Jimmy, due to her inability to provide the level of care he needed. She agreed, and Jimmy was placed in a residential facility that had 24-hour care. Linda maintained guardianship, but Jimmy was moved to a facility that was 40 miles from his home.

Did Jimmy have to be placed in protective custody to receive the level of care that he required? Were there other supports and services that could have been accessed to provide Linda with the support she needed to keep Jimmy at home? Linda was a committed parent who loved her children, including Jimmy. She was forced to make a decision reminiscent of the time before deinstitutionalization, when many parents were advised that the best thing they could do for their children with disabilities was to place them in institutions where their basic physical needs could be met. The results were that the socioemotional needs of these children were neglected and their ability to maximize their developmental potential was compromised. They were condemned to lives of total dependence and an absence of meaningful intimate relationships with family and others. So what could have been done differently for Jimmy and Linda?

PRACTICES THAT EMPOWER STAKEHOLDERS IN CHILD WELFARE

The example above case highlights some shortcomings in both the CPS and the developmental disability system. The needs of children with disabilities and their families are complex and require intervention from multiple disciplines and multiple systems. Therefore, intervention needs to focus on empowering several target populations, including (1) children with developmental disabilities who have been maltreated; (2) biological, adoptive, and foster care families that include children with developmental disabilities; (3) CPS workers; and (4) other professionals and providers that serve children with developmental disabilities.

Empowering Children with Developmental Disabilities

Empowering children with developmental disabilities equates to providing individualized services designed to meet their unique needs and the needs of their caretakers. "Person-centered planning" (PCP; Mercer, 2003; O'Brien, O'Brien, & Mount, 1997) is an approach to service delivery that assists with the development of individualized program plans to meet the unique needs of these children and families. This approach was developed to facilitate effective problem solving, to achieve individualized client-driven outcomes, and to maximize inclusion experiences for each client (O'Brien et al., 1997). Essential features of PCP include open communication; developing a shared understanding; the recognition of all team members (including the child) as equal partners, and a person-driven focus in which the child, not providers, sets the agenda. A child's sense of control in the outcome has been associated with improved adjustment to disability and enhanced motivation in the intervention process (Newman, Christopher, & Berry, 2000). The child's age and ability to participate actively in this process are important to consider. However, the process can also be successful by incorporating the perspectives of those who know the child well, can support the child, and can serve as proxies for determining the child's individual needs and desires. For PCP implementation strategies, see Mercer (2003).

From a systems perspective, maltreatment of young children should be treated as a potential health and development issue as well as a safety issue, because of the potential impact that maltreatment can have on the children's development (National Scientific Council on the Developing Child, 2004). Empowerment from this perspective should emphasize a dual focus on the developmental needs of children and the identification of community-based supports for children and their families. Increasing the focus on the developmental needs of children with disabilities will necessitate strong collaborative ties between the early intervention and developmental disabilities systems and the CPS (Little, 1998).

Implementing a PCP approach also involves ensuring that service providers (e.g., CPS workers) have the skills and knowledge to meet the unique needs of children with disabilities. Children with developmental disabilities can benefit from self-protection education modified to meet their specific needs (Hughes & Rycus, 1998). Children with disabilities often need to receive counseling and mental health services. It is important for them to have access to therapists who can make specific therapeutic accommodations to assist them in coping with the trauma they may have experienced as a result of their maltreatment (Mansell, Sobsey, Wilgosh, & Zawallich, 1997).

Children with disabilities who have been maltreated experience negative behavioral, emotional, and social effects that often require therapeutic intervention (Mansell, Sobsey, & Calder, 1992). For example, Mansell et al. (1992) reported that individuals with disabilities who were victims of childhood sexual abuse experienced anxiety, behavioral problems, depression, emotional distress, inappropriate sexual behavior, loss of housing, low self-esteem, social isolation, and withdrawal. Therapeutic intervention for children with developmental disabilities who have been maltreated presents some unique challenges. For example, children with developmental disabilities often have poor coping skills, poor communication skills, low self-esteem, and poor problem-solving skills, even before maltreatment is taken into consideration (Spackman, Grigel, & MacFarlane, 1990).

Improving access to appropriate treatment is the first challenge that needs to be addressed. A survey of individuals with developmental disabilities revealed that over half of the respondents reported having difficulty finding and accessing treatment (Mansell et al., 1992). In addition, over 80% revealed that the services they received were not appropriate and did not meet their needs. Approximately 80% indicated that they required special accommodations that were not made available. In general, Mansell et al. (1997) have suggested that few professionals have the desire or the ability to individualize counseling services to meet the needs of individuals with developmental disabilities who have been abused and neglected. Developing and researching appropriate treatment approaches for such individuals has been and continues to be slow. However, there are several meaningful steps that professionals can take to better serve these children.

First, access to services can be improved both physically and figuratively. Special physical access improvements such as wheelchair ramps and accessible elevators, and resources such as translation services, telephone devices, and nonprint alternatives to written materials, will enhance access. Second, many traditional therapeutic approaches have been considered inappropriate for individuals with developmental disabilities because of their limited language and conceptual abilities (Mansell et al., 1992). However, these objections may be based on a poor understanding of the abilities of these individuals, as well as on a lack of awareness of modifications (based on individual challenges) to therapy that can improve the appropriateness of techniques to treating these children. Clinicians and researchers have begun to adapt therapeutic techniques to meet the unique needs of children with developmental disabilities. Mansell et al. (1992) have highlighted several such adaptations, based on assessment of level of understanding, developmental level, and social adaptability. Finally, essential elements to appropriate services are the training and education of nonjudgmental professionals who believe in and promote the potential of children with developmental disabilities to learn and grow.

Empowering Biological, Adoptive, and Foster Care Families

The principles of "family-centered practice" (FCP) can be an effective complement to the PCP process. The core of the FCP model is that "people can be best understood and helped in the context of their family of origin and current network of intimate relationships" (Laird, 1993, p. 151). The FCP approach emphasizes (1) helping families to cope with the challenges of having children with developmental delays, (2) empowering families to work collaboratively with service providers, and (3) supporting families as they make decisions about which services will benefit them (Dunst & Deal, 1994; McGonigel, Kaufman, & Johnson, 1991). According to Beckman, Robinson, Rosenberg, and Filer (1994, p. 23), family-centered services must (1) consider the complexity that exists within families; (2) utilize intervention strategies that can accommodate diversity in family beliefs, values, and functioning styles; (3) utilize flexible intervention strategies that can respond to evolving family priorities; and (4) be community-based.

Elsewhere (Shannon, 2003), I have discussed several essential ingredients in an FCP approach to empowering a family that includes a child with a developmental disability. Empowerment should start with family members' identifying and addressing their most basic needs, such as food, clothing, health, shelter, and transportation. Once these needs have been satisfied, educating family members regarding their child's disability and available systems of support becomes a key ingredient in empowerment. However, while education provides the basic knowledge to participate in the FCP team process, it does not necessarily facilitate family participation. Therefore, professionals need to encourage family members to become involved in their child's care; this indicates a responsibility for professionals to provide the family members with the support they need to assume control over decision making. Family members also have a responsibility for their own empowerment. They must be persistent in their exploration of the complexities of the child welfare and developmental disabilities systems. Encouraging family-to-family support may further empower a family. Contact with other families can enhance confidence and self-esteem and can strengthen the working relationship with providers.

As mentioned above, education is a key ingredient in empowering families. Families and caretakers can benefit from training focused on improving their ability to effectively parent children with disabilities (Sobsey, 1994). Parents need to be aware of advances in technology, supportive services, educational opportunities, and employment opportunities for individuals with developmental disabilities, to assist them in gaining a realistic and optimistic view of their children's potential. Linking families with parent support networks can reduce the social isolation that many families of children with developmental disabilities experience (Orelove et al., 2000). Making respite care available to all families caring for children with developmental disabilities is an effective tool for reducing parenting stress (Hughes & Rycus, 1998). Specifically, emergency respite for families in crisis (e.g., loss of housing) is an effective abuse prevention strategy for families at risk (FRIENDS National Resource Center for CBFR Programs, 2004). Connecting with advocacy organizations such as the state's P&A system can support families in dealing with issues that arise with health insurance, education, and entitlement programs (National Symposium on Abuse and Neglect of Children with Disabilities, 1995). Each of the strategies described above is dependent upon comprehensive and effective case management services that involve providers from the multiple service delivery areas families interact with.

Dougherty (2004) cites emerging evidence that several child welfare practices are effective in promoting lasting family reunification, especially for families that include children with concerns such as developmental disabilities. These practices include (1) careful decision making about placement, (2) strong support for parent–child visitation, (3) intensive family-based services, (4) promotion of collaboration between resource parents and birth parents, and (5) sustaining reunification through effective aftercare services. The success of out-of-home care for a child with a developmental disability is dependent upon achieving a good match with a foster care or adoptive family that is knowledgeable about the child's strengths and needs.

Parent–child visitation is considered a crucial variable in successful reunification programs. Burke and Pine (1999) suggest that important parent education can take place if the visits are structured in ways that can take advantage of important learning opportunities. For example, if a child with cerebral palsy requires hands-on personal care to get ready for bed (e.g., bathing), the child's biological parent could benefit from visiting at bedtime to work with the trained resource family to learn effective strategies for bedtime routines with the child. Burke and Pine also suggest involving biological parents in other activities, such as doctors' appointments, school activities, and community events.

Intensive family-based services can be particularly effective for families that include children with developmental disabilities, because of these families' increased stress and needs (Center for Child Health and Mental Health Policy, 2002). Intensive services involve 24-hour staff availability, small caseloads, services provided in families' homes, 5–20 hours of services per week, and services available on weekends (National Family Preservation Network, 2003). Intensive services provide more opportunities for day-to-day learning experiences for parents around the issues that are the most difficult to cope with (e.g., the behavioral challenges posed by a child with autism). Finally, empowering foster care families to become equal members of permanency teams can improve services provided to birth families. Foster care families can be more involved with scheduling parent–child visits and can be more involved with teaching parenting skills, especially related to the unique parenting challenges that children with developmental disabilities present (Dougherty, 2004).

Empowering CPS Workers

Hughes and Rycus (1998) have recommended that CPS programs should provide early developmental screening and identification, interagency agreements with other service providers, case management, respite care, specialized foster and kinship care, preadoption training and support for adoptive families, parent education and training, counseling, and emotional support. Improving identification procedures is an important first step in improving services to children with disabilities who have experienced some form of maltreatment. CPS workers could potentially benefit from training that focuses on improving their observational skills to help identify and distinguish developmental disabilities. CPS workers could also benefit from training to strengthen strategies for interviewing children with developmental disabilities. For example, learning how to conduct an interview with a child who is nonverbal or communicates with a facilitative learning device could be very useful for a CPS investigator. In addition, training focused on understanding the available resources and supports available through the developmental disabilities system would be practical and beneficial for CPS workers.

Empowering Other Service Providers

Preventing and/or alleviating the problems associated with the maltreatment of children with disabilities can be improved by promoting collaboration between parents and other professionals, such as educators, disability professionals, and law enforcement officials (Orelove et al., 2000). As mentioned earlier, Mitchell et al. (1999) have noted that early intervention and developmental disability professionals need training regarding definitions of abuse and neglect, and specific training to distinguish between characteristics of a disability and indicators of abuse or neglect. On a systems level, collaboration is needed among health care providers, developmental disability agencies, schools, university centers on disabilitiers, and public and private child protection agencies.

CONCLUSION

Children with disabilities who have been maltreated are prevalent in child welfare programs. They have many unique needs that present challenges for CPS workers and other professionals who serve them. Services can be designed to meet their unique needs and the needs of their families (adoptive, biological, or foster care) by implementing the strategies of PCP and FCP. Greater collaboration among child welfare, developmental disability, education, and medical care providers is needed to provide more comprehensive and coordinated services that encompass the developmental domains where each child experiences challenges. Finally, treatment of children with disabilities will not change substantially until we change the societal misconceptions and prejudices about people with disabilities that make abuse and neglect tolerable in our society. Children with disabilities experience emotional trauma and pain as a result of maltreatment, just as children without disabilities do. However, their reaction to this trauma may be different, and our responses should be flexible enough to meet their unique needs.

REFERENCES

Administration on Developmental Disabilities (ADD). (2001, February). *The risk and prevention of maltreatment of children with disabilities*. Retrieved from http://nccanch.acf.hhs.gov/pubs/prevenres/focus.cfm

Ammerman, R. T., & Baladerian, N. J. (1993). *Maltreatment of children with disabilities.* Chicago: National Committee to Prevent Child Abuse.

Beckman, P. J., Robinson, C. C., Rosenberg, S., & Filer, J. (1994). Family involvement in early intervention: The evolution of family-centered services. In L. J. Johnson, R. J. Gallagher, & M. J. LaMontagne (Eds.), *Meeting the early intervention challenges: Issues from birth to three* (pp. 1–12). Baltimore: Brookes.

Bonner, B. L., Crow, S. M., & Hensley, L. D. (1997). State efforts to identify maltreated children with disabilities: A follow-up study. *Child Maltreatment, 2*, 56–60.

Burke, B. C., & Pine, B. (1999). Family reunification: Necessary components and skillful practices [Electronic version]. *Permanency Planning Today,* 10–12. Retrieved from www.hunter.cuny.edu/socwork/nrcfcpp/newsletters.html

Camblin, L. D. (1982). A survey of state efforts in gathering information on child abuse and neglect in handicapped populations. *Child Abuse and Neglect, 6*, 465–475.

Capper, L. (1996). *That's my child: Strategies for parents of children with disabilities.* Washington, DC: Child and Family Press.

Center for Child Health and Mental Health Policy. (2002). *Serving children with disabilities: A video series for child welfare workers* [Supporting document]. Washington, DC: Georgetown University Child Development Center.

Cohen, S., & Warren, R. D. (1990). The intersection of disability and child abuse in England and the United States. *Child Welfare, 69*, 253–263.

Crosse, S. B., Kaye, E., & Ratnofsky, A. C. (n.d.). *A report on the maltreatment of children with disabilities.* Washington, DC: U.S. Department of Health and Human Services.

Decouflé, P., Boyle, C. A., Paulozzi, L. J., & Lary, J. M. (2001). Increased risk for developmental disabilities in children who have major birth defects: A population-based study. *Pediatrics, 108*(3), 728–735.

Dougherty, S. (2004). *Promising practices in reunification.* New York: Hunter College School of Social Work, National Resource Center for Foster Care and Permanency Planning.

Dunst, C. J., & Deal, A. G. (1994). A family-centered approach to developing individualized family support plans. In C. J. Dunst, C. M. Trivette, & A. G. Deal (Eds.), *Supporting and strengthening families* (pp. 73–89). Cambridge, MA: Brookline Books.

FRIENDS National Resource Center for CBFR Programs. (2004, March). *Respite in community-based grants for the prevention of child abuse and neglect* (Fact Sheet No. 10). Retrieved from www.friendssnrc.org

Goldson, E. J. (1997). Commentary: Gender, disability, and abuse. *Child Abuse and Neglect, 21*, 703–705.

Hanley, B. (2002). Intersection of the fields of child welfare and developmental disabilities. *Mental Retardation, 40,* 413–415.

Hughes, R. C., & Rycus, J. S. (1998). *Developmental disabilities and child welfare.* Washington, DC: Child Welfare League of America Press.

Laird, J. (1993). Family-centered practice: Cultural and constructivist reflections. *Journal of Teaching in Social Work, 8,* 77–109.

Little, L. (1998). Severe childhood sexual abuse and nonverbal learning disability. *American Journal of Psychotherapy, 52,* 367–382.

Mansell, S., Sobsey, D., & Calder, P. (1992). Sexual abuse treatment for persons with developmental disabilities. *Professional Psychology: Research and Practice, 23,* 404–409.

Mansell, S., Sobsey, D., Wilgosh, L., & Zawallich, A. (1997). The sexual abuse of young people with disabilities: Treatment considerations. *International Journal for the Advancement of Counseling, 19,* 293–302.

McGonigel, M. J., Kaufmann, R. K., & Johnson, B. H. (1991). *Guidelines and recommended practices for the individualized family support plan.* Bethesda, MD: Association for the Care of Children's Health.

Mercer, M. (2003). *Person-centered planning: Helping people with disabilities achieve personal outcomes.* Homewood, IL: High Tide Press.

Mitchell, L. M., & Buchele-Ash, A. (2000). Abuse and neglect of individuals with disabilities: Building protective supports through public policy. *Journal of Disability Policy Studies, 10,* 225–243.

Mitchell, L. M., Turbiville, V., & Turnbull, H. R. (1999). Reporting abuse and neglect of children with disabilities: Early childhood service providers' views. *Infants and Young Children, 11*(3), 19–26.

National Family Preservation Network. (2003). *Intensive family reunification protocol.* Buhl, ID: Author.

National Scientific Council on the Developing Child. (2004). *Working paper number 1: Young children develop in an environment of relationships.* Waltham, MA: Brandeis University, School for Social Policy and Management.

National Symposium on Abuse and Neglect of Children with Disabilities. (1995). *Abuse and neglect of children with disabilities: Report and recommendations.* Lawrence, KS: Beach Center on Families and Disability, University of Kansas, and Erickson Institute of Chicago.

Newman, E., Christopher, S. R., & Berry, J. O. (2000). Developmental disabilities, trauma exposure, and post traumatic stress disorder. *Trauma, Violence, and Abuse, 1*(2), 154–170.

O'Brien, J., O'Brien, L., & Mount, B. (1997). Person-centered planning has arrived . . . or has it? *Mental Retardation, 35,* 480–488.

Orelove, F. P., Hollahan, D. J., & Myles, K. T. (2000). Maltreatment of children with disabilities: Training needs for a collaborative response. *Child Abuse and Neglect, 24*(2), 185–194.

Pearson, S. (1996, September–October). Child abuse among children with disabilities. *Teaching Exceptional Children,* pp. 34–37.

Shannon, P. (2003). Barriers to family-centered care in early intervention. *Social Work, 49,* 301–308.

Sobsey, D. (1994). *Violence and abuse in the lives of people with disabilities: The end of silent acceptance?* Baltimore: Brookes.

Sobsey, D., Randall, W., & Parrila, R. K. (1997). Gender differences in abused children with and without disabilities. *Child Abuse and Neglect, 21,* 707–720.

Sobsey, D., & Varnhagen, C. (1988). *Sexual abuse, assault, and exploitation of Canadians with disabilities.* Ottawa: Health and Welfare Canada.

Spackman, R., Grigel, M., & MacFarlane, C. (1990). Individual counseling and therapy for the mentally handicapped. *Alberta Psychology, 19*(5), 14–18.

Sullivan, P. M., & Knutson, J. F. (2000). Maltreatment and disabilities: A population-based epidemiological study. *Child Abuse and Neglect, 24,* 1257–1273.

U.S. Department of Health and Human Services, Administration for Children, Youth, and Families (1995). *National survey of child and adolescent well-being: State child welfare agency survey report.* Washington, DC: Author.

White, R., Benedict, M. L., Wulff, L., & Kelley, M. (1987). Physical disabilities as risk factors for child maltreatment: A selected review. *American Journal of Orthopsychiatry, 57,* 93–101.

CHAPTER 10

Understanding and Treating the Aggression of Traumatized Children in Out-of-Home Care

DAVID A. CRENSHAW
KENNETH V. HARDY

This chapter reviews some of the theoretical concepts pertaining to traumatized children in the child welfare system, and then presents an in-depth case example. The example is followed by a discussion of selected research. It then describes agency-based programs targeting aggression and violence prevention. The chapter concludes with examples of empirically supported multisystemic treatment programs.

THEORETICAL CONCEPTS

Profound Losses at Three Levels

Children who have suffered injury to their vulnerable inner core or spirit learn to protect themselves from further hurt. Some put on a "gorilla suit" and keep others at a safe distance by aggressive acting out. They are deeply hurting children who have suffered profound losses and have adopted the stance that "I will hurt, reject, or abandon you before you can hurt, reject, or abandon me!" Others withdraw and hide behind a "brick wall" of detachment, where they are very difficult to reach in terms of emotional connection. It is as if they made a pact with themselves that they would never allow anyone to get close enough again for the loss or betrayal of that person to hurt them as in the past. These defenses, while providing protection, also further deprive these children, who live in a context of cumulative emotional deprivation.

Children who put on the gorilla suit or hide behind the brick wall of detachment are children who are defending themselves against a profound sense of loss. Their losses, which have not been grieved or mourned, are often unrecognized by others (Hardy, 2003, 2004). Furthermore, they have nearly always experienced losses at three different levels of their community context:

- Primary
- Secondary
- Cultural

"Primary" losses consist of family (in whatever way "family" is defined for a particular individual); "secondary" losses include the network of extended connections to friends, sports, school, and social/recreational activities (Hardy & Laszloffy, 2005; Hardy, 2003). These extended connections are potentially major positive influences in a child's life. Finally, "cultural" losses refer to messages concerning how the child is perceived by the society at large. For example, if a male African American or Latino teenager goes to a grocery store and finds that he is followed closely by the store manager or security guard as he walks from aisle to aisle, this will be a powerful devaluing message and may be quite incongruous with the young man's self-perception.

Interestingly, disruption of the primary network has the most devastating impact on European American youth, while disruption of the cultural community tends to be the most disturbing to African American and Latino/Latina youth (Hardy, 2003). If a child has a strong link to one or more aspects of his or her community, this represents a strength that can be built upon in therapy.

Children who have experienced out-of-home placement in the child welfare system have typically experienced disruption and loss at all three levels of community described above. In addition, these children often feel devalued, which leads to anger and ultimately to rage. Devaluation, so typically experienced among poor children and children of color in U.S. society, leads to a sense of powerlessness (Hardy, 1998).

Tangible and Intangible Losses

It is also crucial to distinguish between "tangible" and "intangible" losses (Hardy & Laszloffy, 2005). Tangible losses are ones that are easily seen by others, such as loss of a parent, loss of a sibling, or loss of a home. Intangible losses are rarely recognized, but just as profound in their impact. Children who have been marginalized in society because they are poor, or female, or racially/ethnically diverse have suffered multiple *intangible losses–loss of respect, loss of dignity, and loss of hope* (Hardy, 2004).

Disenfranchised Grief of Children

The emphasis on unrecognized and unmourned profound loss is related to the concept of "disenfranchised grief of children" (Crenshaw, 2002). Doka (1989) defined the concept of disenfranchised grief as "the grief that persons experience when they incur a loss that is not or cannot be openly acknowledged, publicly mourned or socially supported" (p. 4). Not only do children experiencing such a loss fail to receive recognition, support, or facilitation of their grief, but they experience no social recognition that they are facing a loss in the first place. Their losses are devalued, trivialized, or simply not acknowledged at all.

Children in the child welfare system face special problems in recognition of their losses (Crenshaw, 2002). Often children in residential treatment not only have separated from their biological parents, but in addition have experienced numerous broken relationships with key attachment figures as a result of failed placements in multiple foster homes. In fact, children in the foster care system have typically experienced so many losses that no one loss receives the attention it deserves. More importantly, the meaning that each loss has for such a child is not understood. "Moreover, the children have no one in their lives who can remember the cute things they did when they were younger, tell stories about the times when they were especially funny, or remind them of the people who were there early in their life to love and care for them" (Crenshaw, 2002, p. 296; see also Webb, 2002). These are the "stories of attachment" that older children love to hear repeatedly, because they remind them and reinforce in their minds that they were much-loved, valued, and wanted children.

Multiple Losses and Trauma

All children are reluctant grievers to some degree (Crenshaw, 1992). Children with multiple losses and trauma are even more so. Such children will often exhibit a more limited developmental capacity to grieve, due to the pervasive impact of repeated trauma on their cognitive and emotional development. Typically, these children will also receive less favorable environmental facilitation of their grieving. Consequently, their grief will often be reflected in behavioral disturbances associated with the predominant affects of anger and fear. Their underdeveloped psychological resources cannot tolerate, without feeling overwhelmed, the powerful, painful feelings of sadness, longing, missing, and guilt associated with grief.

Children with multiple losses and trauma also fear intensely that any new relationship will lead to another painful separation and loss. They not only fear rejection and abandonment by those to whom they are beginning to feel close, but they also experience intense loyalty conflicts. These children maintain their loyalty to their actual parents, regardless of how disappointing or hurtful these relationships may have been. But often this loyalty is directed to idealized images of the parents. In their fantasies they maintain images of how they should have been cared for, even though they never experienced such care in reality. They hold on to these fantasies tenaciously–a phenomenon that has been referred to as "sustaining fiction" (Van Ornum & Mordock, 1988). This sustaining fiction is maintained partly by the erratic and unpredictable presence of their parents in their lives.

Many children in out-of-home placement during the last decade have lost one or both parents to the crack epidemic. It is not unusual during a period of recovery (e.g., upon completing a drug rehabilitation program) for such a parent to reappear and become available to a child. Tragically, these appearances are often brief and not sustained, and the parent may soon relapse into the drug habit and disappear again for long periods. The possibility, nevertheless, that the parent will reappear again at some future time and be magically cured helps to maintain the sustaining fiction. Such children continue to believe that at some future point in their lives they will have the parents they have always longed for, and they relinquish this belief with extreme reluctance after multiple disappointments. The sustaining fiction is not always adequate to protect reluctant grievers from experiencing the pain of their loss, however. The disappearance of a parent who has briefly come back into a child's life is often experienced as a crushing blow, accompanied by much anger, sadness, and depression.

Another confusing and upsetting experience for children in residential treatment is the legal termination of parental rights. When the children become freed for adoption, they are confronted with the full impact of this loss. They can no longer maintain the fantasy that their parents will someday meet their needs. The sustaining fiction is no longer sustaining. This is an occasion for intense grieving even for the most reluctant grievers among children in placement. The stark reality of their loss can no longer be ignored.

A person cannot begin the grieving process until he or she has first accepted the reality of a loss. In the case of very painful or sudden unexpected losses, the need to deny the reality can be very strong–not only for a young child, but for an adult as well (Worden, 1982). In the case of a traumatic death such as a drive-by shooting, the sense of shock, disbelief, and numbing of feeling all serve to block full awareness and the affective impact of the tragic death. Children in the child welfare system live so that the affect from their losses becomes disconnected. This self-protective mechanism is a defensive adaptation that allows them to survive–but at the expense of living their lives in a robot-like manner, with little capacity to feel either the full measure of pain and sadness or even the joys and pleasures of life. Children who are overflowing with anger and rage are often filled inside with many unexpressed tears. They discovered a long time ago that it does no good to cry.

Children who have defended against the possibility of further hurt by putting on the gorilla suit or hiding behind the brick wall of detachment experience closeness with others to be very threatening and disorganizing, even though they long for it. It challenges and undermines the very defensive system that they have relied on to keep them safe. Frequently a "crisis of connection" occurs when someone gradually becomes important to a child and the potential for forming an attachment becomes more real (Crenshaw, 1995). A dramatic increase in acting-out behavior, running away, or other symptoms may be the outcome. Such children are actually retreating from the warmth of the potential attachment figures.

We should never underestimate the degree of anxiety that the prospect of closeness evokes in these children, even though their hunger for connection is intense. This is the paradox encountered over and over by those working daily with such youngsters in residential treatment centers, foster care settings, and other intensive treatment programs.

Miller and Stiver (1997) point out that children who have experienced sexual and physical abuse represent extreme illustrations of the strategies of disconnection. Their defenses protect them from attachment, connection, and intimacy, while also ensuring their isolation and disconnection. Sadly, these children live in an environment of cumulative affectional deprivation, because their rigid defenses now cut them off from any possibility of the emotional sustenance so vital for human well-being. The connection they both crave and fear is not likely to be consummated.

Invisible Wounds and Their Devastating Consequences

Shame and Detachment

Some children bear visible scars from beatings, burns, or stab wounds. In contrast, we have found in our clinical work with violent youth that the most devastating injuries are invisible wounds to their psyches or souls. James Gilligan (1997), based on his extensive work in the prison system with violent offenders, believes that the emotion of shame is the primary or ultimate cause of all violence. Many violent youth would rather die than be "dissed" (Hardy & Laszloffy, 2005). Gilligan (1997) asserts that the purpose of violence, whether toward individuals or toward entire populations, is to diminish the intensity of shame and replace it with pride. Gilligan points out, however, that most people do not commit violent acts even when they experience shame, because most people have nonviolent ways available to them to protect or restore their wounded self-esteem.

The capacity for guilt and empathy, which is typically lacking in a population of violent prisoners, inhibits the violent impulse in other persons.

Dehumanized Loss/Learned Voicelessness

The ultimate manifestation of dehumanized loss is the alarming and always disturbing symptom of cruelty to animals (Hardy & Laszloffy, 2002, 2005). Duncan and Miller (2002) have reviewed the literature regarding the impact of an abusive family on childhood animal cruelty and adult violence. They have concluded that, overall, the literature suggests that an abusive family context may be a better predictor of adult violence than childhood animal cruelty. Other studies, however, support the connection between childhood animal abuse and later violence toward humans (Merz-Perez, Heide, & Silverman, 2001; Felthous & Kellert, 1987; Kellert & Felthous, 1985; Wax & Haddox, 1974a, 1974b). Children in the child welfare system have, at a minimum, experienced disruptions in their relationships with attachment figures; many have been exposed to violence and trauma. The number and extent of the losses that these children have experienced are frequently not recognized by others and often unacknowledged even by the children. At times the children have the cognitive awareness of their losses, but the affect is disconnected. Other children may experience a sinking feeling of despair, but lack any cognitive awareness of the source of their feeling (Hardy & Laszloffy, 2005). In either case, unacknowledged loss creates a disconnection between the intellectual understanding of the loss and the affect associated with it. Silverstein (1995) notes that this disconnection within the self may be the most difficult loss of all, because it is a more confusing loss.

Another useful concept in our understanding of children of trauma and violence is the "voicelessness of oppressed people" as a function of their overwhelming sense of powerlessness (Hardy, 1998). One way to conceptualize therapy with these children is to think of it as helping them to regain their voices. Alice Miller (1997) has stated that persons who have been traumatized have a great need to have their pain witnessed by someone they trust. When these children regain their voices, the degree of rage, pain, and deep sorrow may be so intense that it will threaten to overwhelm both them and their therapists (Hardy, 1998).

Anger, Rage, and the Cycle of Violence

When the repeated losses of children are not adequately responded to, and their grief is unsupported or not recognized, the losses lead to anger and ultimately rage (Hardy & Laszloffy, 2005; Hardy, 2003, 2004). In addition, the losses become dehumanized, and the children lose their capacity to feel. *This has alarming implications for society, because if these children's own losses are not recognized and addressed, and as a self-protective mechanism they become numb to their own losses, then they can feel nothing for the losses of others* (Hardy, 2003). This loss of capacity for feeling and empathy for the pain of others can be viewed as a crucial ingredient in the escalating cycle of violence in children.

Repeated losses that are unrecognized and unmourned become dehumanized, and the rage if not redirected leads to revenge, which in turn leads to pseudoresolution. Revenge and pseudoresolution, however, do not ameliorate the underlying pain of loss; they serve as a temporary distraction that provides balm for the wound but not healing (Hardy & Laszloffy, 2005; Hardy, 2003).

An important distinction also needs to be made between anger and rage: Anger is reactive to a situation that is frustrating, while rage is ongoing and deeper, and is related to an injury to the spirit or soul of the child (Hardy & Laszloffy, 2005; Hardy, 2003). The following case example discusses the challenge of providing therapy for a child who had suffered deep wounds to his soul.

THE CASE OF RASHAWN, AGE 10

Family Information

Father: Mort, mid-30s, part-time mechanic and laborer, dependent on alcohol

Mother: Lida, 31, waitress and homemaker, diagnosed with bipolar disorder

First child: Rashawn, 10, in residential treatment for 3 weeks at the onset of therapy

Second child: Daequan, 8, living in foster home

Third child: Kareem, 7, living in foster home with Daequan

Presenting Problem

Rashawn, an African American child, was 10 years old when one of us (David A. Crenshaw–"the therapist" in what follows) first met him. He bore both physical scars and invisible wounds that cut deep to his soul. He had experienced severe maltreatment at the hands of his psychiatrically disturbed parents. His mother suffered from bipolar disorder and experienced frequent rages during her manic episodes, at which times she would sometimes beat Rashawn, his brother Daequan (who was 2 years younger), and sometimes his youngest brother, Kareem (3 years younger). Rashawn, however, was the primary target of her rage, because Rashawn reminded her by his behavior and even his appearance of her abusive, violent, and alcoholic father. Rashawn's father also drank heavily and came home drunk most nights. His father and mother fought every time his father arrived home late at night, and their loud arguments and sometimes violent exchanges would terrify Rashawn and his younger brothers, who would usually huddle together at such times in Rashawn's bed. During the father's drunken, violent binges, the children would sometimes become the targets of his rage.

Once the father burst into the bedroom that the three boys shared and, finding the three boys cowering together under the covers, pulled Rashawn out of the bed and threw him hard to the floor. The father screamed, "I didn't raise my boy to be no G_ _d_ _ _ faggot!" He then kicked Rashawn in the face. In a moment that Rashawn described late in the therapy as one of the scariest moments of his life, his father then snuffed out a burning cigarette on his bare back, leaving Rashawn screaming in pain. Rashawn still carried the scar from the burn on his back, but perhaps more devastating were the tortuous wounds to his soul. Rashawn since that night had seldom had a night's sleep that was not disrupted by frightening nightmares, in which either he himself or his brothers were usually brutally assaulted. Most often he woke up screaming in a cold sweat, with rapid, shallow breathing and heart palpitations typical of a panic attack.

Placement Setting

Rashawn was placed in residential treatment after four different foster families, with whom he was placed after he and his brothers were removed from his parents' home, were unable to manage him safely due to his episodes of uncontrolled rage. He became separated from his younger brothers in the second foster family. The parents in this family said that they could keep his brothers, but they could no longer deal with Rashawn. In fact, they were afraid of him and asked for his immediate removal.

Upon his arrival in the residential treatment program, which was well known for its emphasis on intensive treatment and expertise in working through trauma (Burke, Crenshaw, Green, Schlosser, & Strocchia-Rivera, 1989; Crenshaw & Mordock, 2004; Crenshaw, Boswell, Guare, & Yingling, 1986; Crenshaw, Rudy, Triemer, & Zingaro, 1986), Rashawn quickly made his presence known. He immediately challenged the boy whom he sized up to be the toughest, most aggressive kid in the group, and landed two hard punches to his head before staff members could separate them.

Early Sessions

In his first meeting with the therapist, Rashawn was extremely hostile, suspicious, and guarded. He said, "I don't need no G_ _d_ _ _ therapy. I am not crazy. Why don't you just leave me the f_ _k alone?" The dialogue below is a sample of the exchange:

THERAPIST: It is not easy coming to a place like this. There is so much that is new, and there's a lot to get used to.

RASHAWN: What the f_ _k do you know?

THERAPIST: I have seen a lot of kids come here, and at first it can be very scary. But we try hard to help the kids feel safe here.

RASHAWN: Is this the same b_ _ _s_ _ _ you give all the kids?

THERAPIST: Some kids take a long time before they realize that we are serious about making this a safe place for them, because they have been told things like this in the past and it turned out not to be true.

RASHAWN: This place is a G_ _d_ _ _ prison to me.

THERAPIST: I am not going to b_ _ _s_ _ _ you. This place is not like the home you would rather be in. Although we work very hard to make this a good place for kids—a place where no one will hurt you, a place where you can learn in school, where you can learn to make friends—it is not home, and we do not pretend to take the place of your family. But it is a place where you can learn some valuable things that will help you get along in the world. In the time that you and I spend together, I will do my best to help you learn all you can about yourself.

RASHAWN: What a crock of s_ _ _!

THERAPIST: I will need your help if I am going to be of any use to you. I've worked with lots of kids. Many of them have been very angry, and they had good reasons to be. Lots of them didn't think much of therapy when we started out, but some of them learned some things about themselves that seemed to help.

RASHAWN: Oh, sure! You are a G_ _d_ _ _ expert, I suppose.

THERAPIST: No, not really. I have been helpful to some kids, but only because they worked with me and helped me to get to know and understand them. I am certainly no expert in helping you, and unless you help me, and we work together, I probably won't be very useful to you. I know you have no reason to trust me. You don't know me, and I don't know you. But I would like to get to know you, and I don't care how long it takes, because I have a hunch we will need to go slow. I hope you will give me a chance, but one thing you should know about me is that I don't give up easily.

RASHAWN: (*Turns his back to the therapist and mumbles something inaudible.*)

In this exchange in the first session, the therapist had no interest in changing Rashawn's hostile and resistant attitudes toward therapy. The therapist understood that a boy with Rashawn's life history is not going to approach therapy with a new person in his life without major skepticism, if not outright hostility. At the same time, the dialogue reveals that while the therapist did not take Rashawn's provocative bait to enter into a debate or power struggle regarding participation in therapy, he also wasn't willing to be controlled by Rashawn's hostility. He honored Rashawn's resistance not only as typical and expected, but as adaptive under the circumstances. He also made it clear that he wanted to work with Rashawn, and that he would need the boy's help and collaboration if anything of value was to happen. Finally, he planted the expectations that change would need to occur slowly, and that the therapist was committed and would not easily be discouraged.

Children with visible and invisible wounds are masters at attacking the sensitive and vulnerable parts (perhaps invisible wounds) of their therapists and others. To respond in a personal way to Rashawn's provocative and sometimes hostile remarks would have been a major setback to the goal of forming a therapeutic alliance. Yet these children are adept at "drawing blood," and their ability to hone in on other people's raw and sensitive parts represents one of the most trying challenges to therapists working with aggressive and violent children in the child welfare system.

The Residential Treatment Program

The residential treatment center that Rashawn was admitted to was well staffed. Two child care workers were on duty in the living group with 10 children in the after-school hours. A full-time clinical psychologist served as clinical coordinator of the unit, and a full-time social worker served as a liaison to the families and to the referring social service agency. A well-organized school program was available, with specialized learning services offered to children who needed remediation in one or more academic areas, as well as speech/language therapy and sensory integration training for those needing such services. A recreational and activity program was also available, with many of the children participating in sports leagues in the surrounding community, as well as a host of on-campus sports, social, and recreational activities. Child psychiatrists were available to consult with the clinical teams, to evaluate children, and (when needed) to prescribe and monitor medications. The agency's mission from its inception has been to serve poor and disadvantaged children and families. Whenever possible, the goal is to reunite children with their families.

In Rashawn's case, this was not a realistic goal, because the parents had not followed through with supervised visits to either him or his brothers while the children were living in foster homes. At the time of Rashawn's admission to the residential center, the county social service agency had initiated legal proceedings to terminate the legal rights of his parents with respect to all three boys. Regular times were set up, however, for Rashawn to have supervised visits with his two younger brothers, who were still residing in the second of the four foster families in which Rashawn had been unsuccessfully placed.

Rashawn's feelings toward his brothers were highly ambivalent. He was pleased to have the continuing contact with the only family members available to him, and at times he seemed to enjoy playing the role of oldest, protective brother. However, he could also be quite hostile toward them and had to be carefully supervised during his playtimes with them, which took place at either the county social service office or the residential treatment center. He was jealous and resentful that his brothers were living with a family that had excluded him because of his rages and high-risk behavior. This deep hurt was at the heart of Rashawn's invisible wounds. He was always the excluded one, the one who "didn't fit"—the one who reminded his mother of her despised, violent father; the one who was targeted by his violent and abusive father for the most severe, punitive treatment; the one who was excluded from four consecutive foster families, where he "did not fit" either. This theme emerged powerfully in the course of Rashawn's emotionally focused individual therapy. The reader is referred to *Understanding and Treating the Aggression of Children: Fawns in Gorilla Suits* (Crenshaw & Mordock, 2005b) and *A Handbook of Play Therapy with Aggressive Children* (Crenshaw & Mordock, 2005a) for guidelines in determining whether children meet the criteria to undertake safely the rigors and demands of emotionally focused trauma work.

In the books cited above, we have developed the Play Therapy Decision Grid (see Figure 10.1) as a model for decision making to determine

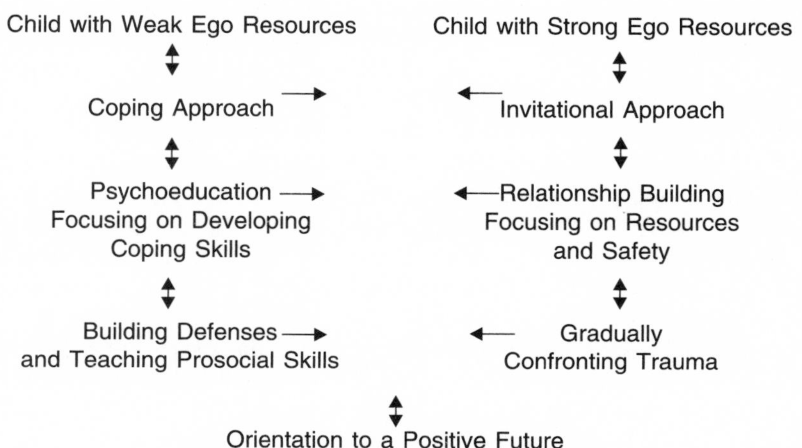

FIGURE 10.1. The Play Therapy Decision Grid. From Crenshaw and Mordock (2005a). Copyright 2005 by Rowman & Littlefield. Reprinted with permission.

whether direct work with trauma material is indicated (the "Invitational Approach") or whether it is necessary to adopt a more psychoeducational approach, with an emphasis on building defenses and developing social and problem-solving skills (the "Coping Approach").

The Treatment Plan

Rashawn, after careful assessment on admission, was diagnosed with posttraumatic stress disorder (PTSD), chronic. His extremely aggressive acting out was considered to be manifestations of "complex PTSD" as described by Herman (1997). He was frequently triggered into trauma reenactments by a multitude of reminders of his early harsh and abusive treatment. A psychological evaluation revealed a Verbal IQ (on the Wechsler Intelligence Scale for Children–Revised) of 91, a Performance IQ of 106, and a Full Scale IQ of 97. On the Woodcock–Johnson, he obtained a Reading Grade Equivalent of 3.9; Math, 3.2; Written Language, 3.2; Knowledge, 3.4; Science, 5.2; Social Studies, 2.5; and Humanities, 2.3. These scores were roughly within his expected cognitive range, with strengths noted in Science.

Rashawn's treatment plan entailed the long-term goal of returning him to a foster family within the community. In order for this goal to be realized, it was important that Rashawn develop more effective self-regulation, including regulation of impulse and affect expression—as evidenced by elimination of violent episodes and rechanneling of angry affect through constructive verbal and motor discharge activities. Educational goals consisted of Rashawn's being able to focus sufficiently to complete classwork and homework assignments, the elimination of bullying and intimidation behaviors with peers, and the extinction of destructive and disruptive episodes within the classroom. These emotional and behavioral changes were to be brought about partly by social reinforcement of positive efforts, and partly by a system of rewards and consequences consistently administered and clearly spelled out both in the classroom and in the living group. Social and recreational activities were focused on the goal of helping Rashawn to participate successfully in such activities, beginning with just one period without a disruptive incident and later gradually expanding to a week without Rashawn's requiring removal due to behavioral disruption.

The goal of the dynamically based individual psychotherapy was to address the repeated, profound, but hidden losses that this child had experienced, due to being "the child who didn't fit." In addition to the need to grieve for these multiple losses, both tangible and intangible, the empirically supported emotionally focused work (Greenberg, 2002; Beutler, Clarkin, & Bongar, 2000) of mastering the maladaptive core emotions and core beliefs associated with the repeated trauma and maltreatment he had experienced was given the utmost priority.

The Coping Approach Phase of Therapy

Rashawn was treated in the initial phase of therapy (the first 8 months) within the Coping Approach, with emphasis placed on helping him develop coping skills, defenses to protect against anxiety, and social skills (including impulse and emotional regulation and modulation). During this period, limit setting and structuring of the sessions were essential in order to provide the firm boundaries that Rashawn needed in order to feel safe. It was a period of relentless testing to see whether the therapist could be strong and competent enough to contain the intensity of Rashawn's primitive aggressive, and sometimes sadistic feelings and impulses. The reader is referred to Crenshaw and Mordock (2005a) for specific strategies to be utilized in the Coping Approach.

One example of a specific technique utilized with Rashawn during the Coping Approach phase was an affect modulation technique adapted from the solution-focused school of therapy (Dolan, 1991). When Rashawn was expressing anger, the therapist would often offer him a foam ball and ask him to show him how angry he was by forcefully throwing it against a wall or down to the floor according to his degree of anger, on a scale of 1 to 100. He would then be asked to identify the degree of his anger on the scale; he might say that his anger was 80 on the scale. The therapist would then ask him to show him what 50 on the scale would look like. He would throw the ball less forcefully. The therapist then would pick another number on the scale, such as 30, and Rashawn would once again demonstrate with a less forceful throw than the one before. The therapist would then engage him in a discussion of the choices and alternatives he would have at each level of anger, in terms of managing and expressing his anger. This was a way of teaching skills in affect modulation, problem solving, and decision making, all in the context of a playful activity that he was able to engage in far more easily then direct discussion of the problem behavior. Rashawn learned that looking for signs of the buildup of his anger and catching it as early in the sequence as possible was empowering, because it left him with more choices as to how to express it. He came to realize that when his anger reached the meltdown point, the anger was in control of him, and he had no choices. Since being in control was very important to him, framing the problem of anger dyscontrol as the anger's taking control of him motivated him to try to develop more reliable internal controls.

Another example of a specific technique involved the rechanneling of anger and rage through artwork. Specifically, Rashawn was instructed to depict the extent of his anger in drawings of volcanos, storms, or angry monsters (Crenshaw & Mordock, 2005a). When the drawings were discussed, opportunities once again arose to discuss what alternatives and options would be available to him if he could notice the anger before it reached the eruption point of the volcano. The drawings themselves

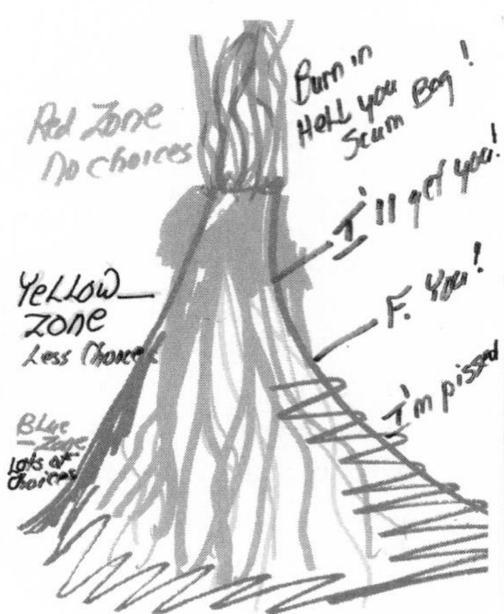

FIGURE 10.2. Rashawn's picture. As anger increased, choices decreased; when anger reached the red zone, his rage replicated the fury of his abusive dad.

offered opportunities for creative expression and sublimation of the rage (see Figure 10.2), and he was sometimes able to use this tool to avoid loss of control.

The Invitational Approach Phase of Therapy

When Rashawn met the criteria for the Invitational Approach (this began at 9 months into the therapy), he was seen twice a week, and the work began to move gradually toward confronting the trauma material. It should be noted that Ricky Greenwald (2002) at the Mount Sinai Traumatic Stress Program has observed that the reason why treatment of children with conduct disorder has often been unsuccessful is that the lives of these children in the child welfare system are replete with loss and trauma, and trauma treatment is not typically included in the treatment programs offered to youth with conduct disorder. Empirical support for this contention comes from a large study of 400 delinquent youth remanded to the Office of Children and Family Services in New York for assault, sexual assault, robbery, or homicide, which revealed that losses and trauma were common in their lives (Crimmins, Cleary, Brownstein, Spunt, & Warley, 2000). In addition, those charged with homicide had often witnessed shootings, knifing incidents, or killings within their own families.

During the Invitational Approach phase of therapy, Rashawn began to show more interest in enacting dramas with puppet characters, who administered violent beatings and sadistic treatment to weaker, helpless puppet characters. The therapist initially responded with reflections of the feelings of the vulnerable, helpless puppets: "Help! Help! Someone please help me! I am scared. I am sorry. Please don't hit me again." Rashawn showed no mercy in response to the reflections of the abused puppets' feelings. In fact, he intensified the sadistic attacks. At that point, the therapist introduced the idea of helpers—police officers, firefighters, or rescue workers who heard the screams of the victimized puppets and quickly gathered at the scene.

The therapist suggested that Rashawn take the Chief of Police puppet, who would take charge of the scene and give orders to all of the helpers. Rashawn was reluctant at first to give up the vengeful, sadistic Alligator puppet, who was terrorizing all the other puppets, but was finally persuaded when told that everyone would follow the orders of the Police Chief, because he was respected by the whole city. This intervention was undertaken because the posttraumatic play as described by Terr (1990) and Gil (1991) had become repetitious and unproductive, and could even lead to harmful effects by reinforcing the maladaptive identification with the aggressor's sadistic use of power. Shifting Rashawn to the role of Chief of Police enabled him to experience the constructive use of power by helping others. The therapist quickly assumed the role of Deputy Chief of Police and reinforced and highlighted the positive leadership of the Police Chief. He also labeled the actions of the sadistic aggressor (Alligator puppet) as very sick and totally unacceptable:

THERAPIST: [As Deputy Police Chief] Chief, as you have told us many times, anyone who beats up on the little guys, like that little Frog (*pointing to the Frog puppet*), is really sick in the head, and you are not going to stand for it. That Alligator is going to have to learn the hard way that you can't treat frogs, turtles, and bunny rabbits that way. He is nothing but a big bully. Shall we take him away, Chief?

RASHAWN: [As Police Chief] Lock him up. He may never see the swamp again! He can just rot in jail for all I care!

THERAPIST: Right, Chief. We'll take care of him.

Children exposed to constant violence sometimes lack a moral compass in determining how to view the normality–abnormality or rightness–wrongness of aggressive acts. By clearly denoting the sadistic actions of the predator Alligator toward the weaker, smaller animals as indicative of being "sick in the head," the therapist bracketed such behavior as abnormal and as a cause for strong intervention.

Since his traumatic experiences had left Rashawn feeling just as powerless and helpless as the beaten-up Frog puppet, the allure of the powerful role of the aggressor Alligator was irresistible. Children like Rashawn, who have felt so helpless, will find such power intoxicating and exceedingly gratifying. Thus the need was for decisive intervention to redirect Rashawn, so he could be empowered by the experience of constructive and effective action on behalf of others.

It was crucial for the therapist to be directive and take charge of these sequences, since Rashawn was inclined to revert to identification with the aggressor. At a pivotal point in the unfolding of the trauma events story, the therapist made the judgment that Rashawn had sufficient ego strengths to confront the trauma more directly. He said to Rashawn, "I've been watching one horrifying thing after another happen to the Frog, Turtle, and Rabbit puppets. I know a lot of scary, awful things happened to you, Rashawn. Can you tell me about it, or show me what happened with the puppets?"

Rashawn pretended he was smoking a cigarette. Then he kicked the Frog puppet across the room and started screaming, "You little b_ _ _ _ _d! I'll show you, you little p_ _s a_s faggot!" He then flipped the Frog over and pushed the cigarette into his back, yelling, "You little s_ _t!" At that point, Rashawn flipped around and started screaming, "That's what he did to me, that son of a b_ _ _h!" He grabbed the Alligator puppet, closed his grip tightly around the puppet's mouth, held it up to eye level, and yelled, "You lousy b_ _ _ _ _d! What did I do? You lousy b_ _ _ _ _d!" He threw the Alligator hard to the floor and kicked it as hard as he could around the room approximately five times. He then fell to the floor and sobbed, "What did I do? What did I do?"

The therapist sat down on the floor next to Rashawn, put his hand gently on his back, and said, "You were just a kid. Rashawn, you were just being a kid. Your dad was sick in the head to do that to you. He was a very angry man, and the alcohol just made it worse, but the only thing you did was just be a kid. No kid should be treated like you were, no matter what they did."

It is difficult for therapists to witness and accompany children through the deep rage and profound sorrow that children like Rashawn experience when they confront the traumatic events of their young lives. Although it is very difficult for therapists to see children in this degree of pain and suffering, we firmly believe that unless such in-depth emotional processing and working through are undertaken, the cycle of violence cannot be broken (Hardy & Laszloffy, 2005; Hardy, 2003, 2004). Anger management alone does not reach the level of the complicated emotional process that is the underbelly of violence in children. "Anger management," as the term implies, helps children to manage their anger—but it does little for the profound unmourned losses and scars to the children's spirits or for the ongoing sorrow and rage that accompany these invisible wounds.

It should be noted that it takes more than one dramatic session to produce lasting changes in these severely traumatized children. Rashawn needed to revisit these horrifying events on multiple occasions until he was able to reprocess them, along with the powerful affects they generated, in a manner that allowed him to move these experiences from "implicit" to "explicit" memory (Siegel, 2003). Implicit memory includes unintegrated trauma fragments that can be triggered or activated by any reminder. Explicit memory allows for processing the event in an integrated manner, so that it can be stored in long-term memory and not intrude in everyday live. It is interesting to note, however, that after the dramatic session described above, Rashawn's nightly terrifying nightmares ceased.

RESEARCH FINDINGS AND CLINICAL IMPLICATIONS

Maladaptive Core Emotions and Beliefs

In a study of core emotions in the treatment of childhood abuse, Greenberg and Paivio (1997) found that the core maladaptive feelings were shame and fear/anxiety. These feelings were in turn coupled with two basic views of the self: feelings of worthlessness and a view of the self as a failure, or feelings of fragility/insecurity and a view of the self as weak. Maladaptive core feelings of shame were linked to the "bad me" sense of self, and fear was intertwined with the "weak me." Greenberg and Paivio (1997) also found that rage can be a core maladaptive feeling, especially when there has been exposure to violence. They noted that rage is often closely connected to fear and related to an underlying sense of vulnerability.

It would be difficult to find a "fawn in a gorilla suit" (a child who is scarred and suffering from invisible wounds), especially one in the child welfare system, who is not struggling with these core maladaptive emotions and distorted views of self as a result of the maladaptive and distorting experiences that have shaped his or her life. Enabling such children to transform these emotions into more positive, life-affirming emotions and positive views of self and others requires intensive emotionally focused therapy. Most of the work involved in turning around the life of a fawn in a gorilla suit requires enormous commitment, perseverance, clinical courage, and conviction. Cognitive distortions such as excessive self-blame often will not yield to logic, because these beliefs are rooted in painful emotional experiences.

Greenberg (2002) observes that destructive anger and rage typically derive from a history of witnessing or suffering violence, and they cause serious relationship problems, including the insecure/ambivalent attachment patterns described by Main and Cassidy (1988). In a study by Main and George (1985) of responses of abused and disadvantaged toddlers to distress in age-mates, they found that not one abused child showed concern in response to the distress of an age-mate. Instead, the abused toddlers often reacted to an age-mate's distress with disturbing behavior patterns, such as physical attacks, fear, or anger. Three of the abused toddlers alternately attacked and attempted to comfort peers found in distress. These responses mirror what have been found in other studies of abusing parents. Disadvantaged but nonabused toddlers in this important study responded to the distress of age-mates with simple interest or with concern, empathy, or sadness. These findings point to the devastating impact evident at an early age on the attachment patterns of children who have been abused; they also point to critical deficits in empathy. The crucial role of empathy in breaking the cycle of violence has been discussed in detail in previous writings (Crenshaw & Mordock, 2005a, 2005b).

The Need to Mourn

Herman (1997) emphasizes that one of a trauma survivor's crucial needs is to mourn his or her losses. Recent research (Greenberg, 2002) provides evidence that in-depth emotional experiencing and working through of these powerful affects are important to the outcome of therapy. These findings are consistent with the emotionally focused work recommended for fawns in gorilla suits and their families if the cycle of violence is to be interrupted.

Fawns in gorilla suits need to feel safe and strong enough to confront what has happened in their lives. They will need to confront the trauma, to grieve their losses, and to experience and express the intense emotions inextricably tied to these events. Once they have been able to face directly the horrors that need to be confronted, the losses that need to be mourned, their shattered dreams and hopes, they will need help in putting the pieces of their lives back together. They will have to work toward developing a sense of meaning and perspective that allows them to view themselves and their world in a new light. Often it means relinquishing self-blame, as well as giving up idealized notions of the parents they always longed for but never had. It also consists of building a sense of virtue and self-worth after taking in repeated negative and devaluing messages. Healing consists of sitting with and containing two of the most painful of all emotions–deep rage and sorrow (Hardy, 2003).

Therapeutic Imperatives

Therapeutic imperatives with these children and their families include placing a premium on validation in contrast to confrontation (Hardy, 1999). They also include recognizing and nurturing their capacity to give. It is through giving that these children and families discover and experience that they have value (Hardy, 2003). The opportunities for contributing to others has typically been sorely lacking for fawns in gorilla suits in the child welfare system.

Islands of Competence

Finally, we need to pursue relentlessly what Brooks (1993) refers to as "islands of competence." In one of the living units in a progressive residential treatment center, the clinical coordinator and child care supervisor joined together in a project to encourage this group of girls to honor the volunteers of the agency. The girls contributed according to their talents: Some baked cookies or cakes; others decorated tables or made up banners and certificates to give to the honored volunteers. Those who were musical practiced songs and dances they could perform for the occasion. The girls experienced the enormous reward that comes from giving to others, and also received much validation and appreciation of their efforts and talents in putting together such an event. This was repeated many times because of the satisfaction the girls received by contributing and giving of themselves in this generous way. We always gain more leverage in the change process with children and families by focusing on strengths as contrasted to an exclusive focus on pathology. Even the most aggressive and violent children are not aggressive and violent all the time, and many have talents or interests that can be nurtured, promoted, and highlighted.

INSTITUTE- AND AGENCY-BASED PROGRAMS AND RESEARCH

The Eikenberg Institute for Relationships: Child and Family Trauma Project

Most of the research to date has focused on trauma and exposure to violence, along with poverty, in explaining the violence and aggression of children; little attention has been directed to the role of profound loss and disenfranchised grief in childhood aggression (Hardy & Laszloffy, 2005; Hardy, 2003; Crenshaw, 2002). The Center for Children, Families and Trauma at the Eikenberg Institute for Relationships in New York City (directed by one of us, Kenneth V. Hardy) focuses on studying the role of trauma and loss in the lives of children and families, and on developing treatment strategies to improve the lives of children and adolescents who have been victims and/or perpetrators of violence.

In addition, the Center for Children, Families and Trauma plans to explore and conduct research on sociocultural trauma, focused on understanding and developing treatment programs for those whose lives have been adversely affected by societal forces such as poverty and racial discrimination. The center also focuses on how profound losses play a pivotal role for children suffering from "dislocation trauma" who share common difficulties as a result of adoption, foster care, migration/immigration, or homelessness.

One innovative program already underway at the Center for Children, Families and Trauma is called Bullies to Buddies. This is a violence prevention and anti-intolerance program involving children, youth, and their families. It is based on the premise that addressing the early warning signs of bullying can deter youth aggression. The program is being implemented at all academic levels in both public and private schools. One of the central tenets of the program is that some prosocial and adaptive life skills coexist with but are overshadowed by a bully's antisocial behavior. The Bullies to Buddies program is focused on developing these prosocial skills and transforming bullies whose social relationships are based on domination and ridicule into buddies whose peer relationships are founded on mutual respect and affiliation. The families of the children are involved along with the children in a minimum of a 10 family therapy sessions; the children also attend biweekly group sessions led by the family therapy team, addressing the emotional/psychological roots of bullying. In-depth assessment and evaluation of the program are ongoing features of the project.

Georgetown University Medical Center: The School-Based Mourning Project

Another very innovative project has been developed at Georgetown University Medical Center. The School-Based Mourning Project: A Preventive Intervention in the Cycle of Inner-City Violence (Sklarew, Krupnick, Ward-Zimmer, & Napoli, 2002) was designed to help children from 7 to 15 years of age to deal with multiple losses and trauma through promoting the work of mourning.

The project takes into account how difficult it is for inner-city children who live in a chaotic environment of poverty, and who are often traumatized by witnessing and enduring violence, to grieve their profound losses. Sklarew et al. (2002) point out that these children are emotionally vulnerable and often developmentally impaired, and are unable to cope with the feelings of helplessness and hopelessness associated with the pain of grief, their violent fantasies, and feelings of guilt.

The project directors explain that children and adolescents try to avoid their underlying depression through aggressive acting-out or destructive behaviors. They fear being overwhelmed and engulfed in their grief. They will sometimes state, "If I ever let myself cry, I will never stop." It is a very hopeful sign that programs like these have been developed to sensitively address the reluctant grief of these children with multiple losses.

EMPIRICALLY SUPPORTED MULTISYSTEMIC INTERVENTION MODELS

The following empirically supported treatment programs to address the aggression and violence of youth in the child welfare system are multisystemic and offer intensive, in-depth treatment. Although this chapter has emphasized the value of in-depth emotionally focused individual treatment to address adequately the trauma issues that so many of these youth have suffered, and that are often neglected in the treatment programs for these children, we have made no claim that this is a comprehensive or stand-alone approach. Work with the families of these children is an absolutely critical aspect of a comprehensive treatment program, as is work with larger systems such as the school, the courts, and the community.

Multisystemic Therapy

Multisystemic therapy (Henggeler et al., 1998) is an intensive family and community-based treatment program addressing the complex network of interconnected factors, both familial and extrafamilial (peers, school, neighborhood), that serve as multiple determinants in serious antisocial behavior (see Crenshaw & Mordock, 2005b, for a detailed description and review). Program evaluation results have demonstrated favorable outcomes across the adolescent age range, for both males and females, and for both African American and European American youth. Of intervention programs evaluated to date, it is the most cost-effective program geared to serious juvenile offenders.

Functional Family Therapy

Functional family therapy is an intervention program for at-risk youth (ages 11–18) presenting with oppositional defiant disorder, substance abuse, or conduct disorder (Alexander et al., 1998). This intensive family intervention program serves clients from a variety of ethnic and cultural groups, both in outpatient clinics and in their own homes. This program's basic tenets are honoring family members' strengths, motivating families to change by uncovering these in ways that enhance self-respect, and offering families specific ways to improve. This program has demonstrated effectiveness in preventing younger children from entering the system of care, including the adult criminal system, and reducing the need for more restrictive, higher-cost services. (For a review of other empirically supported multisystemic programs with aggressive and violent youth, see Crenshaw & Mordock, 2005b).

Prevention Models

We must seriously consider the cautions expressed by Zigler, Taussig, and Black (1992) regarding the multisystemic risk factors that make a child prone to delinquency, including individual, family, and community network factors. This multiplicity suggests that prevention models must address many different levels of intervention. A review of violence prevention programs in the schools (Howard, Flora, & Griffin, 1999) concluded that elementary school interventions and programs focusing on the broader school environment appeared more successful in changing violence-related behavior than single-modality-focused approaches. According to Zigler et al. (1992), longitudinal studies of some early childhood intervention programs suggest that they may help to reduce delinquency. These programs are broad-based in approach and attempt to promote overall social competence at an early age in the many systems in which children are involved. These comprehensive early intervention programs may offer the best hope of averting youth violence.

SUMMARY AND CONCLUSIONS

Far too many children in the child welfare system, especially those who are aggressive and at times violent, are viewed as "bad kids." A frequent diagnosis applied to these children is conduct disorder, childhood-onset type. This diagnosis offers little in the way of capturing the complexity of the underlying emotional processes–the invisible wounds–of these children. No existing diagnostic label elucidates the multidetermined and complicated biopsychosocial factors influencing the children's development, let alone societal and cultural influences that exert a major impact on these typically disenfranchised children and their families. The concept of "complex PTSD" as described by Herman (1997) is a major contribution in the right direction.

Two cultural trends that pertain to the understanding and treatment of aggressive and violent children are of great concern to us. The first is the reductionistic movement in psychiatry toward emphasizing biological explanations and treatments, to the exclusion of other important psychosocial and cultural influences. As far as we know, no drug will heal the hole in the heart of a child whose spirit has been crushed by such oppressive societal factors as extreme poverty; exposure to domestic and community violence; and lack of adequate educational and vocational opportunities or devaluation due to race, gender, class, or sexual orientation. The other disturbing trend is the response to the aggression of youth with increasingly harsh and punitive sentences in the juvenile justice system. A child whose invisible wounds have never been recognized or attended to, and whose tears are still locked secretly inside, will not be helped by a stiff sentence. Nor will society gain from this. These children of wounded spirit are often courageous and inspiring children; they need our profound respect, patience, and caring.

REFERENCES

Alexander, J., Barton, C., Gordon, D., Pugh, C., Parsons, B., Grotpeter, J., Hansson, K., Harrison, R., Mears, S., Mihalic, S., Schulman, S., Waldron, H., & Sexton, T. (1998). *Blueprints for violence prevention: Book 3. Functional family therapy*. Boulder, CO: Center for the Study and Prevention of Violence.

Beutler, L. E., Clarkin, J. F., & Bongar, B. (2000). *Guidelines for the systematic treatment of the depressed patient.* Oxford: Oxford University Press.

Brooks, R. (1993). *Fostering the self-esteem of children with ADD: The search for islands of competence*. Paper presented at the Fifth Annual Conference of CHADD, San Diego, CA.

Burke, A. E., Crenshaw, D. A., Green, J., Schlosser, M. A., & Strocchia-Rivera, L. (1989). Influence of verbal ability on the expression of aggression in physically abused children. *Journal of the American Academy of Child and Adolescent Psychiatry, 28*, 215–218.

Crenshaw, D. A. (1992). Reluctant grievers: Children of multiple loss and trauma. *The Forum, 18,* 6–7.

Crenshaw, D. A. (1995). The crisis of connection: Children of multiple loss and trauma. *Grief Work, 1,* 16–21.

Crenshaw, D. A. (2002). The disenfranchised grief of children. In K. J. Doka (Ed.), *Disenfranchised grief: New directions, challenges and strategies for practice* (pp. 293–306). Champaign, IL: Research Press.

Crenshaw, D. A., Boswell, J., Guare, R., & Yingling, C. J. (1986). Intensive psychotherapy of repeatedly and severely traumatized children. *Residential Group Care and Treatment, 3,* 17–36.

Crenshaw, D. A., & Mordock, J. B. (2004). An ego-strengthening approach with multiply traumatized children: Special reference to the sexually abused. *Residential Treatment for Children and Youth, 21,* 1–18.

Crenshaw, D. A., & Mordock, J. B. (2005a). *A handbook of play therapy with aggressive children.* Lanham, MD: Rowman & Littlefield.

Crenshaw, D. A., & Mordock, J. B. (2005b). *Understanding and treating the aggression of children: Fawns in gorilla suits.* Lanham, MD: Rowman & Littlefield.

Crenshaw, D. A., Rudy, C., Triemer, D., & Zingaro, J. (1986). Breaking the silent bond: Psychotherapy with sexually abused children. *Residential Group Care and Treatment, 3,* 25–38.

Crimmins, S. M., Cleary, S. D., Brownstein, H. H., Spunt, B. J., & Warley, R. M.

(2000). Trauma, drugs and violence among juvenile offenders. *Journal of Psychoactive Drugs, 32*, 43–54.

Doka, K. J. (1989). Disenfranchised grief. In K. J. Doka (Ed.), *Disenfranchised grief: Recognizing hidden sorrow* (pp. 3–11). Lexington, MA.: Lexington Books.

Dolan, Y. M. (1991). *Resolving sexual abuse: Solution-focused therapy for Ericksonian hypnosis for adult survivors*. New York: Norton.

Duncan, A., & Miller, C. (2002). The impact of an abusive family context on childhood animal cruelty and adult violence. *Aggression and Violent Behavior, 7*, 365–383.

Felthous, A. R., & Kellert, S. R. (1987). Childhood cruelty to animals and later aggression against people: A review. *American Journal of Psychiatry, 144*, 710–717.

Gil, E. (1991). *The healing power of play: Working with abused children*. New York: Guilford Press.

Gilligan, J. (1997). *Violence: Reflections on a national epidemic*. New York: Vintage Books.

Greenberg, L. S. (2002). *Emotion-focused therapy: Coaching clients to work through their feelings*. Washington, DC: American Psychological Association.

Greenberg, L. S., & Paivio, S. C. (1997). *Working with emotions in psychotherapy*. New York: Guilford Press.

Greenwald, R. (2002). The role of trauma in conduct disorder. *Journal of Aggression, Maltreatment and Trauma, 6*, 5–23.

Hardy, K. V. (1996, May–June). Breathing room: Creating a zone of safety for angry black teens. *Family Therapy Networker*, pp. 53–59.

Hardy, K. V. (1998) *Overcoming learned voicelessness*. Workshop presented at the Family Therapy Networker Symposium, Washington, DC.

Hardy, K. V. (1999). *Voices at the margin: Therapy with low-income families*. Workshop presented at the Family Therapy Networker Symposium, Washington, DC.

Hardy, K. V. (2003). *Working with violent and aggressive youth*. Workshop presented at the Psychotherapy Networker Symposium, Washington, DC.

Hardy, K. V. (2004). *Getting through to violent kids*. Workshop presented at the Psychotherapy Networker Symposium, Washington, DC.

Hardy, K. V., & Laszloffy, T. A. (2002, Spring). Enraged to death: A multicontextual approach to LGBT teen suicide. *In the Family,* pp. 9–13.

Hardy, K. V., & Laszloffy, T. A. (2005). *Teens who hurt: Clinical interventions to break the cycle of adolescent violence*. New York: Guilford Press.

Henggeler, S. W., Mihalic, S. F., Rone, L., Thomas, C., & Timmons-Mitchell, J. (1998). *Blueprints for violence prevention: Book 6. Multisystemic therapy*. Boulder, CO: Center for the Study and Prevention of Violence.

Herman, J. (1997). *Trauma and recovery: The aftermath of violence–from domestic abuse to political terror* (rev. ed.). New York: Basic Books.

Howard, K. A., Flora, J., & Griffin, M. (1999). Violence-prevention programs in schools: State of the science and implications for future research. *Applied and Preventive Psychology, 8*, 197–215.

Kellert, S. R., & Felthous, A. R. (1985). Childhood cruelty toward animals among criminals and non-criminals. *Human Relations, 38*, 1113–1129.

Main, M., & Cassidy, J. (1988). Categories of response to reunion with the parent at age 6: Predictable from infant attachment classifications and stable over a 1-month period. *Developmental Psychology, 24,* 415–426.

Main, M., & George, C. (1985). Responses of abused and disadvantaged toddlers to distress in agemates: A study in the day care setting. *Developmental Psychology, 21,* 407–412.

Merz-Perez, L., Heide, K. M., & Silverman, I. J. (2001). Childhood cruelty to animals and subsequent violence against humans. *International Journal of Offender Therapy and Comparative Criminology, 45,* 556–573.

Miller, A. (1997). *The drama of the gifted child.* New York: Basic Books.

Miller, J. B., & Stiver, I. P. (1997). *The healing connection: How women form relationships in therapy and life.* Boston: Beacon Press.

Siegel, D. (2003). *Brain-savvy therapy: Lessons of the neuroscience revolution.* Keynote presentation at the Psychotherapy Networker Symposium, Washington, DC.

Silverstein, O. (1995). *Exclusion/inclusion.* Workshop presented at the Ackerman Institute of the Family, New York.

Sklarew, B., Krupnick, D., Ward-Zimmer, D., & Napoli, C. (2002). The school-based mourning project: A preventive intervention in the cycle of inner-city violence. *Journal of Applied Psychoanalytic Studies, 4,* 317–330.

Terr, L. (1990). *Too scared to cry: Psychic trauma of childhood.* New York: Harper & Row.

Van Ornum, W., & Mordock, J. B. (1988). *Crisis counseling with children and adolescents.* New York: Continuum.

Wax, D. E., & Haddox, V. G. (1974a). Enuresis, fire setting, and animal cruelty: A useful danger signal in predicting vulnerability of adolescent males to assaultive behavior. *Child Psychiatry and Human Development, 4,* 151–156.

Wax, D. E., & Haddox, V. G. (1974b). Enuresis, fire setting, and animal cruelty in male adolescent delinquents: A triad predictive of violent behavior. *Journal of Psychiatry and Law, 2,* 45–71.

Webb, N. B. (Ed.). (2002). *Helping bereaved children: A handbook for practitioners* (2nd ed.). New York: Guilford Press.

Worden, J. W. (1982). *Grief counseling and grief therapy: A handbook for the mental health practitioner.* New York: Springer.

Zigler, E., Taussig, C., & Black, K. (1992). Early childhood intervention: A promising preventative for juvenile delinquency. *American Psychologist, 47,* 997–1006.

CHAPTER 11

Animal-Assisted Psychotherapy and Equine-Facilitated Psychotherapy

SUSAN M. BROOKS

Various helping methods, including individual, family, and group approaches, have been employed over the years in working with children in the foster care system (Webb, 2003). In the past 25 years, a growing body of evidence has emerged that demonstrates how psychotherapeutic work within the human–animal bond can uniquely benefit children. Anecdotal vignettes, clinical examples, some doctoral dissertations, and a few research studies have documented the effectiveness of this developing field. Although humans and animals have coexisted for centuries, we have barely begun to explore the myriad benefits of the human–animal interaction. Some of the pioneers who saw the value of bringing people and animals together recognized that animals seemed to provide avenues for building empathy, rapport, feelings of acceptance, nurturing abilities, mental stimulation, touch, socialization and stress reduction (Levinson, 1997; Corson, Corson, & Gwynne, 1975; Ross, 1989a, 1989b; Lee, 1984; Katcher, Friedman, Lynch, & Messent, 1980).

Boris Levinson, a clinical psychologist, is considered to be the father of animal-assisted psychotherapy (see Levinson, 1997). When he discovered by accident with his dog, Jingles, the efficacy of this work, he saw the great diagnostic potential associated with working with animals. As the story goes, Levinson was writing in his office one afternoon, about 2 hours before he was to consult with a mother and her young son, when his office doorbell rang. The mother, quite anxious regarding this consult, had arrived early, confused over the time. In the referral information, the child had been reported as "unrelated" and possibly needing hospitalization. When the child saw Jingles lying under the desk as Levinson was writing, he immediately went down on all fours to be with the dog. The mother wanted the session to begin, and she attempted to yank the child up to sit in a chair and talk to the doctor, but Levinson stopped her. They both watched as the child began to relate to the dog. Levinson agreed to accept the referral, based on the information he obtained from observing the child with Jingles. Jingles's career as a "therapy dog" had begun, together with the field of animal-assisted psychotherapy.

ANIMALS AS TEACHERS: HELPING CHILDREN LEARN RELATIONSHIPS

Today, the incorporation of animals into the healing of people is a burgeoning field. "Animal-assisted therapy" (AAT) is generally viewed as an umbrella term that includes both animal-assisted activities (AAA) and "animal-assisted *therapy*" (AAT) in its traditional meaning.

Animal-Assisted Activities

The Delta Society (www.deltasociety.org), a "leading international resource for the human–animal bond" whose mission is "improving human health through service and therapy animals," defines AAAs as follows: "AAA[s] provide opportunities for motivational, educational, recreational, and/or therapeutic benefits to enhance quality of life. AAA[s] are delivered in a variety of environments by specially trained professionals, paraprofessionals, and/or volunteers, in association with animals that meet specific criteria." (These and the following quotes are all from the www.deltasociety.org website.) According to this definition—and this is an important distinction—AAAs "are basically the casual 'meet and greet' interactions that involve pets visiting people. The same activity can be repeated with many people, unlike a therapy program that is tailored to a particular person or medical condition." An example of an AAA would be visiting elderly persons in a nursing home, making the rounds of each ward, with a dog. Benefits that can occur during a visit of a dog, cat, or rabbit include recollection of past memories while petting the animal, subsequent reinvestment in life, and improved motivation.

Animal-Assisted Therapy

The Delta Society defines AAT as

> a goal-directed intervention in which an animal that meets specific criteria is an integral part of the treatment process. AAT is directed and/or delivered by a health/human service professional with specialized expertise, and within

> the scope of practice of his/her profession. AAT is designed to promote improvement in human, physical, social emotional, and/or cognitive functioning . . . AAT is provided in a variety of settings and may be group or individual in nature. This process is documented and evaluated.

An example of AAT would be a psychotherapy session where an animal was included in the treatment of a child.

Due to the widespread popularity of horses, their species-specific characteristics that enhance the work, and most importantly, the explosion of recent dialogue in the equine world about the therapeutic benefits of horsemanship, therapeutic work with horses is recognized as a discipline separate from AAT with other animals; it has an independent status and its own terminology. Kruger (see Kruger, Serpell, & Trachtenberg, 2004) elaborates:

> Although the Delta Society lists horses as being animals eligible for certification through their PetPartners® program, interventions involving the use of horses typically fall under the jurisdiction of a separate group of agencies. Prominent among these is the North American Riding for the Handicapped Association (NARHA) and its sub-section, the Equine Facilitated Mental Health Association (EFMHA), which provides a separate definition for the term "equine facilitated psychotherapy" (EFP).

NARHA (www.narha.org) sets the standards for working with horses both in general activities (equine-assisted activities), and therapeutically (equine-assisted therapy, equine-facilitated psychotherapy and hippotherapy). Working with animals in a therapeutic milieu, particularly work with equines, requires specialized training and usually the inclusion of an animal handler.

As I discuss in detail later, AAT can involve either a triangular relationship (between animal, client, and clinician) or a diamond-shaped relationship (when a fourth person, an animal handler, also assists in the work). The therapist establishes the boundaries that connect humans and the animal as part of the AAT process. During the session, the therapist as the coordinator of the clinical work takes account of the behavior and personality of the animal, as well as of the client.

Current trends in the field of AAT include calls for more extensive critical research, both quantitative, and qualitative, to help AAT gain credibility among other mental health professionals. There also continues to be much discussion of the terminology for how we work in the field and what we call what we do. In lieu of the aforementioned AAA/AAT definitions, some professionals have suggested, or are even currently using, terms such as "animal-assisted interventions." Others define what they do as "animal-assisted psychotherapy" (the term I personally prefer due to its specific clinical reference) or "therapeutic animal-assisted activities." Unfortunately, these inconsistencies lead to confusion among the clients, other professionals, and the public at large. For AAT to be seriously regarded as a viable treatment modality, the language of AAT must become much more standardized. Lastly, although many workshops and college courses are being conducted by professionals who have worked within the human–animal bond for many years, there remains a need for more accredited AAT certificate training programs. Such specialized training is essential, because professionals who are interested in incorporating this treatment modality into their practice require not only knowledge of human behavior, but also an extensive knowledge of animal behavior.

We are all learning every day by working in various aspects of AAT. This is an exciting and challenging time for the field. The debate about these topics adds freshness to the work and creates potential for growth in the children and adults who are served.

Since 1994, I have had the privilege of working at Green Chimneys Children's Services for at-risk youth, in Brewster, New York. Green Chimneys (www.greenchimneys.org) has been a pioneer in the field of AAT for many years. I function as the clinical psychologist at the Green Chimneys Farm. My role involves creating innovative programs for the 170 children in the center. These children have difficulties being maintained safely either in a traditional classroom setting, at home, or in the community. Many of the children have histories of trauma. In my work with these children, I utilize AAT as an alternate and effective treatment modality.

In this chapter, I focus specifically on clinical sessions in which I work with equines and other animals. These sessions were conducted with at-risk children who have been in the foster care system for several years, who now reside at a residential treatment facility, and who have histories of trauma. Some recent investigations show that AAT is helpful when used with traumatized children (Ascione, Kaufmann, & Brooks, 2000; DePrekel & Walsh, 2000; Moreau, 2001; Brooks, 2001).

ASSESSMENT

Assessment is always the first and foremost concern to the therapist who uses AAT as a treatment modality. In the case of AAT, the assessment pertains to both the client and the animal involved. The animal's temperament, behavior, and willingness to work must be thoroughly assessed on a daily basis. With regard to the child, the assessment includes not only a mental status examination, but an evaluation of the child's past and present responses to animals. Specifically, in addition to the child's mood, affect, and cognitive functioning, both the client's history with animals and current reactions to them are assessed. Since animals are integrated into almost all our program areas, we need to know details about each child in regard to them.

As we walk around with each child outdoors at the farm, we ask him or her specific questions. These include the question of loss through the death of a pet or seeing an animal die. Many children describe painful situations. For example, one child had an experience in which his father, in a drunken rage, threw the family dog down the cellar stairs, and the child listened to the dog howl in pain until it died. Observing the death of an animal or experiencing the loss of a pet may make it difficult for the child to attach to an animal, or this memory may repeatedly trigger unresolved painful feelings.

Another important area to assess involves animal abuse or aggression toward an animal. We ask each child directly whether he or she has ever hurt or killed an animal, or whether he or she has seen another person do so. We assess both *what* the child says and *how* the child answers these questions.

Assessing a child's moral level of development is another aspect of this assessment. This refers to the child's understanding of "right" and "wrong" behavior regarding the treatment of living creatures. We take note of any differences between the chronological age of the child and the developmental level at which he or she is functioning. If a child were to have an incident of animal aggression, this knowledge would be helpful in assigning consequences for the behavior. Knowing the child's level of functioning, both morally and cognitively, helps to formulate the appropriate intervention.

We also ask whether a child likes animals, understanding that some children do not. Each child's preference is honored, and we assess this on a continuing basis. The child will never be forced to participate in extracurricular animal-related activities.

Many children come into placement frightened of animals. For some children, their connection to animals has been through observing cockfighting, or watching others train a dog to be aggressive. Children who come with fear of animals often change and do well in an AAT program. It is gratifying to watch their fearful behavior change into joyfulness, as a result of the therapist's thoughtful interventions and patience. Both from being with an animal, and in overcoming fearful behavior, the child's sense of self-efficacy is enhanced.

Assessing how an undernurtured child touches an animal is an excellent diagnostic indicator. I discuss this further in the next section. Due to the importance of assessing a child for AAT, and the space constraints of this chapter, I refer readers who wish more information about this topic to Levinson (1997).

TOUCH AS A DIAGNOSTIC INDICATOR

Touch is a very good diagnostic indicator for children who struggle with issues of neglect or trauma, and for those who are undernurtured. Observing how a child touches an animal gives us information about how the child has been touched, how the child has been nurtured (or not), and whether the child has experienced some form of intimacy. We look at *whether* the child attempts to build a relationship with an animal, and *how* the child does this. We look at whether the child holds the animal like an inanimate object or like a living being, and whether this behavior changes over the assessment session (and, if so, how). Does the child talk only to the animal, or only to the assessor, or to neither? Does the child know how to hold an animal? Does the child have good boundaries while holding the animal, neither smothering it nor holding it too far away? Does the child barely notice the animal, due to being overstimulated by everything else going on around him or her? Is the child afraid? If so, how does the child deal with this fear? Is there a difference between how the child touches an animal and what the child says about touching animals? These are all important questions to be answered while assessing touch. We invite a child to touch many different animals, both small and large, because there is often a difference in the child's reaction to animals of different sizes and species.

Another key piece of assessing the child is how the animal reacts to the touch. Does the animal move away, act fearful, or pull its head back quickly? Does the animal come to the child or not? All aspects of this engagement are important for the assessment. Animals respond to their sense of a person's energy, smell, and speed of approach. They are wonderful partners in diagnosing how children relate, particularly when children move too fast or when their actions and words are incongruent. One child who came with a history of animal aggression, while walking around the farm, approached one of our mares. The child reached out to touch her, and the mare pulled back quickly in an unusual response. Although the energy of the child was not abusive in that moment, the animal sensed the child's underlying aggression. Animals were only objects to this child, to be manipulated and moved, out of his own needs.

There is often a difference in how a child touches different-sized animals, as suggested above, and the assessment data can reflect this. Sometimes a child likes to ride a horse, but is afraid to touch a horse in its stall. Touching a lamb or a goat may give the child an opportunity to lie down with, hug, kiss, and look deeply into the eyes of an animal. Such interactions are healing for the child and can provide much clinical information for the therapist who is treating the child. When a child is being assessed in this way, however, safety concerns must be paramount to protect both the child and the animal.

Children who have been undernurtured have a second chance to experience being wanted through touching and hugging large animals who can "hold" them. Many of us have had a big grandmother who, when she pulled us to her and enveloped us in her big hug, allowed us to feel love and security. Animals, in many ways, can provide such a "hug"; they can certainly give undernurtured children a second chance to feel a sense of security and love.

Many children in the foster care system are under chronic stress from years of being moved within the system and from continually facing the consequences of their negative behavior toward others. Touching and holding animals can allow such children to relax and feel less lonely. Katcher, Freidman, Lynch, and Messent (1983) conducted a research study on this concept, monitoring subjects' blood pressure as a measure of tension versus relaxation. They found that a subject's blood pressure stayed the same or went down while petting a dog, although it stayed the same or went up when the subject was talking to a person. James Lynch (2000), in his book, *A Cry Unheard: New Insights into the Medical Consequences of Loneliness*, states that loneliness is one of the most deadly problems undermining our physical health. Animals can help children relax and feel less alone.

CONSIDERATIONS FOR CONDUCTING PSYCHOTHERAPY WITH ANIMALS

The role and involvement of the animal are essential in conducting animal-assisted psychotherapy in general and equine-facilitated psychotherapy in particular. The animal included in a psychotherapy session is considered a partner in the work and is especially selected and trained by knowledgeable professionals. The animal is not included as an object manipulated for the betterment of the person, but is included into the session as another living being respected and chosen for its nature, behavioral characteristics, or temperament. An uninformed professional who is working with an animal in the treatment process for the betterment of the child (or adult), and *not* also for the betterment of the animal, risks stressing the animal (which will also have poor effects on the client). Moreover, such a professional is an inadvertent role model, teaching the client that "power over" an animal is all right, or that animals are here only for the use and enjoyment of people. Safety concerns for both the client and the animal require knowledge of the animal's limits in any given session. The therapist must understand animal behavior to understand the animal's limits in any session. I have seen professionals new to working in the human–animal bond excited about this new "tool." However, the animal is not a tool in this work, but a living being with its own limitations, fears, and gifts. We must, as therapists, employ self-reflection about animals before we begin this work. If we treat animals as expendable, or carry even the subtlest "power over" mentality, our clients will inevitably assume this attitude themselves. For this reason, we must be mindful as therapists about what we unconsciously convey through our verbal and nonverbal behavior about the care of others different from ourselves.

To conduct the most ethical clinical work, we must know enough about animal behavior to be able to see the subtle signs of stress an animal may experience in doing this work. Also important to consider is the ability of the therapist to explain the behavior of the animal to the client. Furthermore, does the animal *want* to do this work? A thorough knowledge of animal behavior is essential. Not all animals make good therapy animals. A pet dog may be a good companion, but not a good therapy animal. Knowledgeable and specially trained people should evaluate a particular animal to determine whether the animal can be included in a psychotherapy session. Organizations such as the Delta Society, NARHA, and the Human–Animal Bond Association of Colorado and its partners are specifically set up to do this type of evaluation.

Including animals in a psychotherapy session must also be planned with regard to the client. Does the client have allergies to animals? Is the client fearful of animals, or does the client even like animals? Does the client have painful memories regarding animals that may emerge in the session, before the client has developed internal resources to handle these? Many psychotherapists consider animals as wonderful "icebreakers" in beginning to build a therapeutic relationship. However, if some clients are inadvertently opened up too soon, this can add a complication to the psychotherapy and interfere with the treatment plan. Similar to including a client's sibling or parent in a session, adding an animal to a treatment session must be thoroughly discussed and planned for ahead of time and should not be a surprise. At all times, we must use our clinical judgment and work within our theoretical backgrounds, as well as remain mindful of the relationship we have with our clients (including transference or countertransference feelings). Including an animal in a session can change the relationship with the client in either positive or negative ways. The timing of when to include an animal must be thoughtfully considered, since it may be inappropriate at certain times.

The therapist should be clear about the reasons for including an animal into a psychotherapy session and about how to achieve a positive outcome for the animal and the client. The therapist should have training in animal behavior, and in methods for bringing humans and animals together for the benefit of both. The following case example illustrates what can happen when the therapist does not know how to include animals into a psychotherapy session.

Kitty, a 17-year-old, had been in psychodynamic psychotherapy with her male therapist for 1 year prior to entering the foster care system. The therapy appeared to be at a standstill. The therapist had heard that including a dog in a treatment session could assist a client in feeling more open. The therapist thought that perhaps including his dog in a few sessions would assist Kitty in opening up and trusting him more, in order to facilitate her being able to verbalize and explore more intimate and intense material about the abuse she had suffered at her father's hands when she was younger.

The therapist brought in his dog, but over the next 2 months Kitty managed to deflect her issues to an even greater degree. In fact, she actually used the dog as a way to avoid opening up even more; she did this by constantly focusing on the dog and its behavior. Rather than focus on her own issues, and what was generated within her from being with the animal, she merely played with the dog without reflection. The therapist was aware of his own countertransference issues coming up as Kitty poured all her affection into his dog. He felt pushed out. The therapist saw what was happening and approached the client with his thoughts, causing Kitty to shut down even more. They discussed having the dog in the sessions and agreed to have the dog stop coming. Shortly after this, Kitty said she did not want to continue treatment.

A well-meaning attempt to help a client with a new "tool" boomeranged. A more informed decision, made after the therapist received training in AAT, could have had a different therapeutic outcome.

TWO MODELS FOR INCLUDING ANIMALS IN CLINICAL SESSIONS

Over the years at Green Chimneys, two models have emerged in the process of conducting AAT. The "triangle model" (Figure 11.1) developed from working independently with an animal and a child. The "diamond model" (Figure 11.2) evolved from my work with an animal handler, and further emerged from a discussion with my colleague Leslie Moreau, MSW. These models have become useful in teaching others how to think about including animals in a clinical session, in either psychotherapy, physical therapy, occupational therapy, or recreation therapy. These models serve as ways to facilitate animals in a therapy session within a professional framework.

The triangle and diamond models depict the potential of each participant in a session to ultimately enhance or hinder the connection between the child and animal. Each part of the model influences the others. Clinical work with children and animals focuses on the interaction of all aspects of these models.

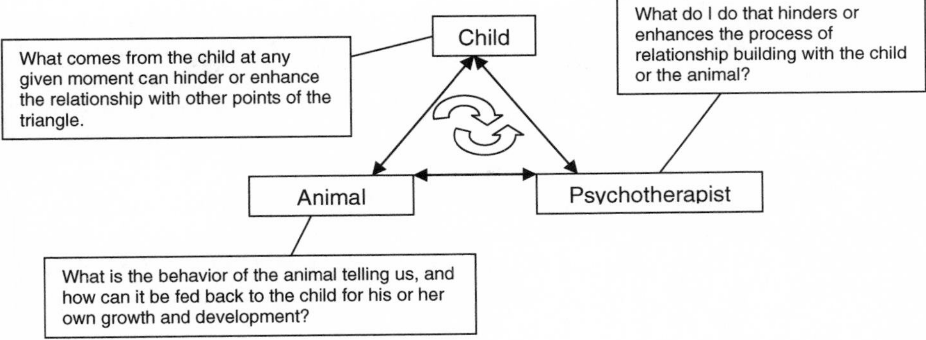

FIGURE 11.1. The triangle model. Copyright 2005 by Green Chimneys Children's Services, care of Dr. Susan M. Brooks. Reprinted by permission.

One aspect of either the triangle or the diamond model considers what the therapist brings to the relationship at any given moment. The therapist's response can enhance or hinder the connection the child is making with the animal, as well as the animal's own behavior. Is the therapist only present physically, while worrying about other things? Animals, like children who carry a chronic trauma history, are attuned to and respond to incongruent behavior. In particular, equines will pick up and be affected by this discrepancy between intent and behavior.

Another aspect of both these models considers what the animal brings at any given moment that can be interpreted to the child for his or

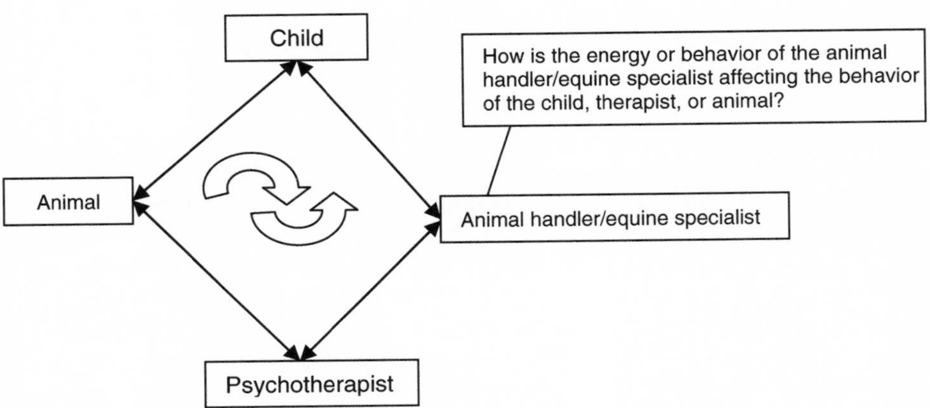

FIGURE 11.2. Copyright 2005 Green Chimneys Children's Services, care of Dr. Susan M. Brooks. Reprinted by permission.

her own growth and development. It is impossible to work clinically in this area, without having a keen knowledge of animal behavior and being a continuous student of animal behavior. The essence of this work necessitates that the therapist knows how to feed back the animal behavior to the child, so that the child can learn about how his or her own behavior affects others.

The third aspect of both these models is what the child brings that can be shared with the child vis-à-vis the animal's reaction, to enhance the child's knowledge about him- or herself. We must understand the behavior of the child and have an understanding of what underlies this behavior.

In the diamond model (Figure 11.2), the animal handler's energy and presence can also influence the session, in positive or negative ways.

Considerations in using these models in psychotherapy include the following:

1. Knowledge of how to build a therapeutic relationship with animal and client.
2. Self-examination regarding the therapeutic process and what the therapist may unconsciously bring to it.
3. Concerns about the client's energy or behavior and how that might affect the behavior of the animal.
4. Concerns about the behavior of the animal and how this might affect the behavior or feelings of the client.
5. Factors related to the other animal handler (Figure 11.2): What does this person need to know to assist in keeping the session therapeutic?

These issues are dynamic and interactive. An example using the diamond model is as follows: In an equine-facilitated psychotherapy session, a child on a horse becomes frightened, and the horse balks or stops. There may be a wealth of reasons why the horse balks. Either the therapist's body language or that of the animal handler may be at odds with the therapist's verbalization. This may cause the child with a trauma history to feel fearful on the horse, because he or she may not know what to respond to—the therapist's (or handler's) body language, or the therapist's words. The child, feeling fear, may cause the horse to balk or stop. In other words, incongruent behavior in the human helpers can cause the child to be fearful, and the child's fear response may be communicated to the animal.

In addition, what is the role of the equine (let's assume it's a male) in ensuring his own safety and well-being, and therefore the well-being of all? Let's continue the example above by saying that the horse balks, flattens his ears, swishes his tail, and tries to bite the handler. Was the horse asked to participate in too many sessions recently? Was the horse reacting in this manner because he was bored with walking around and around the indoor ring? Or has the animal handler been pulling too heavily down on the lead rope, causing the horse to walk with his head too low? Or perhaps the horse has felt the child's fear and stopped moving. At any given moment, the dynamics will shift back and forth among all the participants in the session. The therapist should reconsider the important questions mentioned above throughout each stage of the session. Is the therapist's body language congruent with what is being said? Does the therapist's body language generate confidence or fearfulness in the traumatized child?

Each aspect of these models can affect the other. Animal-assisted psychotherapy is present-centered work for the therapist. Attending to both the subtlest and the most overt aspects of animal and child communication gives the therapist the knowledge needed to assist the child in making a change in his or her behavior.

Bessel van der Kolk (see van der Kolk, McFarlane, & Weisaeth, 1996) has stated that some people who have been chronically traumatized have had to relearn how to engage in authentic relationships. Some people who have not dealt with their own past trauma issues can be hypervigilant to the subtle nuances of another in terms of their personal safety. Relearning safety cues, and learning to decrease responding from fear in an interaction through affect modulation, are aspects of learning how to be in a relationship and truly meet another. These are skills that can be directly addressed in clinical human–animal interactions.

CASE EXAMPLES

The first clinical vignette is an example of how animal-assisted psychotherapy can be useful in helping children relearn safety cues and affect modulation. In this case, Sam needed to understand the behavior of the animal and to respond directly to that behavior. The behavior of therapy animals is usually untainted by humans' meaning making. Animals do not carry ulterior motives. What you see is what you get, once you learn the behavior of that species and the behavioral nuances of particular individuals. When children learn how to *relate* to an animal, they can transfer this knowledge to human relationships. Trust and confidence develop as children learn to relate to the animal's behavior. When an animal does not respond to a child, the therapist helps the child to see immediately how his or her behavior contributed to the animal's response. This is valuable knowledge. It can be fed back to the child and discussed in terms of problems he or she is having relationally with others. The child learns the reciprocity of being in a relationship. After learning and practicing with animal behavior in each session, parallels are drawn back to the humans in the child's life and how the child is relating to them.

Fear of Rejection: Case of Sam, Age 13

Background

This clinical example presents an animal-assisted psychotherapy session with a 13-year-old youth I worked with for 1½ years while he was at a residential treatment center. He had grown up in a family of violence. He had watched repeated episodes when his father kicked and hit his mother. His two older sisters, victims of child sexual abuse from their father, had run away from the home. Sam might have been sexually abused by the father as well.

Sam appeared as a smart, sensitive young man who covered his vulnerabilities with constant swearing, spitting, and gang slang. He had a swagger when he walked. Sam anticipated rejection and had built up a rough façade of indifference and arrogant imperviousness, using scorn as a defense. This was manifested in comments and attitudes such as "He had the nerve to walk away from me," whether Sam was referring to an animal or a person. Sam did not trust anyone. He covered his anxieties with this rough exterior, and because of this, he had difficulties making friends and pushed most people away with his constant swearing. His whole modus operandi was protecting his sensitivities so that no one could see how desperate and fearful he actually was. Sam had been involved in AAAs at the farm for a year, mostly doing chores at the wildlife center and in the horse barn. His behavior worsened after his stepmother refused to take him home. He was then referred for animal-assisted psychotherapy.

First Session with an Animal

Below, I describe our first session working with an animal, and our fourth session in Sam's treatment. Our first three sessions consisted of just "hanging out" at the farm—that is, walking around and looking at all the different animals. I wanted to see whether Sam had any particular feel for any specific animal. I also was evaluating which animals he showed interest in, how he did this, whether or not he attempted to pet any animal, and (if so) what his touch looked like as he attempted to pet the animals. He spent somewhat more time with Raisin, a 1-year-old llama, because "man, is he weird-looking." However, overall, Sam did not appear to be particularly interested in any animal, but appeared to enjoy being out of his classroom.

I chose to work with an animal and Sam, because animals can teach children about energy, boundaries, how we move our bodies, and the intensity of purpose we bring to others. These are all particular components of what we naturally bring or do not bring to our relationships with people. Animals can teach this, because they are very sensitive to our energy and how we move around them. If we move too fast or *want* to touch animals, they often move away from the intensity of the energy we convey. (For readers who may be unfamiliar with llamas, it is worth noting that llamas are particularly responsive to human movements of this sort. They are very independent animals and are generally careful about maintaining their personal space. However, they are also very curious and will usually approach a human who remains calm and unaggressive.) Sam was referred to me for animal-assisted psychotherapy to assist him in beginning to see how his behavior actually pushed people away. His violent verbalizations and his rapid body movements, which stemmed from his fear of rejection, did not elicit behaviors that would bring people close to him. And, of course, he desperately wanted to feel close to someone, and safe. Here now is a present-tense description of our first session with Raisin.

Sam spits on the ground, and as he does the young male llama walks away, keeping a wary eye on the young man who has just spit. Completely oblivious to this movement of the llama walking away, Sam says in a loud, gruff voice, "In this book I'm writing, Cheetaman is evil! He goes after everyone!" This sudden verbalization illustrates to me that for Sam, being in a pasture with an animal is a nonrelated experience. Sam volunteers information to me, someone he already trusts, because of a deep desire to establish a connection. However, because Sam perceives the animals around him as objects more than beings, he ignores them and initiates an unrelated conversation topic. Sam starts wildly swinging around the lead rope he is holding, trying to tell me yet another violent episode from his personal writing project. The llama stands in the corner of the paddock, and inches his way to the part of the fence that separates him from the male alpaca, which stands on his own side of the fence. They touch noses. Sam is completely unaware of the llama, or of the impact his own actions are having on the animal.

I ask Sam to describe to me what he sees going on in this paddock. Sam looks around and says, "Whatdya mean?" I repeat the question and he looks around, laughs, and says in an exasperated tone, "We're standin' in here, and there's the llama."

"Yes," I say. "What might the llama be aware of right now? Do you think he is happy we are in here?" Sam looks at the llama. Raisin is still near his buddy, the alpaca, but is facing us.

"I don't know," Sam says as he begins walking over to the llama, which quickly walks away from him. Sam begins to follow the llama, with his hand outstretched as if he had food or a treat in his hand. Raisin keeps walking away, and Sam begins to chase the llama around the paddock slowly (at a fast walk), attempting to touch it.

"What's happening now?" I ask.

Sam, continues to follow the llama around with one outstretched hand and the other in his pocket. He states, "He won't let me pet him."

Sam runs a little at the llama, stops, spits, then slowly swaggers over to me. He spits again. The llama moves as far away from Sam as he can. Raisin continues to look at his buddy, the alpaca, who is on the other side of the fence. He wants to get closer to the alpaca for protection, but to do so would mean moving closer to Sam. Sam says, "Can we work with another animal? This one doesn't like me!"

"Why do you think he doesn't like you?" I ask, attempting to determine whether Sam can see that his own behavior is pushing the llama away.

"Hell, who knows," says Sam and spits again.

Sam has very few friends. He is unable to see that his behavior actually pushes people away from him. He is obsessed with violent video games and movies. He has also been referred to me because he has experienced some traumatic situations in his home and has been verbally aggressive toward some animals. Sam seems unable to see that the manner in which he expresses himself can actually determine whether people move toward him or away from him. We hope that Raisin's behavior will teach Sam something about himself.

Sam slumps against the fence, picks up a stalk of hay, and puts it in his mouth, sucking on it.

"You attempt to get closer to the llama, and all he does is walk away," I say in a slow and calm way. Sam says nothing and starts to walk toward the llama, again in a fast and purposeful manner, making direct eye contact with the llama. The llama begins to move away quickly, and again Sam begins his slow chase around the paddock. Sam soon gets angry and scares the llama by lifting up his arms aggressively and shaking them at the llama, which quickly moves away. The llama stops and looks at Sam. They stand looking at each other, neither moving, facing off. I am ready to intervene when necessary, should Sam's anger escalate toward the llama. They continue to face off, when Sam's body begins to relax. Sam looks down, and as he does, Raisin stretches out his neck toward Sam.

I say to Sam, "Did you just see what Raisin did?"

Sam spits. Raisin moves away, and Sam says, "Yeah," in a "So what?" tone of voice.

"He tried to reach toward you a little," I said. "At first you were pushing him away by your energy. Then what happened?"

Sam spits and says, "I stopped running after him."

"Yeah that's right," I say, "and do you know what you did to let Raisin feel less scared?"

"No." he says. I role-model what I saw. "When you stopped chasing him, and just stood looking at each other, what were you feeling?" I asked.

"I don't know," Sam says. "I wanted to get him to let me touch him."

"Yeah," I said, "I saw that the 'I want to touch him' had a lot of 'Aggressive—I want to touch him' energy, right?"

"Yeah," he says.

"Then I saw you change that," I said. "Did you see it yourself, what you did?"

Sam says, "I just stopped running after him. I was tired. It was going nowhere."

"That's right," I say. "What were you feeling, though?" Sam shifts his position and looks at Raisin out of one eye, with his head cocked. Raisin is now nibbling hay a short distance away.

"I wasn't angry any more. I didn't care if I touched him or not."

"So something as small as just letting go of anger in your body, relaxing a little, allowed Raisin to reach out a little to you! Let's see if Raisin would let you touch him or get close if *you* were more relaxed and didn't have that 'Aggressive—I want to touch you' energy."

Sam spits and acts as if he is bored.

"Try not to make eye contact, and see if you can approach him relaxed and at an angle toward his withers [the high point of the animal's back]," I say.

Sam starts to walk slowly to Raisin. Raisin stops eating and looks up. Sam continues to walk toward Raisin, approaching near his withers, and Raisin begins to walk slowly away.

"What is Raisin's behavior telling you now?" I ask.

"He still doesn't like me," Sam says.

"How do you know that?" I ask.

"Because he walks away still."

"OK," I say. "Good read of the behavior. He does walk away. Could it be Raisin might be feeling something else besides not liking you? What did his behavior tell you? Think about how you were walking toward him for most of this hour."

Sam says, "Maybe I scared him?"

"Yeah, could be," I say.

Sam seems to become a little interested, challenged maybe. He is beginning to see that he has some control over how the llama behaves around him. Sam again tries to walk toward Raisin, who is again nibbling at a pile of hay in the corner of the paddock. Sam walks very slowly, almost nonchalantly, toward the back of the llama, not making eye contact. Raisin looks up, and Sam stops walking.

"Why'd you stop, Sam?"

"I thought it might scare him if I kept walking," Sam replies.

"Good for you!" I say. "Good read on what Raisin might feel or need from you."

Sam has not spit on the ground for at least 15 minutes. Raisin keeps looking at Sam as Sam approaches slowly. Sam stops and just stands there, looking more relaxed. He begins to talk to Raisin like you might talk to your dog.

"Good boy, Raisin!" he says. "Come on, boy, come on." Raisin just stands by his hay. Sam stops about 3 feet before Raisin, who has not moved away, or eaten any more food. Sam looks up slowly and Raisin slowly, reaches out his neck to sniff Sam. I see Sam become excited, and he quickly reaches to pet Raisin. Raisin quickly moves his head away, but does not run away.

"Aww!" Sam stomps over to me. "See, it doesn't work! Stupid llama, who cares about this stupid llama anyway!" Sam spits and comes over to me. " Come on, let's get out of here. I want to go pet something!"

"What did you see happen?" I ask. "You did great!"

"Stupid llama wouldn't let me touch him . . . who cares anyway?"

"You do!" I say. "Did he run away from you?"

"No, but he's playing with me, making me look like a fool."

"I saw him feel more comfortable with you. Up until the end, you were doing great," I say. Sam spits.

"He's playin' with my head," he says. "He lets me come close and then won't let me touch him."

"Llamas can't play with your head," I say. "But their behavior can teach us something about ourselves if we really listen to it and understand it. You did great right up to the end. What happened at the end?"

"I thought I could just pet him," he says.

"Yeah, and in the intense energy of 'I want to touch him *now*,' what happened?"

"He moved away."

"That's right. Try it again, and at the end keep the same slow energy you had prior to just touching him."

Sam spits and eyes Raisin, who is eating again–a signal of less stress. Sam slowly walks over to Raisin. He walks at an angle toward the llama's withers without making eye contact. Raisin looks up. Sam stops. Sam then begins to walk very slowly to Raisin. Raisin lifts his head and lets Sam touch the tip of his nose. Raisin sniffs his hand. Sam just stands there with his hand out. Raisin sniffs again and puts his head down to eat more hay, still looking up at Sam while he chews. Sam slowly backs away and then grins at me.

"Hey! Good work!" I say. "What made it work this time?" I ask.

Sam looks down and says, "I didn't try to scare him."

"Yup," I say, "but what behavior did you have that wasn't scary?"

"I was slow, I didn't make eye contact. I know *that's* aggressive!" he says.

"Raisin wanted to reach out to you then," I said.

"Yeah . . . "

"Sam, with other kids your age, do you think you come on too strong?" I ask.

"Ya mean, do I try too hard?" he says.

"Yeah. What makes it hard for you to make friends? What might you be doing that pushes people away, like it did Raisin in the beginning?"

"I don't know," Sam says. "Maybe I scare them, too."

"How might you do that? What happened with Tom the other day?" I ask.

Sam thinks. "Tom thought I was going to hit him 'cause I was mad at something."

"Yeah, that's right. I bet if you could deal with your anger better, you wouldn't have kids push you away all the time. Do you see how, when you changed your behavior with Raisin, he let you touch him? If you can be less aggressive to your peers, I bet they wouldn't exclude you so much. Why don't you try it?"

Sam and I have continued to work with Raisin. Sam has begun to learn llama behavior and to see what aspects of his human behavior make Raisin come close or move away from him. In working with the llama over time, Sam is becoming able to translate what he is learning about his own behavior back into his peer relationships.

Discussion

From this clinical example, we can see that Sam appears as a narcissistically injured young man whose adolescent ego-centered ways of being were intensified by his deep fear of rejection. Through these psychotherapy sessions, he could slowly, over time, begin to understand how he could more easily get his needs met interpersonally. His bravado, as an interpersonal protection could slowly lessen, and he could begin to make more direct eye contact with me. Through the immediate feedback from the llama's behavior, he could see what it was he was doing that pushed the llama away—and then, as we translated this behavior back to his relationships with people, could see what he did to push his peers away.

A critical point for Sam was when he became a little engaged in the session. This can be a crucial moment for children, when they start to see that, in fact, they do have control over themselves and how the animal responds. The point is crucial: The children have to learn that this control is control of themselves and not control over the animal. This is a vital piece of the therapy. Otherwise, for a child who holds anger as Sam did, it can be translated to power over an animal as the only way to have control. For this reason, having well-established clinical skills is vital—as is conceptually understanding animals as living, breathing beings, and not tools in treatment for the betterment of children.

Building Resilience Case of Susanna, Age 6

In this second case, an example of mounted equine-facilitated psychotherapy according to the diamond model is presented.

Background

Susanna was referred to equine-facilitated psychotherapy to assist her in building a sense of self. She was quite limited cognitively, as indicated by the Wechsler Intelligence Scale for Children–Revised; her Full Scale was 69 at the age of 6 years. Her referral to equine-facilitated psychotherapy stated that she had difficulty with attachment. She had witnessed violence in her biological family before being removed from the home. She was also emotionally and physically abused in foster care. She regressed easily secondarily to becoming overwhelmed. She did not feel safe.

When Susanna was referred to me, she was acting out most of her feelings. This can be associated with not having a sense of self to assist in mediating the emotional ups and down that all of us face throughout a day. She was having to be restrained physically almost every day. The hope from her team in referring her was that as part of her team, I could help her begin to develop an internalized sense of self–or at least, given her limited cognitive ability, could help her develop more emotional controls. Susanna's diagnoses were posttraumatic stress disorder, chronic type, and oppositional defiant disorder.

Self psychology, especially Kohut's work (Kohut, 1977; Kohut & Wolff, 1978) emphasizes the importance of self-objects in development. I rely on this theory and employ object relations theory in my clinical work (Winnicott, 1992, 1965/1996, 1971/1996). We all need self-objects to help us build a sense of self. "Mother" is thought to be the first self-object that we utilize as she nourishes, soothes, and mirrors back to us, helping us grow and develop acceptance and trust. Susanna did not have this "mother" mirror in a "good-enough" way, in Winnicott's terms. In designing a series of clinical sessions, I wanted to create opportunities for her to begin the task of experiencing this "good-enough" mothering.

The Rationale for Bodywork and the Diamond Model

Somatic techniques can help to ameliorate traumatic effects such as anxiety and dissociation. In setting up clinical sessions for Susanna, I wanted to include bodywork for the following reasons: She was undernurtured, very cognitively limited, and in need of positive physical holding. In making the decision to include bodywork, I decided to put my hand in the center of Susanna's back during the session described below, as she sat astride a pony. Mothers hold their infants supporting their backs; this allows the infants to feel secure and emotionally held. I felt that putting the flat of my open hand on Susanna's back was a way Susanna could take in "good-enough" mothering. Although touching a client during a session may be misunderstood or misused, in this case it felt appropriate. Susanna was beginning to develop an attachment to the animal handler and sidewalker. Together, we hoped to create an environment where Susanna could accept healthy touch and our comments to help build her self-esteem. We attempted to create a therapeutic "holding environment," in Winnicott's terms, in order for Susanna to grow and feel nourished.

In choosing to work with the diamond model, I took the behavior of the animal, the conformation of the animal, and the animal handler's equine expertise into consideration. I chose to work with Breeze, a pony, for several reasons. Susanna liked Breeze. In addition, Susanna was short and young, and Breeze was the correct width for optimal comfort in the sitting position. Yet Breeze was also stocky and strong enough that Susanna could lean forward and relax on his neck, increasing the sensation of being "held" by his size and warmth. We used a bareback pad so Susanna could feel the movement of Breeze more directly as he walked around the indoor ring. The sessions, each lasting 30 minutes from mount to dismount, occurred over a year and a half. The example below is from our 10th session, and our 3rd session working in this way.

A Session with an Equine

As we circled the indoor ring one more time, Susanna's body relaxed more over the neck of Breeze, the pony. The sun was flooding in, and the smell of sweet hay wafted up to us as I sang a lullaby with the palm of my hand flat down, gently, in the center of Susanna's back. We circled slowly at a walk, around and around the ring. Breeze seemed to enjoy the peaceful feeling, walking attentively and without stress. Susanna closed her eyes and made a gurgling sound with her mouth as she lay over the neck of the pony. The equine specialist and I made eye contact. Likewise, the sidewalker and I connected above the child on the pony. Nonverbal communication between the humans involved in the session can be an important way to facilitate the child's focus on the feeling created from the experience of being with her pony. I began to croon to Susanna, much as a mother does while holding her infant. I spoke about how relaxed she seemed, what a beautiful day it was, how relaxed Breeze was while "holding" her, and how happy he was to be spending time with her. As we circled the indoor ring, Susanna's eyes opened and she smiled in a dreamy way, her body relaxed, moving gently with the movement of Breeze. As the end of our 30 minutes of mounted work approached, I gave her prompts that we would be stopping soon, every 3–4 minutes. I did this to prepare her to come back and be with us, and to have her return slowly from this dreamy, relaxed state. At the end of the session, Susanna was asked to sit up on Breeze. When asked whether there was anything she wanted to say, she smiled shyly. With a prompt, she gave Breeze a hug; then she hugged the equine specialist. Finally, Susanna helped to take the bareback pad off Breeze and helped to walk Breeze out to the pasture to join his buddies.

Discussion

We are still working together. Susanna has moved from needing reminders to reach out and pat Breeze, to spontaneously giving Breeze a hug or offering a carrot. These sessions are also helping to build Susanna's capacity for empathic responses. Over time, Susanna has been able to internalize these positive self-objects and integrate them into a more balanced sense of self. This is permitting her to gradually build a sense of resilience to manage her daily ups and downs.

In this clinical example, the diamond model was utilized, because it was important to have an equine specialist assist in this session. Each person working in this type of session can enhance or hinder the work. While a psychotherapist is leading the session, he or she has to be aware of what each person is bringing to the work, including proper boundaries, energy, and attitude. In this case, communication, especially nonverbal communication, was essential to ensure safety and comfort for all participants in the session, in order to provide what Winnicott would call a safe "holding environment" for the client.

SUMMARY

The foregoing clinical case examples of children with severe traumatic issues demonstrate clinical work in an animal-assisted psychotherapy session and an equine-facilitated psychotherapy session. The models presented offer a theory of how to assist in building a relationship between a person and an animal.

In these types of clinical sessions, knowledge about animal behavior is as important as knowledge about the client. The nuances of the interaction between the animal's behavior and the nature of the child's responses, create a milieu in which the child's growth and development can proceed.

Safety is paramount for all concerned in this work, based on a thorough knowledge of the behavior of humans and animals. As with all forms of psychotherapy, this is not a treatment intervention for everyone. A thorough assessment of the child and the animal is essential in order to determine whether this therapy is appropriate and necessary. Furthermore, the therapist must be trained and knowledgeable about the intricate interactions of all involved in this challenging and rewarding work.

If you would like more information on anything regarding this chapter please contact www.greenchimneys.org.

ACKNOWLEDGMENTS

The case of Sam is adapted from Brooks (2004). Copyright 2004 by Greenwood Press. Adapted by permission.

REFERENCES

Ascione, F., Kaufman, M., & Brooks, S. (2000). Animal abuse and developmental psychopathology: Recent research, programmatic and therapeutic issues. In A. Fine (Ed.), Handbook on animal-assisted therapy: Theoretical foundations and guidelines for practice (pp. 343–353). San Diego, CA: Academic Press.

Brooks, S. (2001, Winter). Working with animals in a healing context. *Reaching Today's Youth*, 19–22.

Brooks, S. (2004). Animal-assisted psychotherapy. In M. Bekoff (Ed.), *Encyclopedia of animal behavior* (Vol. 1, pp. 135–138). Westport, CT: Greenwood Press.

Brown, S. E. (2004, Winter). The human–animal bond: Self psychology offers special insight. *Psyeta News*, pp. 2, 4.

Deprekel, M., & Welsch, T. (1999). *Educational and therapeutic animal-assisted activities and animal-assisted therapy lesson plans. Phoenix Process Consultants, and Minnesota LINC–Linking Individuals Nature & Critters*. Minnetrista, MN: Authors.

Katcher, A., Friedman, E., Lynch, J., & Messent, P. (1983). Social interaction and blood pressure: Influence of animal companions. *Journal of Nervous and Mental Disease, 171*,461–465.

Kohut, H. (1977). *The restoration of the self*. New York: International Universities Press.

Kohut, H., & Wolf, E. S. (1978). The disorders of the self and their treatment. *International Journal of Psycho-Analysis, 59*, 413–425.

Kruger, K., Serpell, J., & Trachtenberg, S. (2004). *Animal-assisted interventions in adolescent mental health: A review of the literature*. Unpublished manuscript, Center for the Interaction of animals and society, University of Pennsylvania School of Veterinary Medicine.

Lee, D. (1984). Companion animals in institutions. In P. Arkow (Ed.), *Dynamic relationships in practice: Animals in the helping professions* (pp. 229–236). Alameda, CA: Latham Foundation.

Levinson, B. M. (1997). *Pet-oriented child psychotherapy* (2nd ed., rev. by G. P. Mallon). Springfield, IL: Thomas.

Lynch, J. J. (2000). *A cry unheard: New insights into the medical consequences of loneliness*. Baltimore: Bancroft Press.

Moreau, L. (2001, Winter). Outlaw riders: Working with equines and court adjudicated youth. *Reaching Today's Youth*, pp. 14–18.

Ross, S. B. (1989a). Children and animals: Many benefits–some concerns. *New York State Outdoor Educational Association, 3*, 2–13.

Ross, S. B. (1989b). Thoughtful wisdom on PFT from the perspective of Green Chimneys. *The Latham Letter, 2*, 5–6.

van der Kolk, B. A., McFarlane, A. C., & Weisaeth, L. (Eds.). (1996). *Traumatic stress: The effects of overwhelming experience on mind, body and society*. New York: Guilford Press.

Webb, N. B. (2003). *Social work practice with children* (2nd ed.). New York: Guilford Press.

Winnicott, D. W. (1992). *The child, the family, and the outside world* (2nd ed.). Reading, MA: Addison-Wesley.

Winnicott, D. W. (1996). *The maturational processes and the facilitating environment: Studies in the theory of emotional development.* London: Karnac Books. (Original work published 1965)

Winnicott, D. W. (1996). *Therapeutic consultations in child psychiatry*. London: Karnac Books. (Original work published 1971)

CHAPTER 12

Treating Traumatized Adolescent Mothers

A Structured Approach

RUTH R. DEROSA
DAVID PELCOVITZ

Exposure to trauma is one of our most urgent public health issues, and adolescents are more likely to be victims of trauma than any other age group (Menard, 2002). Approximately 8.8 million adolescents witness severe interpersonal violence, 3.9 million are severely physically abused/assaulted, and 1.8 million are sexually assaulted (Kilpatrick, Saunders, & Smith, 2003). The majority of this violence is perpetrated by someone an adolescent knows (Kilpatrick et al., 2003). Exposure to trauma can have profound effects on behavioral self-regulation, self-concept, academic achievement, and interpersonal functioning, and can permanently alter biology and life course.

Adolescent victims face tremendous demands when successful negotiation of developmental tasks is compromised by the overwhelming helplessness, the loss of safety, and the alterations in identity that trauma can bring (Marans & Adelman, 1997). It is estimated that more than one in eight 17-year-olds meet lifetime diagnostic criteria for posttraumatic stress disorder (PTSD), with adolescent girls at particular risk (Kilpatrick et al., 2003). However, the International Consensus Group on Depression and Anxiety has reported that the "pure" form of PTSD occurs rarely; the typical clinical presentation of PTSD includes multiple comorbid diagnoses (Ballenger et al., 2000). The clinical presentation of abused and neglected youth is often characterized by a constellation of pervasive problems with attachment, attention, emotional regulation, and the management of physiological arousal; this constellation is commonly referred to as "complex PTSD" (Berenbaum, 1996; Cicchetti & Toth, 1995; Cook, Spinazzola, Ford, Lanktree, Blaustein, Cloitre, et al., 2005; Putnam, 2003; Rodriguez, Ryan, Vande Kemp, & Foy, 1997; Ursano & Fullerton, 1999).

This chapter presents a 22-week, manualized, evidence-based group intervention for chronically traumatized adolescents. Exposure to the "hurricane" of chronic trauma leads to adaptations and alterations in social, emotional, physiological, and cognitive functioning. Although these adaptations may serve them well some of the time, approximately 60% of adolescent trauma survivors struggle with the painful psychological sequelae of trauma (Kelley, Thornberry, & Smith, 1997). As these young survivors begin to forge new attachments and negotiate intimate relationships with others for the first time, they may be especially vulnerable to dating abusive partners, initiating violent conflict, and engaging in high-risk impulsive behaviors (Pelcovitz & Kaplan, 1994)—all of which heighten the risk for continuing the cycle of violence into the next generation. Therefore, the intervention presented here is specifically designed to address the needs of traumatized adolescents currently living with or soon returning to chaotic, stressful environments, who would benefit from stabilization and increased coping strategies. This intervention is described in detail after a review of the literature on the impact of chronic trauma, especially in adolescence.

COMPLEX PTSD: CHRONIC DYSREGULATION AND ADAPTATIONS

The treatment described in this chapter was developed to address the construct of "complex PTSD," as described in both the *International Classification of Diseases*, 10th revision (ICD-10; World Health Organization, 1992, p. 112) and the *Diagnostic and Statistical Manual of Mental Disorders*, fourth edition, text revision (DSM-IV-TR; American Psychiatric Association, 2000, p. 465). In the ICD-10, the diagnostic category of "lasting personality changes following catastrophic stress" is defined as an "impairment in interpersonal, social and occupational functioning," including "a hostile or mistrustful attitude towards the world, social withdrawal, feelings of emptiness and hopelessness, a chronic feeling of being 'on edge' and constantly threatened and chronic sense of estrangement" (World Health Organization, 1992).

In the "associated features and disorders" section for the PTSD diagnosis, the DSM-IV-TR (American Psychiatric Association, 2000, p. 465) describes a similar set of symptoms associated with early, chronic, interpersonal trauma. The following problems are described, " . . . impaired affect modulation, self destructive and impulsive behavior, dissociative symptoms, somatic complaints, feelings of ineffectiveness, shame, despair or hopelessness, feeling permanently damaged, loss of previously sustained beliefs, hostility, social withdrawal, feeling constantly threatened and impaired relationships with others." This group of symptoms, though not formally labeled in the DSM-IV-TR, is commonly referred to as "Complex PTSD." Empirical research establishing the prevalence and consistent co-occurrence of these alterations in functioning in a number of traumatized populations has grown in recent years (e.g., Ford & Kidd, 1998; Roth, Newman, Pelcovitz, van der Kolk, & Mandel, 1997; Zlotnick et al., 1996, 1997), and they have been documented in children (Hall, 1999; Praver, DiGiuseppe, Pelcovitz, Mandel, & Gaines, 2000). Complex PTSD includes the following six types of alterations in functioning:

- Difficulty with affect modulation and behavioral control.
- Alterations in attention or consciousness.
- Alterations in self-perception.
- Alterations in relations with others.
- Somatization.
- Alterations in systems of meaning.

Components of Chronic PTSD

Difficulty with Affect Modulation and Behavioral Control

"Affect dysregulation" is defined as having high-intensity emotional reactions to minor stresses, followed by a slow return to baseline state (van der Kolk et al., 1996). This hallmark symptom can be expressed in a variety of ways, including frequently experiencing overwhelming emotional distress; engaging in impulsive aggressive actions in response to minor provocations (Kaplan et al., 1998; Singer, Anglin, Song, & Lunghofer, 1995); suicide attempts, ideation, and self-mutilation (Lipschitz et al., 1999; Kaplan et al., 1999); risky sexual behavior and substance use (Brown, Lourie, Zlotnick, & Cohn, 2000); and dissociative responses (see below) even to minor stresses. Victims of interpersonal trauma are particularly vulnerable to having difficulty with affect modulation and impulse control (e.g., Gleason, 1993). For example, adolescents who experience child maltreatment have a twofold to threefold greater risk of abusing their own children (Ross, 1996) and are at greater risk of using threatening or physical abuse against their dating partners (Wolfe, Scott, Wekerle, & Pittman, 2001).

Alterations in Attention or Consciousness

The relationship between trauma and dissociative symptoms has been well established (van der Kolk et al., 1996, Ogawa, Sroufe, Weinfield, Carlson, & Egeland, 1997). Although dissociation may initially serve a protective function, dissociation during the trauma has been found to be one of the most robust predictors of PTSD (Shalev, Peri, Canetti, & Schreiber, 1996). Long-term use of dissociative coping may lead to numerous negative consequences, including problems with focusing on and completing tasks, difficulty in paying attention to one's own needs or the needs of others, chronic numbing, depersonalization, and potentially disorganized attachment between a mother and her baby.

Alterations in Self-Perception

Identity formation is a central developmental task of adolescence. Therefore, adolescent trauma survivors struggling with feeling ineffective, damaged, ashamed, and guilty may be at particularly high risk for experiencing long-term maladaptive changes in their identities and sense of self. Alterations in self-perception have been shown to have a significant impact on mental health outcome (Celano, Hazzard, Webb, & McCall, 1996; Feiring, Taska, & Lewis, 2002; McGee, Wolfe, & Olson, 2001).

Alterations in Relations with Others

Childhood maltreatment is a significant predictor of both intimate partner violence and dating violence victimization (Wekerle et al., 2001), as well as disrupted peer and parent–child relationships in the form of excessive dependence and compliance, or domineering and intimidating ways of dealing with interpersonal conflict. As supportive relations with others have repeatedly been shown to be a protective factor in buffering against the detrimental impact of interpersonal trauma, disruptions in interpersonal relationships carry significant long-term risk. Socially isolated mothers are more likely to interpret their children's behavior as oppositional and deviant than are to mothers with more social support (Wahler, 1990).

Somatization

In recent years, a close association between somatization and trauma has been noted (Saxe et al., 1994; van der Kolk et al., 1996). In a study of 99 women diagnosed with somatization disorder, over 90% reported histories of abuse (Pribor, Yutzy, Dean, & Wetzel, 1993). Similarly, somatic complaints in the absence of organic findings have been reported in several studies of traumatized children and adolescents (Rimsza, Berg, & Locke, 1988; Hexel & Sonneck, 2002; Lipschitz et al.,1999).

Alterations in Systems of Meaning

The final type of altered functioning in complex PTSD consists of how trauma survivors make meaning, or understand why and how trauma has affected their lives, both the positive and the negative. It refers to fundamental beliefs and schemas about self and the world at large that are changed by facing terror and helplessness. Some schemas may be adaptive in the short run or in the face of imminent threat; however, in the long term, they may significantly impair an individual's sense of empowerment and ability to plan for the future. Survivors of chronic trauma often struggle to understand why bad things happen, whether there is justice in the world, and whether they have a future–be it in school, in their careers, or in their ability to find happiness in love relationships. Some literature suggests that establishing a sense of meaning is a key ingredient in the process of recovery from trauma (e.g., Davis, Nolen-Hoeksema, & Larson, 1998; Krupnick, 2002; McCann & Pearlman, 1990; Park & Blumberg, 2002; Roth, DeRosa, & Turner, 1996).

Chronic Trauma: Intervention Needs in Adolescence

Traumatized adults are most likely to seek treatment for problems caused by chronic dysregulation of their emotional, behavioral, physiological, and interpersonal functioning, as described above (van der Kolk et al., 1996). Interventions specifically targeting these symptoms in adolescence may therefore be expected to prevent the long-term emotional, social, and financial costs of childhood trauma. In addition, intervention during the teen years may minimize the potentially harmful alterations in biological stress response systems and brain development found in adult survivors of chronic maltreatment (DeBellis, 2002; van der Kolk, 2003). In her work with adult trauma survivors, Cloitre (2003) found that group members repeatedly wished aloud that they had learned the coping skills taught in therapy when they were teens; it might have changed the course of their lives, choices, and opportunities.

Trauma and Adolescent Motherhood

Adolescent parenthood has been described as a "dual development crisis" (Sadler & Catrone, 1983), as young mothers must cope not only with the developmental challenges of adolescence, but with the physical and emotional strains of pregnancy, followed by the competing needs of their newborn children. Traumatized adolescent mothers with the associated features of PTSD may experience a significant decrease in the emotional, physiological, and cognitive resources available to them, *just* as they are faced with the demands of motherhood. Teenagers in general are at greater risk for abusing and neglecting their children (Herrenkohl, Herrenkohl, Egolf, & Russo, 1998), and are more likely to treat their babies roughly and have unrealistic expectations of their children's capacities (Tamis-Lemonda, Shannon, & Spellmann, 2002; Musick, 1993). Lyons-Ruth and Block (1996) have found that mothers with a history of child abuse are also more likely to engage in hostile and negatively instrusive behaviors with their babies, or, alternatively, in passive and withdrawn behaviors when their babies are in need. Traumatized adolescent mothers are thus particularly vulnerable, as are their children.

Although welfare reform in some states has attempted to improve resources for young mothers, Kalil and Danziger (2000) found that despite new welfare rules regarding living arrangements, school attendance, and financial support, teen mothers continued to fare poorly on dimensions of psychological well-being and parenting stress. Eckenrode et al. (2000) demonstrated great success with an early intervention program for young disadvantaged mothers, which significantly decreased the risk for child abuse among those who received monthly visits from a public health care nurse. However, 20% of the mothers did not benefit from their early intervention program—those young women living with ongoing chronic domestic violence. Therefore, addressing traumatic stress and the adaptations to chronic abuse or neglect, as well as enhancing coping strategies, is critical: It has the potential to influence the developmental course not only for these young mothers, but also for the next generation.

STRUCTURED PSYCHOTHERAPY FOR ADOLESCENTS RESPONDING TO CHRONIC STRESS: A TRAUMA-FOCUSED GUIDE

Verb Spark 1) To set in motion; activate.
2) To rouse to [mindful] action; spur (www.dictionary.com)

Active coping can be a powerful antidote to helplessness. Structured Psychotherapy for Adolescents Responding to Chronic Stress (SPARCS; DeRosa et al., 2004) is an adolescent group treatment intervention guided by a manual that is designed to "sparc" participants to mindful action in the face of helplessness, in a way that builds on their strengths and enhances resilience. SPARCS targets the associated features of PTSD described in the preceding section—that is, the alterations in functioning that frequently occur after chronic trauma (American Psychiatric Association, 2000, p. 465). SPARCS is present-focused and strengthens the group members' ability to cope with a range of complex trauma symptoms, including difficulties with modulating affect; problems in negotiating interpersonal relationships; problems with attention, concentration, dissociation, and somatic complaints; and problems of shame, self-hatred, and hopelessness. The 22-week manualized SPARCS approach is based on three other empirically validated interventions, which were adapted and integrated in an effort to address the topics specifically relevant to exposure to chronic trauma among adolescents:

- The Trauma Adaptive Recovery Group Education and Therapy (TARGET) treatment program for complex PTSD (Ford, Mahoney, & Russo, 2003).
- Dialectical Behavior Therapy (DBT) for adolescents (Miller, Rathus, & Linehan, in press).
- The School-Based Trauma/Grief Group Psychotherapy Program (Layne et al., 2001).

Each of these approaches provides a unique contribution while also complementing the others, allowing for flow and integration along with useful repetition of concepts.

Group Format and Structure

The participants in the SPARCS group described in this chapter were eight adolescent mothers between the ages of 12 and 17, living in a group home. Although such adolescents may appear to have survived the hurricane of interpersonal trauma in their lives, one could argue that residential placement is but the eye of the storm. In the eye of a storm, skies are often clear, and winds are calm and light. In other words, group homes may provide a momentary safe haven for intervention. However, one must keep in mind that many residents of group homes will return to their families and/or communities–a return that may mirror travel through the "eye wall" of a real hurricane, the ring of the heaviest thunderstorms and turbulence. Therefore, the current treatment is a present-focused, non-exposure-based approach designed to enhance coping strategies and teach young mothers how to make choices mindfully, even in the face of potential danger. Although the group described in this chapter was specifically for adolescent mothers, the SPARCS intervention has also been conducted with other traumatized adolescent populations.

Group members attend 45-minute weekly sessions for approximately 5 months. Since a core skill thought to spark resilience is learning better ways to manage stressful moments, each session begins with a check-in and mindfulness exercise. This is followed by the topic of the day, activities (including role plays, movie clips, and discussion) and a final check-out. Many sessions include colorful handouts that cover practice exercises for group members to try between group sessions. During check-in and check-out for every session, participants are asked to practice Ford et al.'s (2003) "SOS." This acronym stands for "*S*low down, *O*rient yourself, and do a *S*elf-check." As part of the self-check, participants and group leaders all rate how stressed out they are feeling and, separately, how in control they are feeling in the moment, using a visual thermometer on a scale from 1 to 10 for each rating (see Figure 12.1). This exercise is useful for a number of reasons:

PERSONAL THERMOMETER

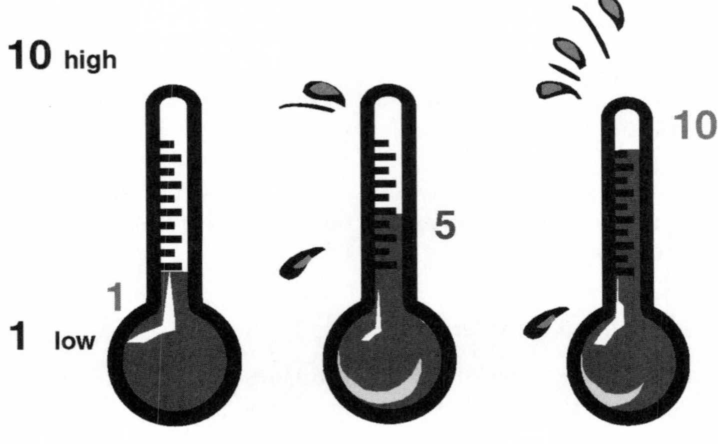

Personal Distress Right now I feel ...

1 2 3 4 5 6 7 8 9 10
Completely Calm — Most Distressed

Personal Control Right now I am ...

1 2 3 4 5 6 7 8 9 10
Completely In Control — Totally Out of Control

FIGURE 12.1. A form for self-check ratings of distress and control. Adapted from Ford, Mahoney, and Russo (2004). Adapted by permission of Julian Ford.

- The act of self-rating helps participants experience and learn to identify a range of intensity. All stress is not always a 10.
- There is reason to celebrate when those who tend to minimize report feeling above a 2.
- Being "present in the moment" and identifying how and what one feels are the first steps in effective coping.
- Participants learn that their distress level is not always tied to the amount of control that they have over their behavior. They learn that they can be very upset and have intense urges, but can still maintain control over what they do or say.

- Not only do group members begin to rate themselves spontaneously; they often begin to rate the staff: "After dealing with that fight in the hall, you look like you're about an 8 and a 5—right?"

The broad goals of treatment, as described below, are to help group members master the following four "Cs":

- *Cultivate* mindfulness.
- *Cope* more effectively.
- *Connect* with others.
- *Create* meaning.

Cultivate Mindfulness

As proposed by the developers of DBT for Adolescents (Miller et al., in press), each session includes mindfulness exercises designed to help participants practice paying attention in a particular way: "Mindfulness means moment-to-moment, non-judgmental awareness" (Kabat-Zinn & Kabat-Zinn, 1997, p. 24). "Awareness" can refer to noticing internal experiences (thoughts, feelings, physical sensations, and urges) as well as external experiences (events in the environment and with other people). Therefore, group members practice not only focusing and concentrating, but also observing, describing, and fully participating in the moment without judging themselves, others, or the situation. Several treatment outcome studies have demonstrated that mindfulness is a powerful intervention (see Rathus & Miller, 2000, 2002; Robins & Chapman, 2004; Teasdale et al., 2002). Teasdale et al. (2002) hypothesize that clients improve not because they are changing their negative thought content or belief system, but because becoming aware of their thoughts as separate from themselves changes their relationship to negative thoughts. Therefore, practicing mindfulness changes the *way* that the negative thoughts (and feelings) are experienced. As articulated by both Linehan (1993a) and Teasdale et al. (2002), mindfulness practice teaches acceptance and tolerance, together with the experience of self as separate from one's thoughts, feelings, and actions.

Adolescents have the opportunity to practice mindfulness in a number of engaging ways—for example, blowing bubbles, mindful eating, listening to music without judging it, and noticing urges to move *without acting on those urges* (e.g., the urge to shift in their seats, scratch their noses, etc., see Table 12.1). It is anticipated that teaching adolescents mindfulness skills will address several complex PTSD symptoms, including alterations in regulation of affect and impulses, somatization, attention, and self-perception.

- Mindfulness can have a powerful influence on *affect dysregulation and impulsivity*, because being observant and working to describe one's experiences requires that one slow down, and consequently respond to situations less impulsively.
- Mindfulness can facilitate recognition and labeling of the link between emotions and the body; this link often becomes disconnected in traumatized adolescents, who simply report frequent *somatic complaints* (headaches, stomachaches, etc.).

TABLE 12.1. Sample Mindfulness Practices

Description	Comments
Snap, Crackle, Pop[a]	
First, leaders ask group members to stand around in a circle. The person who starts the game moves her left or right hand over her head to point to her neighbor (to her left or right), and says "Snap." The neighbor pointed to then moves her hand across her chest (in either direction) pointing to a neighbor (to left or right), and says "Crackle." The person pointed to can then point straight to anyone in the circle whom she chooses, and says "Pop." That person then starts the cycle over again with the "Snap" gesture. When group members miss the right gesture or word, they are out of the circle, and can distract the remaining players (by yelling "Snap," "Crackle," or "Pop," or doing these gestures). The idea is to stay really mindful, to focus on one thing in the moment, and to let go of distractions to do this successfully! After 3 minutes or so, leaders should ask whether anyone would like to share their observations. Volunteers are asked to describe any observations, thoughts, and feelings about the exercise.	If participants are fully present in the moment, not only will they be more successful at the game; they will also have more fun! Leaders explain how practicing mindfulness will help them to identify why they are feeling stressed and to communicate more effectively (if they are mindful and focused, they are more likely to get what they want). Leaders discuss how being on "automatic pilot" in life—not being in the moment, especially when things are stressful—may lead to impulsive behavior that causes problems. It may also lead to being disconnected from their true goals/needs and make it less likely that they will get what they want.
Urges to Move	
This mindfulness exercise is about noticing urges to move. Leaders tell group members: "Sit straight in the chair, shoulders back, and arms in your lap or folded. Notice any urges to move, to change position or scratch. Instead of giving in to the urge, resist it. Instead, notice it, and observe how some urges come and go like a wave. From time to time, everyone acts on urges to do or say things that may make a situation worse, so it is helpful to practice simply noticing our urges and realizing that we can have urges without acting on them, even if we are uncomfortable."	Despite very strong impulses to move, scratch, laugh, or look around the room, group members are asked to be statues. Then they have the opportunity to practice not acting on impulse while being fully aware of how it feels—fully aware instead of distracting themselves. This may provide an opportunity to discuss maladaptive coping strategies to avoid pain.

[a]Jill Rathus and Alec Miller (personal communication, 2003).

- Mindfulness practice includes several active games, such as sound ball, line dancing, and "Snap, Crackle, Pop" (see Table 12.1) which require focused *attention* in order to succeed. During quieter practice, group members are asked to observe and describe their thoughts or feelings, while repeatedly refocusing their attention on the present moment as their minds drift to the past or their plans for the weekend.
- Mindfulness practice is the key to accessing one's "wise mind" (Miller et al., in press), otherwise known as one's "intuition." The adolescents learn that this wisdom is something everyone has access to; they just need practice getting there. This concept can be empowering and runs counter to trauma survivors' negative *self-perceptions* as permanently damaged and ineffective. Interestingly, adolescents have rated these skills, which are linked to developing acceptance, as the most helpful skills they learned (Miller, Wyman, Huppert, Glassman, & Rathus, 2000).

After group members become familiar with mindfulness practice, the leaders begin to discuss the ways that participants have begun to use mindfulness in their daily lives. The following excerpt describes the first time we asked for some examples in the group of young mothers we are describing in this chapter.

Description	Rationale
LEADER: That was a great [mindfulness] practice. Jackie, your description was very specific. I really got a sense of what you were feeling and thinking. Would anyone be willing to describe a time that they recently thought about getting into "wise mind" or being mindful—even if it didn't turn out that way?	Simply remembering the skills in the moment is an important first step.
GROUP MEMBERS: (*No response. Little eye contact.*)	
LEADER: If you think back now, see if you can remember a time that it might have been helpful.	We wait, but still no response.
GROUP MEMBERS: (*Shift in their seats. Some shrug their shoulders. Others look around as if to see who might speak first.*)	Most group members were uncomfortable when we first began describing our own experiences after practicing

mindfulness. We modeled describing our own observations during the practice for several weeks as more and more group members volunteered spontaneously. So we try asking for a volunteer now.

LEADER: I have a little example of something that happened over the weekend. I try to practice being mindful, too. Sometimes I can do it; sometimes it's extra hard; and sometimes I just can't do and need some help.

Everyone looks up and is more engaged.

We were having pizza with the kids, and they were having a *really* hard time sitting still. They were poking each other, being way too loud, and it felt like they were constantly whining. I felt like pulling my hair out! I snapped at them when it would have been better to find something for them to do while we were waiting for the food. Can anyone guess what state of mind I was in?

Lots of smiles and giggles.

GROUP MEMBER: I think you were in "emotion mind," cause they were all over the place.

We often refer to a poster one of us made (adapted from Linehan, 1993b) that depicts the three states of mind: "emotion mind," "reasonable mind," and "wise mind." (See Figure 12.2.)

LEADER: That's exactly right. I was in emotion mind. Suddenly my son has to go potty *now*, so we race to the bathroom. He abruptly stops in his tracks in the back hallway as some salsa music comes blaring through the speakers overhead. He immediately breaks into a cha-cha dance (*leader demonstrates*). OK, given everything that had happened up until now, guess what I might have done next?

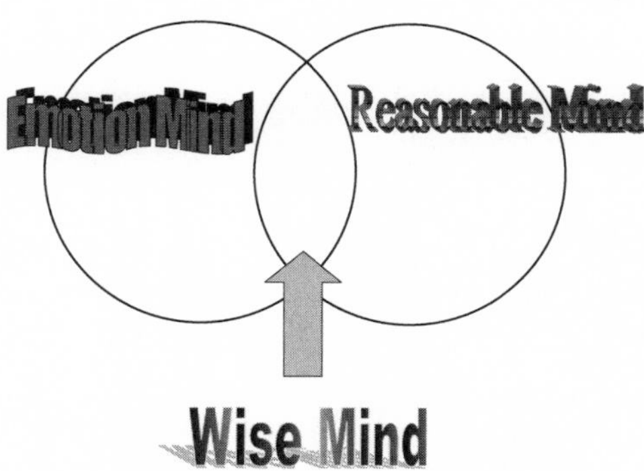

FIGURE 12.2. The "states of mind" poster. Adapted from Linehan (1993b). Copyright 1993 by The Guilford Press. Adapted by permission.

GROUP MEMBER: Yell at him to cut it out and get his butt into the bathroom.

LEADER: Yes. But in that split second, a waitress came by and started dancing too! So instead, I decided to "fully participate" in the moment, and we all danced in the hallway for a couple of minutes. And the more we danced, the harder we laughed. The rest of the dinner went much smoother. Can anyone guess why?

"Fully participating" means being spontaneous, "becoming one" with the activity, without being self-conscious (Linehan, 1993a).

GROUP MEMBER: You felt better.

LEADER: By being more mindful and letting myself fully participate in the moment, I was able to have more fun and move from emotion mind into wise mind. Being in wise mind helped me pay better attention to what my children needed in the moment, instead of just my frustration.

We repeatedly remind the group why we practice mindfulness and use examples from their lives. Mindfulness is the path to wise mind where we can better access our intuition to make better decisions and parent more effectively.

[Then a group member volunteers:]

GROUP MEMBER: Well, I think I might have an example, maybe.

LEADER: Great. Go ahead.

GROUP MEMBER: I was in the bathroom, you know, and I was changing my daughter, and she spit up all over her clothes. There were all these other mothers there. There were all these older women, and they were, you know, looking at me like "Does she know what she's doing?" I was upset that I didn't bring the baby bag with her change of clothes, and she was soaking wet. One of them asked me, "Do you need some help?" I don't need their help.

LEADER: You felt like they were judging you?

GROUP MEMBER: Yeah, people act like I'm stupid just because I'm young. I just didn't want to walk around with the big bag of stuff. My sister was right there–she usually brings it, but she didn't bring it this time.

Feeling alienated is a common response to trauma that was heightened by previous reactions to her early pregnancy.

LEADER: How did you feel with all of this going on?

GROUP MEMBER: I was mad that they were acting like I didn't know what to do. I'm a mother too, you know. I was mad at myself too, because I should have brought her extra clothes. (*Pause*) I was kinda mad at her too for spitting up all over the place, but I know that she's just a baby and can't help it.

Exploring the possibility that not all of the other mothers may have been judging her was addressed at a later time. Instead, the focus remained on her ability to access wise mind while coping with a stressful situation and meet her baby's needs.

LEADER: So in that moment it sounds like you were being very mindful of all of the different thoughts and feelings that you were having. Being embarrassed, mad–at them and yourself and the baby all at the same time.

GROUP MEMBER: Yeah, when I was telling myself that she can't help it, she smiled at me (*member smiles*). How could I be upset now?

LEADER: By being fully present in the moment, you were able to appreciate that smile without being distracted by all of the other stress you were feeling.

GROUP MEMBER: Yeah, and then I figured out how to get her home quick as possible and keep her happy.

Cope More Effectively

SPARCS presents many types of skills and coping strategies in order to help participants enhance their ability to manage ongoing extreme stress. These include psychoeducation; identifying emotions and thoughts and their connection to somatic complaints; identifying PTSD triggers; anger management; and problem-solving strategies.

As an example, one of the psychoeducation exercises from the SPARCS manual (DeRosa et al., 2004) is included below. This exercise illustrates the impact of extreme posttraumatic stress on the body. As countless studies have shown across a wide range of problems, it is critical that clinicians not underestimate the power of providing basic information regarding the impact and nature of traumatic stress (Pelcovitz & Kaplan, 1994). Doing this provides teens not only with a common language, but also with validation and knowledge, which foster empowerment–the first step toward freedom to address the problem in a different way.

"Bottle about to Burst" Stress Exercise

A few materials are needed in preparation for the exercise, including two seltzer bottles filled with seltzer, an identical bottle filled with water, and paper towels. A leader explains that one way to think about chronic stress is that all of the feelings get bottled up inside of us. The leader then asks for three volunteers to shake each of the seltzer bottles, while the group members list stressful events they have experienced (e.g., "I've had practically no sleep in the past few days staying up with the baby," "People in my house were fighting a lot," "Something embarrassing happened at school," "My baby is sick," "Someone close to me is having problems"). The first volunteer then quickly opens up the first bottle (one of the seltzer bottles). The group discusses what happened inside the bottle and the parallel process that sometimes occurs when they respond to chronic stress. Group members identify how they themselves or people close to them have "exploded" when the pressure builds in their lives.

Next, the volunteer with the seltzer bottle that actually contains only tap water opens the bottle. This time nothing happens. Leaders explain how sometimes when people keep things bottled up inside, they feel numb, as if they don't have any feelings at all. They feel flat. After the group has had time to discuss this reaction to stress, the final volunteer opens the second seltzer bottle very slowly. With each turn, leaders ask group members to list and discuss possible coping strategies that will decrease the likelihood of an explosion (e.g., "Write in my journal," "Talk to a friend," "Go for a walk," "Watch TV," etc.). Discussing and processing this activity can be a validating and educational intervention to examine how the mind and body work together to manage stress, as well as the power group members have to respond effectively.

Things That "Mess 'U' Up"

Another piece of trauma psychoeducation includes helping participants to identify both adaptive and maladaptive coping strategies they are currently using on a regular basis. Group members are asked to generate a list of ways they cope that cause problems, including things like drinking, doing drugs, spending too much money, driving too fast, going to places that aren't safe, and so on. We call these maladaptive coping strategies "MUPS," for things that "*M*ess '*U*' *Up*." Ford et al. (2003) describe the vicious cycle (see Figure 12.3) that frequently happens among teens struggling with the impact of extreme stress: something stressful happens that triggers unfinished emotional business, which leads to additional stress and using MUPS. MUPS may then in turn cause additional stress and make teens more vulnerable to additional stress and trauma. Group members often report that they were unaware how much they respond automatically to stress when the MUPS take over.

Connect with Others

Enhancing communication skills and increasing perceived social support are critical components of treatment among chronically traumatized ado-

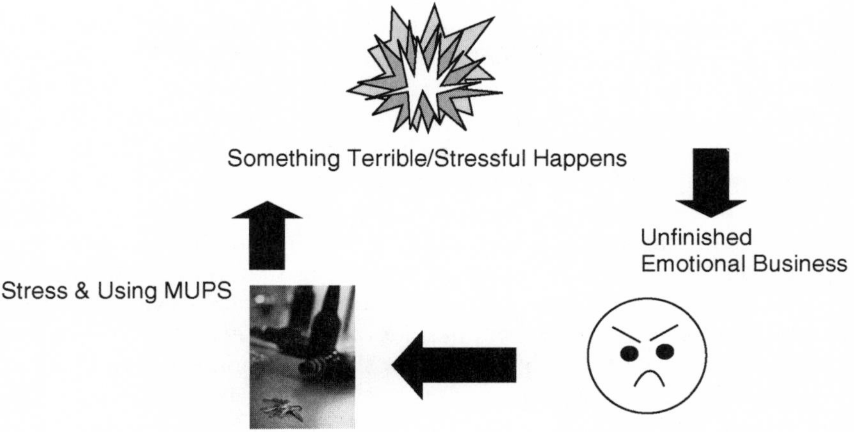

FIGURE 12.3. The MUPS vicious cycle.

lescents in general, and especially among the subgroup of teen mothers, who often feel alienated, unable to trust anyone, and sometimes too ashamed to let others really get to know them. This emotional isolation and distress significantly increase the risk of child abuse among adolescent mothers (Budd, Heilman, & Kane, 2000). SPARCS includes (1) role plays for group members to practice asking for what they want and listening skills for relationships (Miller et al., in press); (2) specific, concrete ways for teens to reach out to others for different kinds of support; and (3) tips for managing triangulation that may occur in their families, in residential care or among friends (Layne et al., 2001). Based upon feedback from group members, the original interpersonal effectiveness skills (Miller et al., in press) were adapted and shortened to one acronym. In order to "keep a relationship or get what you want," it is important to "MAKE A LINK" with that person:

[Be] Mindful.
Act confident.
Keep a calm and gentle manner.
Express your feelings.

A

Let them know you get their point of view.
[Act] Interested.
Negotiate–give to get.
Keep your self-respect.

Over the course of several sessions, group members practice these skills, using scenarios from group members' lives. If participants are initially reluctant to try, group leaders role-play an escalating conflict *without* using the skills, and then ask for group feedback and suggestions. Particularly shy or reluctant participants can initially be given the role of directors to start and stop the role-play action. Examples of role plays include negotiating with one's roommate, assertively but nonaggressively approaching someone in the house for not cleaning up the kitchen, or *gently* confronting a friend who may have disclosed something shared in confidence.

The "L," "*L*et them know you understand their point of view," is often the most challenging. Validation does not require agreeing with other persons; however, letting other people know that their point of view is heard and understood is often experienced as agreeing or giving in. Repeated discussions and debriefing after the role plays are helpful: "How did it feel when the other person really heard you without saying 'but'? Were you more or less likely to hear the other person's point of view then?"

Create Meaning

SPARCS is a strength-based approach that incorporates two elements of meaning making. On the one hand, "meaning making" refers to understanding the impact of the trauma—examining maladaptive expectations, beliefs, and feelings (e.g., helplessness, self-blame, and a sense of injustice) that affect one's worldview and sense of self. Examining these themes may foster choices for the future that are not bound by the trauma narrative. On the other hand, "meaning making" also refers to finding a way to own what has happened, honoring the strength it took to survive and figuring out how to find the benefits of having survived.

Every session devotes some time to Ford et al.'s (2004) "FREEDOM" steps, which specifically address meaning making. FREEDOM is a mnemonic for a "deceptively simple" sequence of skills that enhances the group participants' ability to address the traumatic material in the here-and-now. These skills (see the left-hand column of Table 12.2) are as follows: *F*ocus (i.e., the SOS procedure described earlier); *R*ecognize stress triggers; identify true *E*motions (in the wave of emotional flooding); *E*valuate automatic thoughts; *D*efine goals; articulate *O*ptions, reorienting to a position of strength; and recognize the ways in which one is already *M*aking a meaningful contribution to others and "making a difference" in the world. The group leaders cover the FREEDOM skills in every session—spending from 2 to 15 minutes on them, depending on the needs of the group. This flexibility is important for times when a group member may discuss coping with a current crisis; the therapist can spend more time on the FREEDOM steps to help the adolescent navigate the current situation. There are also sessions dedicated entirely to the FREEDOM steps.

TABLE 12.2. The FREEDOM Steps and Their Application to Allie's Example

Freedom Steps	Description	Comments
Focus (SOS): Slow down Orient yourself Self-check	"I actually did that. I took a breath before I did anything."	Although group members were skeptical at first, Allie was able to explicitly describe taking a breath. The group recognized that she had not "Oriented herself" and in that moment was probably reliving a previous attack and was on automatic pilot.
Recognize trigger	"She attacked me."	The trigger might be from past trauma or the present
Emotions	"Shock, confusion."	Allie's initial response was anger. Continued discussion revealed she was primarily shocked that someone would attack her unprovoked.
Evaluate thoughts	"What's her problem? How could she do this?"	Again, she was trying to make sense out of what was happening.
Define goals: Immediate goal True Goal	"Kill, kill, kill!" "I wanted her to think about this—why would she do this to someone. Maybe then she won't hurt anyone else."	Initially, all Allie wanted to do was retaliate. With further discussion, she explained that her true goal was not revenge but to prevent that student from hurting anyone else—especially those more vulnerable, like her baby.
Options	"Defend myself; strongly say something about her behavior; press charges; get security."	This was also difficult, and other group members helped to identify options.
Make a Contribution	Addressing injustice; heeding[a] her protective instincts	

[a]One of the most important aspects of this exercise is to help volunteers identify the ways in which they were *already* making a personal contribution—not what they should have done in that situation or could do next time, but in what ways they helped others, supported particular values, or established principles *at the time*. In this example, once we had identified that Allie's contribution was to support the value of addressing injustice in the world and the value of protecting those she loved, her entire stance and mood shifted. Once she had been helpless in living with domestic violence; now Allie's response to injustice in the world and her desire to protect others, especially her baby, was immediate and paramount. Discussing the fight in this way shifted the focus from what she did wrong to what she was doing that *did* have value and meaning. This shift allowed her to hear much more than would have been possible with the traditional problem-solving approach. Instead of speaking from a place of numbness and bravado, Allie was moved to tears as group members started to discuss some of the values that she held most dear.

The group leaders ask for a volunteer to discuss a recent stressful event. This might be a conflict with someone or a difficult time with the baby, for example. The group leaders and participants alike help the volunteer to identify each of the FREEDOM steps as they relate to her particular situation. As an example from our group, Allie described a fight that took place at school (see the "Description" column of Table 12.2). She explained that she was attacked, unprovoked, by another girl in the house who (she later found out) wanted to date Allie's boyfriend. Although she initially responded in self-defense, Allie's aggression soon escalated; she physically assaulted the other student and was suspended from school. Both the leaders and group members worked together to help Allie to identify each component of the FREEDOM steps. The "Comments" column of Table 12.2 describes the group's step-by-step process with Allie.

SUMMARY AND CONCLUSIONS

What Went Well

Preliminary data on the group of adolescent mothers who participated in the group described in this chapter suggest a high level of satisfaction with the group process. At intake, the majority of students enrolled in the groups were experiencing significant psychological distress, with 73% scoring in the clinically significant range on the total score of the Youth Outcome Questionnaire (a measure of adolescent emotional and behavioral adjustment). The posttreatment group scores, relative to the pretreatment group scores, on this questionnaire are presented in Figure 12.4. As can be seen, there was a clear trend toward improvement after the group, although this was not statistically significant.

On the Self Satisfaction Survey (a measure of group satisfaction), the adolescents overwhelmingly endorsed statements indicating that they found the group to be helpful. Specifically, 80% felt that they had made progress in achieving their goals; all group members felt hopeful about the group's potential to help them and endorsed a view of the group as cohesive. Anecdotally, the enthusiasm that the adolescent mothers had for the group was indicated by their spontaneously approaching the group home's administration to request permission that the group meet for a longer period of time. Seventy-seven percent of the group members stayed as active members of the group, yielding only a 23% dropout rate. Considering the chaotic nature of these young women's lives, this was a remarkably low dropout rate.

Interviews with the staff indicated that among the positive changes noted several months after the group started were increased cohesiveness and support among the group members. Staff members reported a num-

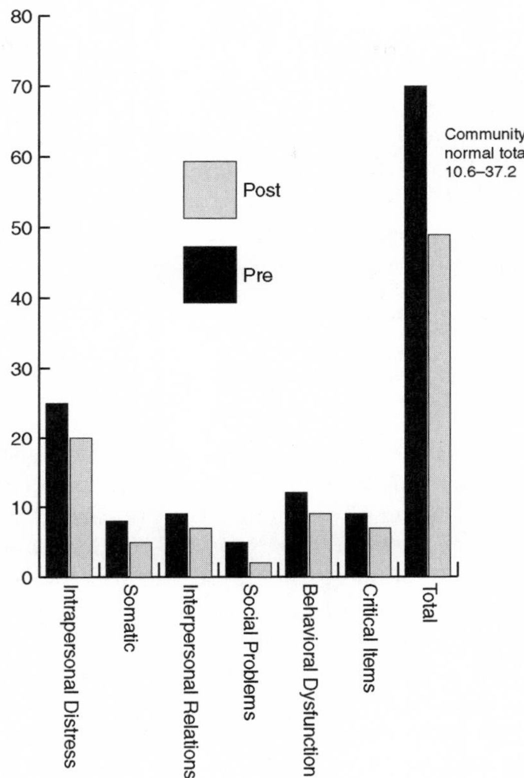

FIGURE 12.4. Pre- and posttreatment scores on the Youth Outcome Questionnaire for our group of adolescent mothers.

ber of incidents where the students found the coping mechanisms taught in the group helpful for themselves and their friends in dealing with difficult situations. In an unexpected outcome, the program's staff told us that since the group started there had been a significant reduction in the number of physical fights between the girls in the program. Although this outcome cannot be directly linked to the group, the perception was that the girls' ability to regulate their affect and solve problems more effectively had improved to such an extent that there were fewer fights.

Challenges

A number of challenges presented themselves during the course of the group. Awareness of these difficulties should facilitate realistic planning and future implementation of this intervention.

Staff Members' Perception of Adolescent Difficulties

The traumatic antecedents of the adolescents' difficulties were quite painful for some staff members to accept. A gradual process of education was necessary to help staff members recognize and respond to the often horrifying histories of physical, sexual, and emotional abuse suffered by the adolescent mothers. The paradigm shift that accompanied viewing complex PTSD behaviors as signs of suffering rather than as behaviors that needed to be suppressed or punished was arrived at only gradually; in several cases, it was met with resistance.

Working with Child Protective Services: Balancing the Need to Protect with the Need to Build Trust

On a number of occasions, the adolescents reported situations that warranted filing a report of suspected child abuse with the local child protective services agency. Although we therapists were careful at the outset of treatment to let the girls know the limits of confidentiality, the group members felt betrayed and angry when information they divulged about their caretakers necessitated a report. Even though intellectually group members were aware that they had to be protected from adults who put them in danger, the adolescents understandably wanted to be in control of how abusive situations in their lives would be handled. When on several occasions during the course of the group it was necessary to file an abuse report, the sense of group cohesiveness and trust suffered. Once feelings of anger and betrayal were addressed and validated, a sense of equilibrium was gradually regained, and ultimately the group recovered.

Training Needs

As the year progressed, it became increasingly clear that the entire staff should have been more actively included in the training for the group. Among the many potential advantages would have been to promote generalizability by having the entire staff reinforce the girls for using the skills taught in the group. In fact, at one point a staff member who had become familiar with the skills taught in the group requested a copy of the manual, so that she could incorporate some of the techniques into her work with the girls. An additional benefit would have been to facilitate making the group a priority in the home's busy schedule. All too often, group sessions were canceled because of competing pressures on the calendar. Had a more inclusive training made the benefits of the group more evident to the entire staff, it is likely that the slot the group filled in the weekly schedule would have been more consistently respected.

Final Thoughts

A beautiful parable is told of a king who greatly valued a diamond that was at the center of his crown. An insecure man, the king took inordinate pleasure in knowing that he owned the largest diamond in the world. One morning he woke up to discover that a flaw had developed right down the center of the diamond. The king was extremely upset, seeing the flaw as a bad omen that threatened his sense of power and invulnerability. He put out a call to the kingdom saying that anybody who was able to fix the crack would be made wealthy beyond his wildest dreams. Jewelers came from around the world to work on the flawed diamond, but were unable to fix the damaged jewel. Ultimately, a wizened old man came and used his engraving tool to carve leaves around the flaw—which now became the trunk of a tree that made the diamond even more magnificent than it was before.

Trauma survivors cannot erase what has happened during the ongoing "hurricane" of chaos and trauma in their lives. However, we hope that this intervention will teach traumatized adolescents skills that enhance their sense of mastery and resilience, and that therapists can help them to make meaning out of their lives as creatively as the wizened old man carved the king's diamond.

REFERENCES

American Psychiatric Association. (2000). *Diagnostic and statistical manual of mental disorders* (4th ed., text rev.). Washington, DC: Author.

Ballenger, J. C., Davidson, J. R. T., Lecrubier, Y., Nutt, D. J., Foa, E. B., Kessler, R. C., McFarlane, A. C., & Shalev, A. Y. (2000). Consensus statement on posttraumatic stress disorder from the International Consensus Group on Depression and Anxiety. *Journal of Clinical Psychiatry, 61*(Suppl. 5), 60–66.

Berenbaum, H. (1996). Childhood abuse, alexithymia and personality disorder. *Journal of Psychosomatic Research, 41*(6), 585–595.

Brown, L., Lourie, K., Zlotnick, C., & Cohn, J. (2000). Impact of sexual abuse on the HIV risk related behavior of adolescents in intensive psychiatric treatment. *American Journal of Psychiatry, 157,* 1413–1415.

Budd, K. S., Heilman, N. E., & Kane, D. (2000). Psychosocial correlates of child abuse potential in multiply disadvantaged adolescent mothers. *Child Abuse and Neglect, 24*(5), 611–625.

Celano, M., Hazzard, A., Webb, C., & McCall, C. (1996). Treatment of traumagenic beliefs among sexually abused girls and their mothers: An evaluation study. *Journal of Abnormal Child Psychology, 24*(1), 1–17.

Cicchetti, D., & Toth, S. (1995). A developmental psychopathology perspective on child abuse and neglect. *Journal of the American Academy of Child and Adolescent Psychiatry, 34*(5), 541–565.

Cloitre, M. (2003). *Treatment for traumatized adolescent girls: Skills training in affective and interpersonal regulation (STAIR)*. Workshop presented at Boston University School of Medicine and The Trauma Clinic's conference, Psychological Trauma: Maturational Processes and Therapeutic Interventions, Boston.

Cook, A., Spinazzola, J., Ford, J., Lanktree, C., Blaustein, M., Cloitre, M., et al. (2005). Complex trauma in children and adolescents. *Psychiatric Annals, 35*(5), 390–398.

Davis, C. G., Nolen-Hoeksema, S., & Larson, J. (1998). Making sense of loss and benefiting from the experience: Two construals of meaning. *Journal of Personality and Social Psychology, 75*(2), 561–574.

DeBellis, M. D. (2002). Developmental traumatology. *Psychoneuroendocrinology, 27,* 155–170.

DeRosa, R., Pelcovitz, D., Rathus, J., Ford, J., Habib, M., Sonnenklar, J., Mahoney, K., Turnbull, A., Sunday, S., Labruna, V., & Kaplan, S. (2005). *Structured Psychotherapy for Adolescents Responding to Chronic Stress (SPARCS): A trauma-focused guide*. Manhasset, NY: North Shore University Hospital.

Eckenrode, J., Ganzel, B., Henderson, C. R., Jr., Smith, E., Olds, D. L., Powers, J., Cole, R., Kitzman, H., & Sidora, K. (2000). Preventing child abuse and neglect with a program of nurse home visitation: The limiting effects of domestic violence. *Journal of the American Medical Association, 284*(11), 1385–1391.

Feiring, C., Taska, L., & Lewis, M. (2002). Adjustment following sexual abuse discovery: The role of shame and attributional style. *Developmental Psychology, 38*(1), 79–92.

Ford, J. D., & Kidd, P. (1998). Early childhood trauma and disorders of extreme stress as predictors of treatment outcome with chronic posttraumatic stress disorder. *Journal of Traumatic Stress, 11*(4), 743–761.

Ford, J. D., Mahoney, K., & Russo, E. M. (2003). *TARGET: Trauma Adaptive Recovery Group Education and Therapy. Nine-session version of participant handouts.* Unpublished manuscript, University of Connecticut Health Center.

Gleason, W. J. (1993). Mental disorders in battered women: An empirical study. *Violence and Victims, 8*(1), 53–68.

Hall, D. K. (1999). "Complex" posttraumatic stress disorder/disorders of extreme stress in sexually abused children. *Journal of Child Sexual Abuse, 8*(4), 51–71.

Herrenkohl, E. C., Herrenkohl, R. C., Egolf, B. P., & Russo, M. (1998). The relationship between early maltreatment and teenage parenthood. *Journal of Adolescence, 21*(3), 291–303.

Hexel, M., & Sonneck, G. (2002). Somatoform symptoms, anxiety, and depression in the context of traumatic life experiences by comparing participants with and without psychiatric diagnoses. *Psychopathology, 35*(5), 303–312.

Kabat-Zinn, J., & Kabat-Zinn, M. (1997). *Everyday blessings: The inner work of mindful parenting.* New York: Hyperion.

Kalil, A., & Danziger, S. K. (2000). How teen mothers are faring under welfare reform. *Journal of Social Issues, 56*(4), 775–798.

Kaplan, S., Pelcovitz, D., Salzinger, S., Mandel, F., Weiner, M., & Labruna, V. (1999). Adolescent physical abuse and risk for suicidal behaviors, *Journal of Interpersonal Violence, 14*(9), 976–988.

Kaplan, S., Pelcovitz, P., Salzinger, S., Mandel, F., Weiner, M., Lesser, M., &

Labruna, V. (1998). Adolescent physical abuse: Risk for adolescent psychiatric disorders. *American Journal of Psychiatry, 155*, 954–959.

Kelley, B. T., Thornberry, T. P., & Smith, C. A. (1997, August). *In the wake of child maltreatment (Juvenile Justice Bulletin)*. Washington, DC: U.S. Department of Justice, Office of Juvenile Justice and Delinquency Prevention.

Kilpatrick, D. G., Saunders, B. E., & Smith, D. W. (2003). *Youth victimization* (Research in Brief). Washington, DC: U.S. Department of Justice, National Institute of Justice.

Krupnick, J. L. (2002). Brief psychodynamic treatment of PTSD. *Journal of Clinical Psychology, 58*(8), 919–932.

Layne, C. M., Pynoos, R. S., Saltzman, W. R., Arslanagic, B., Black, M., Savjak, N., et al. (2001). Trauma, grief-focused group psychotherapy: School-based postwar intervention with traumatized Bosnian adolescents. *Group Dynamics: Theory, Research and Practice, 5*(4), 277–290.

Linehan, M. M. (1993a). *Cognitive-behavioral treatment of borderline personality disorder*. New York: Guilford Press.

Linehan, M. M. (1993b). *Skills training manual for treating borderline personality disorder*. New York: Guilford Press.

Lipschitz, D. S., Winegar, R. K., Nicolaou, A. L., Hartnick, E., Worlfson, M., & Southwick, S. (1999). Perceived abuse and neglect as risk factors for suicidal behavior in adolescent inpatients. *Journal of Nervous and Mental Disease, 187*(1), 32–39.

Lyons-Ruth, K., & Block, D. (1996). The disturbed caregiving system: Relations among childhood trauma, maternal caregiving, and infant affect and attachment. *Infant Mental Health Journal, 17*(3), 257–275.

Marans, S., & Adelman, A. (1997). Experiencing violence in a developmental context. In J. D. Osofsky (Ed.), *Children in a violent society* (pp. 202–222). New York: Guilford Press.

McCann, I. L., & Pearlman, L. A. (1990). *Psychological trauma and the adult survivor: Theory, therapy, and transformation*. New York: Brunner/Mazel.

McGee, R., Wolfe, D., & Olson, J. (2001). Multiple maltreatment, attribution of blame, and adjustment among adolescents. *Developmental Psychopathology, 13(4)*, 827–846.

Menard, S. (2002, February). *Short- and long-term consequences of adolescent victimization* (Youth Violence Research Bulletin). Washington, DC: Office of Juvenile Justice and Delinquency Prevention and the Centers for Disease Control.

Miller, A. L., Rathus, J. H., & Linehan, M. (in press). *Dialectical behavior therapy for adolescents*. New York: Guilford Press.

Miller, A. L., Wyman, S. E., Huppert, J. D., Glassman, S. L., & Rathus, J. H. (2000). Analysis of behavioral skills utilized by suicidal adolescents receiving dialectical behavior therapy. *Cognitive and Behavioral Practice, 7*, 183–187.

Musick, J. S. (1993). *Young, poor and pregnant: The psychology of teenage motherhood*. New Haven, CT: Yale University Press.

Ogawa, J. R., Sroufe, L. A., Weinfield, N. S., Carlson, E. A., & Egeland, B. (1997). Development and the fragmented self: Longitudinal study of dissociative symptomatology in a nonclinical sample. *Developmental Psychopathology, 9*(4), 855–879.

Park, C. L., & Blumberg, C. J. (2002). Disclosing trauma through writing: Testing the meaning making hypothesis. *Cognitive Therapy and Research, 26*(5), 597–616.

Pelcovitz, D., & Kaplan, S. J. (1994). Child witnesses of violence between parents: Psychosocial correlates and implications for treatment. *Child and Adolescent Psychiatric Clinics of North America, 3*(4), 745–758.

Praver, F., DiGiuseppe, R., Pelcovitz, D., Mandel, F. S., & Gaines, R. (2000). A preliminary study of a cartoon measure for children's reactions to chronic trauma. *Child Maltreatment: Journal of the American Professional Society on the Abuse of Children, 5*(3), 273–285.

Pribor, E. F., Yutzy, S. H., Dean, J. T., & Wetzel, R. D. (1993). Briquet's syndrome, dissociation, and abuse. *American Journal of Psychiatry, 150*(10), 1507–1511.

Putnam, F. W. (2003). Ten-year research update review: Child sexual abuse. *Journal of the American Academy of Child and Adolescent Psychiatry, 42*(3), 269–278.

Rathus, J. H., & Miller, A. L. (2000). DBT for adolescents: Dialectical dilemmas and secondary treatment targets. *Cognitive and Behavioral Practice, 7,* 425–434.

Rathus, J. H., & Miller, A. L. (2002). Dialectical behavior therapy adapted for suicidal adolescents. *Suicide and Life-Threatening Behavior, 32,* 146–157.

Rimsza, M. E., Berg, R. A., & Locke, C. (1988). Sexual abuse: Somatic and emotional reactions. *Child Abuse and Neglect, 12*(2), 201–208.

Robins, C. J., & Chapman, A. L. (2004). Dialectical behavior therapy: Current status, recent developments and future directions. *Journal of Personality Disorders, 18*(1), 73–89.

Rodriguez, N., Ryan, S. W., Vande Kemp, H., & Foy, D. W. (1997). Posttraumatic stress disorder in adult female survivors of childhood sexual abuse: A comparison study. *Journal of Consulting and Clinical Psychology, 65*(1), 53–59.

Ross, S. M., (1996). Risk of physical abuse to children of spouse abusing parents. *Child Abuse and Neglect, 20*(7), 589–598.

Roth, S., Newman, E., Pelcovitz, D., van der Kolk, B., & Mandel, F. (1997). Complex PTSD in victims exposed to sexual and physical abuse: Results from the DSM-IV field trial for posttraumatic stress disorder. *Journal of Traumatic Stress, 10,* 539–555.

Roth, S. H., DeRosa, R., & Turner, K. (1996). Cognitive-behavioural interventions for PTSD. *Balliere's Clinical Psychiatry, 2*(2), 281–296.

Saltzman, W. R., Pynoos, R. S., Layne, C. M., Steinberg, A. M., & Aisenberg, E. F. (2001). Trauma and grief focused intervention for adolescents exposed to community violence: Results of a school-based screening and group treatment protocol. *Group Dynamics: Theory, Research and Practice, 5*(4), 291–303.

Sandler, L. S., & Catrone, C. (1983). The adolescent parent: A dual developmental crisis. *Journal of Adolescent Health Care, 4*(2), 281–296.

Saxe, G. N., Chinman, G., Berkowitz, R., Hall, K., Lieberg, G., Schwartz, J., & van der Kolk, B. A. (1994). Somatization in patients with dissociative disorders. *American Journal of Psychiatry, 151*(9), 1329–1334.

Shalev, A. Y., Peri, T., Canetti, L., & Schreiber, S. (1996). Predictors of PTSD in injured trauma survivors: A prospective study. *American Journal of Psychiatry, 153*(2), 219–225.

Singer, M. I., Anglin, T. M., Song, L. Y., & Lunghofer, L. (1995). Adolescents' exposure to violence and associated symptoms of psychological trauma. *Journal of the American Medical Association, 273(6)*, 477–482.

Tamis-Lemonda, C. S., Shannon, J., & Spellmann, M. (2002). Low-income adolescent mothers' knowledge about domains of child development. *Infant Mental Health Journal, 23*(1–2), 88–103.

Teasdale, J. D., Moore, R. G., Hayhurst, H., Pope, M., Williams, S., & Segal, Z. V. (2002). Metacognitive awareness and prevention of relapse in depression: Empirical evidence. *Journal of Consulting and Clinical Psychology, 70(2)*, 275–287.

Ursano, R. J., & Fullerton, C. S. (1999). Posttraumatic stress disorder: Cerebellar regulation of psychological, interpersonal, and biological responses to trauma? *Psychiatry, 62*(4), 325–328.

van der Kolk, B. A. (2003). The neurobiology of childhood trauma and abuse. *Child and Adolescent Psychiatric Clinics of North America, 12*(2), 293–317.

van der Kolk, B. A., Pelcovitz, D., Roth, S., Mandel, F., McFarlane, A., & Herman, J. L. (1996). Dissociation, affect dysregulation and somatization: The complexity of adaptation to trauma. *American Journal of Psychiatry, 153*, 83–93.

Wahler, J. (1990). Some perceptual functions of social networks in coercive mother–child interactions. *Journal of Social and Clinical Psychology, 9*(1), 43–53.

Wekerle, C., Wolfe, D. A., Hawkins, D. L., Pittman, A. L., Glickman, A., & Lovald, B. E. (2001). Childhood maltreatment, posttraumatic stress symptomatology, and adolescent dating violence: Considering the value of adolescent perceptions of abuse and a trauma mediational model. *Developmental Psychopathology, 13*(4), 847–871.

Wolfe, D. A., Scott, K., Wekerle, C., & Pittman, A. L. (2001). Child maltreatment: Risk of adjustment problems and dating violence in adolescence. *Journal of the American Academy of Child and Adolescent Psychiatry, 40*(3), 282–289.

World Health Organization. (1992). *International classification of diseases* (10th rev.), Geneva: Author.

Zlotnick, C., Shea, T. M., Rosen, K., Simpson, E., Mulrenin, K., Begin, A., & Pearlstein, T. (1997). An affect-management group for women with posttraumatic stress disorder and histories of childhood sexual abuse. *Journal of Traumatic Stress, 10*(3), 425–436.

Zlotnick, C., Zakriski, A., Shea, M., Costello, E., Begin, A., Pearlstein, T., & Simpson, E. (1996). The long-term sequelae of sexual abuse: Support for a complex posttraumatic stress disorder. *Journal of Traumatic Stress, 9*, 195–205.

CHAPTER 13

Eye Movement Desensitization and Reprocessing with Traumatized Youth

RICKY GREENWALD

This chapter provides an overview of how eye movement desensitization and reprocessing (EMDR) may be used to treat trauma/loss memories and related symptoms in children and adolescents. The literature on EMDR indicates not only that it works well, but that it may be more efficient than other methods. The reasons for its effect are unclear. Several cases are presented. It is important that clinicians receive formal training to use EMDR, and that it is integrated into a comprehensive trauma-informed treatment approach.

TRAUMA-INFORMED CHILD TREATMENT

A Clinically Relevant Definition of Trauma

There is no question that trauma exposure is ubiquitous among youth in the child welfare system (see Maluccio, Chapter 1, this volume), and that the impact is considerable (see Webb, Chapter 2, this volume). For present purposes, "trauma" will be broadly defined to include any memory of trauma or loss that continues to engender vulnerability, reactivity, and other symptoms, such as unwanted thoughts, emotions, or problem behaviors (Greenwald, 2005). This is a clinically relevant definition, because the focus is not on whether the event itself meets some arbitrary criteria, but whether the clinical *impact of the event* calls for a trauma-informed treatment approach.

Trauma-Informed Treatment: A Phase Approach

When we think of trauma treatment, we tend to focus on the trauma resolution method—perhaps exposure, cognitive processing therapy, or EMDR. However, there is much more to trauma treatment than that. In fact, the trauma resolution component occurs at a late stage in trauma treatment, and is unlikely to be effective unless the earlier tasks have been completed. The following outline and discussion present a data-based comprehensive phase approach to trauma-informed child treatment (Greenwald, 2005).

Note that some phases, such as evaluation, can be accomplished in a set amount of time, whereas other phases may move slowly or quickly, depending on the client and situation. For example, many youth in the child welfare system have been exposed to such significant trauma and loss that they may be cautious about developing a trusting relationship with a therapist, and they may be cautions about getting their hopes up and endorsing personal goals. They may also have difficulty developing effective self-management skills, and they may be reluctant to discuss emotionally challenging content such as trauma memories. Therefore, the phase approach to treatment specifies the tasks that must be accomplished in a certain order, but not how long each task may take.

1. *Evaluation,* including history of trauma/loss, strengths/successes, and circumstances in which the problem symptoms/behaviors occur. The development of the therapeutic relationship begins here, builds steadily, and is critical to further progress.

2. *Trauma-informed case formulation and psychoeducation.* Based on the evaluation, the therapist communicates this understanding to the client. It is important to convey the findings in a sympathetic way that does not focus on blame, but on deeper understanding. This can be accomplished by telling the child's story, describing his or her responses to trauma/loss as typical of kids facing overwhelming events, and explaining how these responses lead to the reactivity and behavior associated with the presenting problems. This explanation opens the door to possible solutions.

3. *Motivational interviewing/goal setting and treatment contracting.* It takes a lot of work, persistence, and courage to overcome trauma-related problems. Children and adolescents are not likely to commit to this process unless we can help them to identify their own goals—things they want for themselves—and to understand how doing these treatment activities can help them to achieve their goals. This is the motivational component; most kids won't do all this work just because someone else says they should.

The treatment contracting involves coming to an agreement to pursue specific activities in service of the young client's goals. These activities typically include doing things to become more safe and stable, to gain better self-control skills and emotional strength, and to face/work through the trauma memories.

4. *Case management* for safety and other needs. It is very difficult to focus on building up strength and skills when an ongoing threat or danger remains in a child's life. If we want to help youth to get over their trauma memories, we have to first make sure that the trauma is not ongoing. We also have to make sure, to the best of our ability, that their basic needs are being met. Otherwise, they will be too distracted by daily survival to focus on trauma recovery.

5. *Parent/caregiver training* for physical and psychological safety and security. We often work with parents and other caregivers to help them provide a more predictable and supportive environment–for example, by becoming more consistent in their discipline style. This helps kids to feel more safe and secure, so they can relax and concentrate on their treatment tasks.

6. *Self control skills training* for stability and improved affect regulation. Training youth in various self-management and self-control skills contributes to their sense of safety and security, because the more they are able to control themselves, the better they are treated by others and the more supportive their environment becomes. Over time, they become more competent and confident, and are able to handle progressively greater challenges.

7. *Trauma resolution.* Once a child feels safe enough and strong enough, the next step is to face the trauma memories and integrate or resolve them. In treatment, this typically involves thinking and talking about these memories over and over again in a structured, systematic way.

8. *Consolidation of gains.* Once the trauma is resolved, the other problems may melt away, but sometimes they don't. The child may have some bad habits or may be missing some skills. Now that the trauma is no longer driving the problem, the child is in a better position to respond positively to other interventions, to solve remaining problems, and to get firmly on a better track toward his or her goals.

9. *Relapse prevention and harm reduction.* It is not enough for a child just to recover from the trauma and get on a better track in life. It is better if the child can also learn from this experience and take measures to prevent a trauma recurrence. This is the time to work with the child and others in his or her life to identify potential risks and take specific actions to mitigate those risks. This makes other bad things less likely to happen in the future. And since no one can guarantee that trauma will never recur, this is also the time to anticipate a possible recurrence and to make specific action plans for recognizing and addressing it when it does happen, so as to minimize the damage.

TRAUMA RESOLUTION METHODS

Although the literature on trauma treatment supports the treatment approach outlined above, there is plenty of room for therapists to make clinical decisions within that model. One of the most important decisions a trauma therapist can make is the selection of a trauma resolution method. The research is very clear on one thing: Structured, focused trauma treatments work better than other approaches (Chemtob & Taylor, 2002). The structured, focused approaches–such as exposure, cognitive processing therapy, and EMDR–all share some important features:

1. A trauma-informed case formulation.
2. A treatment plan that includes a rationale for facing and working through the trauma memory.
3. Specific tasks to help the client prepare to face and work through the trauma.
4. Specific tasks to guide the client in facing and thinking/talking about the trauma memory, in detail and for some extended time period.

Compared to other popular child treatment methods, such as play therapy, active listening, art therapy, psychodynamic therapy, and eclectic treatment, the structured, focused trauma resolution methods offer superior performance in trauma resolution (Chemtob & Taylor, 2002; Cohen, Berliner, & March, 2000). Therapists who rely only on the less structured methods have much smaller chances of providing the best help to their clients. Unless a structured, focused trauma resolution method is used, trauma resolution is likely to occur more slowly (if at all) and less completely.

This does not mean that therapists should totally abandon the other approaches. In fact, for younger children, the structured, focused trauma resolution methods often have to be modified in ways that incorporate other child therapy techniques. For example, when exposure is used with younger children, it may entail using play therapy methods in a structured, focused manner (e.g., Gil, 1991; James, 1989) or creating a "book" with the child, using pictures and words, to tell and retell (i.e., work through) the story of the trauma memory (Deblinger & Heflin, 1996).

Although it is clear that appropriate treatment for kids' trauma/loss memories should include a structured, focused trauma resolution method, there is not yet an obvious front-runner among such methods. There are two main methods to consider: exposure and EMDR. Exposure is the more traditional method, and there is more research on using exposure for trauma/loss resolution with youth (Taylor & Chemtob, 2004). There are many variants of exposure, but the core of the method is that it guides a child to tell the trauma story over and over again in a systematic way. Many of the exposure variants involve homework as well—for example, listening each day to the cassette tape recording of the story told in the exposure session, or writing down the whole story again each day. The research on exposure for children and adolescents has shown it to be efficacious, especially when other treatment components such as psychoeducation, parent training, and self-control skills training are included (Cohen et al., 2000; Taylor & Chemtob, 2004).

EYE MOVEMENT DESENSITIZATION AND REPROCESSING

The other major trauma resolution method for kids is EMDR, the focus of this chapter. EMDR is a recently developed method that is best known as a treatment for traumatic memories and their psychological sequelae. In 1987, a psychology graduate student named Francine Shapiro noticed that her own upsetting thoughts faded when her eyes spontaneously moved rapidly from side to side. Over the next several years, she and her colleagues developed and refined this discovery into a systematic therapeutic approach.

Brief Description

EMDR is a complex method that combines elements of behavioral and client-centered approaches. To oversimplify, the client is asked to concentrate intensely on the most distressing segment of a traumatic memory while moving the eyes rapidly from side to side, by following the therapist's fingers moving across the visual field. (Other methods of alternating bilateral stimulation, including tones in alternating ears, taps on alternating hands, etc., are used when eye movements prove difficult for a client, but these methods have not yet been formally evaluated.)

Following the initial focus on the memory segment, after each *set* of eye movements (of about 30 seconds), the client is asked to report anything that came into awareness—whether this was an image, thought, emotion, or physical sensation (all are common). The focus of the next set is determined by the client's changing status. For example, if the client reports, "Now I'm feeling more anger," the therapist may suggest concentrating on the anger in the next set. The procedure is repeated until the client reports no further distress and can fully embrace a positive perspective. This method has been presented in detail (Greenwald, in press; Shapiro, 2001). Like other methods, EMDR can be modified in various ways to work with children at different developmental levels (Greenwald, 1999).

Research Review

A recent review of randomized treatment studies, published as part of the International Society for Traumatic Stress Studies' treatment guidelines, found EMDR to be an empirically supported efficacious trauma treatment (Chemtob, Tolin, van der Kolk, & Pitman, 2000), with the reservation that EMDR had not yet been directly compared to other validated focused treatments for posttraumatic stress disorder (PTSD) such as prolonged exposure. Since the publication of that review, several studies meeting most of Foa and Meadows's (1997) "gold standard" criteria have directly compared EMDR to validated cognitive-behavioral therapy (CBT) treatments (including an exposure component) for PTSD. Findings across studies indicate that both treatments were, in general, comparably efficacious (Ironson, Freund, Strauss, & Williams, 2002; Lee, Gavriel, Drummond, Richards, & Greenwald, 2002; Power et al., 2002; Taylor et al., 2003). One study (Taylor et al., 2003) found a greater effect for prolonged exposure; the others slightly favored EMDR. Two of the studies (Ironson et al., 2002; Power et al., 2002) suggested that the therapeutic effect may have occurred more quickly for EMDR than for CBT. One study (Ironson et al., 2002) found that the level of distress both during and between sessions was lower for EMDR; this study also found a lower dropout rate in the EMDR group.

These findings suggest that EMDR may be at least equal to other CBT approaches in efficacy and acceptability, while being more efficient (i.e., with EMDR, much less homework is required, and the treatment effect may be achieved in fewer sessions). However, it would be premature to draw this conclusion. There are many CBT approaches, not all of which were compared; furthermore, such findings need to be replicated and elaborated. Also, one study found that EMDR fared much worse than CBT in terms of dropout rates as well as outcomes for treatment completers (Devilly & Spence, 1999). Unfortunately, significant methodological problems make that study difficult to interpret (see Chemtob et al., 2000; Lee et al., 2002).

There is less research on EMDR for children and adolescents as compared than on EMDR for adults. Early case reports were positive and consistent with findings on similar treatment of adults, except that child treatment appeared to be even more rapid (e.g., Cocco & Sharpe, 1993; Greenwald, 1993, 1994; Pellicer, 1993; Shapiro, 1991). For example, one report (Greenwald, 1994) described the one- to two-session treatment of five children traumatized by a hurricane, and found that all returned to pretrauma functioning, with gains maintaining or increasing at a 1-month follow-up.

Case studies in which EMDR was incorporated into a comprehensive trauma-informed treatment approach have also been positive (Greenwald,

2000, 2002). One such study (Greenwald, 2002) reported on the treatment of six teens with school-related problems, and found that all had reduced posttraumatic stress symptoms, reduced discipline problems, and improved academic performance. However, EMDR's specific contribution to this outcome cannot be determined, since other interventions were also used.

Several controlled studies testing EMDR for youth have also been reported. These are of varying quality. One study of 10 adolescents institutionalized for sex offenses found that three EMDR sessions (focusing on the participants' own trauma) led to decreased disturbance, increased sense of cognitive control, and increased empathy for their victims, as well as some spontaneous attempts at victim restitution (Datta & Wallace, 1996). Generally improved behavior in the school and the community was also reported, up to a year after treatment. Limitations include the use of nonequivalent control groups and lack of established validity for the primary outcome measure. Given these problems, this study is probably best viewed as a case series.

Another report (Puffer, Greenwald, & Elrod, 1998) described a wait-list design study of 20 children and adolescents who were nonrandomly assigned (according to convenience of scheduling) to EMDR treatment or delayed treatment. Treatment was a single session; the focus was a single trauma or loss. Puffer conducted all treatment and assessment (using several measures) at pretreatment, posttreatment, and a 1- to 2-month follow-up. There was no change during the 1-month no-treatment delay, and significant improvement between the first and last scores on all measures. On the best measure of trauma symptoms (the Impact of Event Scale), of the 17 participants starting in the clinical range, 11 moved to nonclinical levels and 3 others dropped 12 or more points, while the other 3 stayed the same. Problematic design features included lack of randomization, lack of independent assessment (although no subjective scoring was involved), and use of a therapist with only partial EMDR training. Also, 3 participants had ongoing sources of distress, making recovery unlikely. Still, the results were quite positive, although somewhat more variable than in other studies.

Several studies have compared EMDR to "standard care" or to a nonspecific treatment. One such study (Soberman, Greenwald, & Rule, 2002) compared standard care plus three sessions of EMDR to standard care for 29 boys ages 10–16 with serious conduct problems who were in either residential or day treatment. They found that EMDR led to significant reductions in both reactivity to the targeted memories and severity of the primary identified problem behaviors. Limitations included use of a single therapist and lack of independent assessment.

Scheck, Schaeffer, and Gillette (1998) compared two sessions of

EMDR with two sessions of active listening (AL). Participants were 60 females between the ages of 16 and 24, who were actively pursuing high-risk behaviors (substance abuse, unsafe sex, criminal acts, suicide attempts, etc.) and who had histories of trauma. This study included random assignment, 24 well-trained therapists, independent blind assessment, and multiple standardized measures. Although both groups improved at posttreatment, EMDR outperformed AL on all five measures, with significant differences on four of the five. The posttreatment gains for the group receiving EMDR were also clinically significant, with mean scores falling within one standard deviation of the nonclinical norms on all measures, whereas for the group receiving AL, only one of the measures was in the nonclinical range. Two measures readministered at a 90-day follow-up showed maintenance of gains for the group receiving EMDR. This study found no differences between the responses of the young adults and those of the older adolescents (J. Schaeffer, personal communication, November 1996), in that EMDR was equally effective. This study was limited by failure to assess behavioral outcomes.

Rubin et al. (2001) reported only nonsignificant trends favoring EMDR with a challenging child guidance center population (n = 39, ages 6–15). Participants in each treatment group had the same therapists, and randomization determined which children would have EMDR included in their otherwise similar eclectic treatment. Reasonable efforts were made to ensure treatment fidelity for EMDR. Unfortunately, the researchers relied on a single outcome measure (the Child Behavior Checklist) that does not assess posttraumatic stress, and that is known to be relatively insensitive to change.

There are only three studies in which EMDR has been compared to a credible alternative trauma treatment for youth. Chemtob, Nakashima, Hamada, and Carlson (2002) reported very positive results in using EMDR with 32 children and adolescents traumatized by Hurricane Iniki in Kauai. Only those who did not respond to a generally effective previous CBT small-group program were offered EMDR. The design featured a delayed-treatment control group, independent assessment with several standardized measures, and five therapists with varying levels of EMDR training and experience. The treatment protocol was clearly specified, and a number of efforts were made to ensure treatment fidelity. The participants averaged a 58% reduction on the primary trauma measure following three sessions, with these results holding several months later. The primary limitation was the lack of an alternative-treatment control group at the time that EMDR was being delivered. Thus, although EMDR did work for these youth who did not respond to the prior treatment, we still don't know how the participants might have responded to additional sessions of the other treatment.

An Iranian study (Jaberghaderi, Greenwald, Rubin, Zand, & Dolatabadi, 2004) compared EMDR to CBT for 14 sixth-grade girls who had been sexually abused and who suffered from clinically significant posttraumatic stress symptoms. Participants were randomly assigned and received up to 12 sessions of either CBT or EMDR treatment. Assessment of posttraumatic stress symptoms and problem behaviors was completed at pretreatment and 2 weeks posttreatment. Both treatments showed large effect sizes on the posttraumatic symptom outcomes, and a medium effect size on the behavior outcome, all statistically significant. A non-significant trend on self-reported posttraumatic stress symptoms favored EMDR over CBT. Treatment efficiency was calculated by dividing change scores by number of sessions; EMDR was significantly more efficient, with large effect sizes on each outcome. Limitations included small *n*, a single therapist for each treatment condition, no independent verification of treatment fidelity, and no long-term follow-up.

Finally, a Dutch study (de Roos, Greenwald, de Jongh, & Noorthoorn, 2004) compared EMDR to CBT for 38 children (ages 4–18) who had been affected by the Enschedde fireworks disaster in the Netherlands and who presented for treatment at the local community mental health center. Participants were randomly assigned to eight therapists who were trained in both methods, and then again randomly assigned to treatment condition. Participants were assessed on posttraumatic stress, related symptoms, and problem behaviors at pretreatment, posttreatment, and 3 months post-treatment. Both treatments were highly effective, with no significant differences on outcomes. EMDR was significantly more efficient than CBT in achieving termination criteria, with an average of 3.17 sessions for EMDR as compared to an average of 4 sessions for CBT.

In sum, the child/adolescent literature on EMDR is basically consistent with the adult literature. It is clear that EMDR works well, probably about as well as the other proven-effective trauma treatments. It is possible that EMDR works better than other trauma treatments, and likely that EMDR works more quickly. However, the literature is only suggestive on these latter points, and more research needs to be done.

Meanwhile, there is no evidence that there is any reason to avoid using EMDR for the portion of treatment that involves helping the client to resolve trauma/loss memories. Negative "side effects" (e.g., clients' becoming more upset) have been reported, but mainly by those attempting to use EMDR in ways that were clearly inappropriate (see Greenwald, 1996a). Clinicians formally trained in EMDR generally agree that EMDR is less risky than alternative trauma resolution methods (Lipke, 1994/1995)—perhaps because clients can more easily tolerate EMDR as compared to exposure, and/or because with EMDR, so much resolution occurs within the session.

Pending further research findings, many clinicians have chosen to obtain EMDR training because of the "word of mouth" reports as well as personal experience. Many therapists and clients will describe their experiences with EMDR as being qualitatively different from, and more effective than, any other therapy experience they have had. Although the research literature has not yet established EMDR as the trauma/loss treatment of choice, it has at least established EMDR as a responsible choice.

Why Does EMDR Work?

The underlying mechanism or mechanisms of EMDR are not known at this time. Shapiro (2001) has suggested that the procedure somehow induces adaptive information processing, whereby "stuck" traumatic material can be accessed and rapidly integrated in a healthy way. Along these lines, others have speculated that the purported information-processing effect may be related to rapid-eye-movement dreaming (see Greenwald, 1995; Stickgold, 2002). Taking a different tack, and not addressing the possible effect of the eye movements, others (Hyer & Brandsma, 1997; Sweet, 1995) have pointed out that the EMDR procedure is quite comprehensive in incorporating many elements believed to be effective in trauma therapy.

The question of how EMDR works is far from resolved, and in particular the role (if any) of the eye movements remains a mystery. One possible role for the eye movements is that they force the client to concentrate on something in the room (the therapist's moving fingers) at the same time as concentrating on the trauma memory. This dual focus may help to keep the trauma memory from becoming overwhelming (Kavanagh, Freese, Andrade, & May, 2001), so that it can be "digested" in manageable doses. It is likely that multiple components of EMDR each contribute some portion of the treatment effect.

CHILDREN HELPED WITH EMDR

There are several published sources providing detailed case reports of children who have been helped with EMDR (Cocco & Sharpe, 1993; Greenwald, 1994, 1998, 1999, 2000b, 2002; Lovett, 1999; Pellicer, 1993; Tinker & Wilson, 1999). Several cases are now presented here from my own caseload, to portray how EMDR might be used and the different types of children who might benefit from EMDR. Identifying information has been altered to protect the privacy of the children and families. The first vignette includes a lot of detail to illustrate the process; the others are briefer.

Jennie

Jennie was a 10-year-old girl who, at age 6, had been raped and tortured daily for a week by a small group of older boys in school, until she finally told her mother. When the school failed to respond, Jennie was removed to prevent recurrence, and tutored at home. She developed PTSD with numerous symptoms, including intrusive memories, bedwetting, nightmares, social withdrawal, and poor personal hygiene. Since the torture experience had involved orders to read aloud and perform in certain ways, Jennie later had a very hard time with structured academic activities, which triggered the torture memories. She received 2 years of psychotherapy, but made only slight improvement. She continued to experience an appropriate and supportive family environment.

Four years after the trauma, with symptoms unabated, Jennie's mother enrolled her in a pilot study involving EMDR. Just prior to EMDR treatment, she was assessed with the Parent Report of Posttraumatic Symptoms (PROPS) and the Child Report of Posttraumatic Symptoms (CROPS), covering a broad spectrum of posttraumatic symptomatology (Greenwald & Rubin, 1999). She was also assessed with the Subjective Units of Distress Scale (SUDS), a 0–10 self-report scale of current reactivity to the traumatic memory (Wolpe, modified by Shapiro, 1989), and the Problem Rating Scale (PRS), a parent rating of the present severity of the problems that the parent has identified as being of greatest concern (Greenwald, 1996b). She had one introductory and five treatment sessions over a 2-month period, and was reassessed at 2 months after the end of treatment.

Jennie expressed considerable discomfort at the prospect of deliberately facing her traumatic memories. Therefore, the therapist practiced having Jennie call out "Stop!" to make the therapist's hand stop moving, to emphasize that Jennie could be in control in this situation. Then the therapist helped Jennie to select images that might help her to begin to gain some sense of mastery over the memory (Greenwald, 1999). She chose to imagine herself as more powerful—first by wielding a baseball bat, and then by becoming a bear. With each image in turn, she was asked to concentrate intensely on the image ("Notice how heavy the bat is, how you feel when you hold it . . . ") while moving her eyes back and forth as described above. Following this exercise, she did indeed report feeling stronger and more confident, and was finally willing to begin to face the memory.

Jennie was asked to select the most upsetting segment of the memory that she was willing to think about. She was asked to concentrate on the visual image (being held at knife point), along with the associated self-statement ("I'm helpless"), emotion (scared), and physical sensation (sick to her stomach). She was instructed to maintain this focus during about

20–30 seconds of eye movements–but also to allow spontaneous changes in focus, should any occur. Then she was asked to take a deep breath, rest a moment, and report on anything she may have noticed. This routine was repeated perhaps a dozen times, with her previous response generally serving as a starting point for the new set of eye movements. Although at first she reported that the image became more vivid, along with a stronger sense of terror, after a few sets she began to report a steady decrease in the potency of the image. As rated with the SUDS, the image began at 7 (on a 0–10 scale with 10 being the highest level of distress), moved up to 9, and eventually went down to 5.

After about 35 minutes, Jennie said she felt very tired and wanted to stop. Before completing the session, she was asked to concentrate again on the positive images (with eye movements), and then (also with eye movements) was asked to imagine packing the memory into a secure container where it could stay until the next meeting. This type of exercise is often done at the end of a session, to consolidate gains and facilitate recomposure (Greenwald, 1999).

The next two sessions generally followed this routine and lasted about an hour each. The same positive images were routinely introduced, and sometimes Jennie would spontaneously inject the positive image into the memory–for example, by imagining beating the boys up with the bat. She was able to master several disturbing parts of the memory in each session.

On a technical note, even when the SUDS rating goes down to 0, work on that memory segment is not over. The client is then asked to select an adaptive reframe related to the memory, such as "I'm safe now," or "It wasn't my fault." If the client cannot endorse this view wholeheartedly, the obstacles to that endorsement are identified and treated with EMDR until no obstacle remains. Finally, the client is asked to notice any residual body tension or discomfort, which must also be treated to full resolution.

Once the memory itself appeared to be worked through, EMDR was applied to related targets, such as the location of the trauma and the faces of the perpetrators. EMDR was then applied to current triggers, such as seeing one of the perpetrators on the street, or being told by her tutor to read aloud. Jennie was also able to fully endorse, at this and later sessions, the following statements: "It's over now," "I can keep myself safe," "It wasn't my fault," "I'm a good person," and "I'm pretty."

The fourth EMDR session lasted only 15 minutes, and involved reviewing previously addressed material and applying EMDR to anything that still seemed to carry any degree of distress greater than 0. There was an additional memory segment that had been missed before, and there was more work done on current triggers related to personal attractiveness as well as educational activities. The fifth and final session was also short, and involved additional work on a few targets that still carried minuscule reported levels of distress.

Jennie's pretreatment combined score on the CROPS and PROPS (broad-spectrum posttraumatic symptoms) was 54, for over the suggested "clinical" cutoff of 36. At the 2-month posttreatment follow-up, her combined score was 26, well below the cutoff. The SUDS (current reactivity to the memory) began at 7 and was 0 at follow-up. The PRS (parent rating of biggest problems, using a similar 0–10 scale) included the following items: refusal to learn on command; self-worth (posture, dress, hygiene); and sleep problems (nightmares, bedwetting). The pretreatment PRS scores were, respectively, 10, 9, and 5; at follow-up, the respective scores were 1, 1.5, and 0.

Jennie's responses to this course of treatment were fascinating. On the physiological level, her mother reported that Jennie experienced a severe facial rash for a couple of days following the fourth session, and that she grew several inches taller within the 4 months following the beginning of treatment. Her mother also reported occasional emotional volatility between sessions, and then generally improved mood and functioning—as well as some turbulence and confusion in the family, as Jennie was apparently "suddenly catching up on 4 years of her development." She worked with her tutor with increased comfort, and also began venturing outside her home for education, at first by attending a course with her mother at the local community college. Jennie herself, who had only grudgingly participated in the treatment, later made a work of art for a community exhibit on the theme of interpersonal violence. Her piece featured the following statement: "If you are raped, try EMDR. I did, and I feel good now."

An informal follow-up occurred 2 years later, when Jennie and her mother read a draft of this report. Jennie was still occasionally bothered by the memory, but seemed to cope well when it comes up. She was also able to discuss it with ease. Jennie was now very active in her Girl Scouts group and had won several awards for athletics, in addition to continued academic success. Her mother told me, "I don't think you conveyed how much of an impact [EMDR] had. She's done so many things she could never have done otherwise. It has opened up all of our lives—she's no longer a handicapped child."

Angela

Angela was an 11-year-old girl living with her grandmother, who had recently adopted her. When Angela was 7, she disclosed that her stepfather had been molesting her regularly. Her mother refused to ask the stepfather to leave, so she gave up Angela instead. Angela's grandmother brought her to treatment at a child guidance center because of concerns about Angela's bossiness with peers, her extended temper tantrums following her weekly visit with her mother, and her fears about testifying in court regarding the abuse she had experienced in her original home.

Treatment began with relationship building, working with the grandmother to help her feel better about how she managed Angela during the challenging times, and helping Angela with some problem-solving skills regarding peer interactions. It took 3 months for the therapist to try EMDR with Angela, and even then the first focus was not on the major trauma memories, but on a recent upsetting event: her mother's failing to show up for a scheduled visit. The EMDR session took less than 10 minutes, and follow-up conversations with the grandmother indicated that Angela's visit-related tantrums were much less severe following this brief EMDR session than previously.

This small success gave Angela a positive experience with EMDR, making her more willing to try the procedure with more emotionally challenging memories. Over the next couple of months, Angela was able to get through six more EMDR sessions, focused on the abuse memories as well as the rejection by her mother. A final EMDR session focused on a feared future event: testifying in court about the abuse. When EMDR is used with a feared future event, it is done pretty much the same as with a past event–going over and over the distressing parts until there is no more distress and the child has developed a more self-confident perspective.

After 6 months of treatment had passed, the EMDR portion was completed (even during this time period, relatively few sessions had included EMDR). Angela's tantrums were much less intense and prolonged, and the district attorney was so impressed with Angela's ability to discuss the abuse that he finally initiated prosecution. Angela also seemed to have become happier and was in a good mood more of the time. There was still more work to do in treatment; for example, Angela had a long-standing vulnerability to coercion, so the next focus was on assertiveness training. However, the trauma-related problems had been substantially addressed, and no longer seemed to interfere with the efforts she was making in various areas.

Charles

Charles was a 15-year-old boy who had recently been incarcerated for several months and was still legally in state custody, even though he was living with his family again. He had been in trouble for a variety of charges related to fighting, robbery, and selling drugs. His parents cared about him and were supportive, but there were a variety of stresses at home, in school, and on the street. Charles expressed a deep desire to stay out of trouble and live a good life. However, he was not all that hopeful, because

"My problem is my anger. I get mad, and I can lose everything. I have a lot of anger; it's just the way I am, and it's always going to be that way." His trauma/loss history included the following: age 6, the death of a younger brother; age 10, death of a grandparent; age 11, witnessing an older sister buying crack cocaine; age 12, witnessing an uncle commit a murder.

A trauma-informed treatment approach was used (see Greenwald, 2002), including motivational interviewing and self-control skills training as a lead-up to trauma resolution work. Charles missed many sessions, but seemed to be engaged when he did attend, and gradually was getting more control over his life (e.g., doing better in school, using better restraint when provoked). He came to appreciate the opportunity to talk to his therapist and felt that he was getting something out of it.

After 5 months, Charles had attended eight sessions. At this point EMDR was introduced as a way to reduce the piled-up stress related to the trauma/loss memories, with the hope of reducing the anger as well. In session 9, he did EMDR with the memory of the death of his younger brother. This session lasted about 40 minutes. At first, Charles reported feeling sad, angry, and to blame. Rather quickly he recognized that he was not to blame, that it was no one's fault, and that these things just happen. After that, he went over and over certain parts of the memory, with the sad and angry feelings gradually fading. By the end of the session, he reported no further distress related to the memory.

He showed up the following week and did EMDR with two other significant memories. These went quickly, and by the end of a 30-minute session he reported no further distress from either of these. When he returned again 2 weeks later, he reported no distress on the final memory either (witnessing the murder) but agreed to do EMDR with it anyway, just in case. With repeated sets of eye movements, he reported that he became progressively more comfortable with the memory, even though it hadn't been bothering him in the first place. (It is not unusual for other trauma memories to lose much of their power once the first major trauma has been resolved.)

In subsequent sessions Charles reported that he was able to think of any of these memories without getting upset. He also reported that he was not getting angry as strongly or as frequently as before, and that his anger did not overwhelm him any more: "When I get mad now, I have time to think before I just do something stupid."

There were four more sessions over the 2 months following completion of EMDR. These focused further on coping skills and on anticipating future challenges. Charles was feeling more confident about his ability to succeed in life, and he was doing well on a daily basis. He was avoiding high-risk situations, handling provocation without getting himself into trouble, doing well in school, and starting to get involved in organized sports again.

SUMMARY AND CONCLUSION

Since so many youth in child welfare have problems that are related, at least in part, to their trauma/loss history, it is important to use a trauma-informed case formulation and treatment plan. This treatment plan should also incorporate other effective interventions. When the trauma is addressed and resolved, there is a better chance that the other interventions will be effective.

A central component of trauma treatment is a trauma resolution activity that helps the client face and work through the trauma memory. This should be accomplished with a structured, focused trauma treatment method that has been empirically validated, such as exposure or EMDR. Available evidence indicates that these treatments seem to be about equal in effect, and that EMDR may be more efficient.

EMDR is a complex intervention, and those using it should obtain formal training as well as follow-up supervision. EMDR should be used within the context of a comprehensive trauma-informed treatment approach. Use of such an approach, including a structured, focused trauma resolution method such as EMDR, can enable therapists to become more effective in helping children and adolescents.

ACKNOWLEDGMENTS

The case of Jennie was first published in Greenwald (1998). Copyright 1998 by Sage Publications. Adapted by permission.

REFERENCES

Chemtob, C. M., Nakashima, J., Hamada, R., & Carlson, J. G. (2002). Brief treatment for elementary school children with disaster-related posttraumatic stress disorder: A field study. *Journal of Clinical Psychology, 58,* 99–112.

Chemtob, C. M., & Taylor, T. L. (2002). The treatment of traumatized children. In R. Yehuda (Ed.), *Trauma survivors: Bridging the gap between intervention research and practice* (pp. 75–126). Washington, DC: American Psychiatric Press.

Chemtob, C. M., Tolin, D. F., van der Kolk, B. A., & Pitman, R. K. (2000). Eye movement desensitization and reprocessing. In E. B. Foa, T. M. Keane, & M. J. Friedman (Eds.), *Effective treatments for PTSD: Practice guidelines from the International Society for Traumatic Stress Studies* (pp. 139–154). New York: Guilford Press.

Cocco, N., & Sharpe, L. (1993). An auditory variant of eye movement desensitization in a case of childhood posttraumatic stress disorder. *Journal of Behavior Therapy and Experimental Psychiatry, 24,* 373–377.

Cohen, J. A., Berliner, L., & March, J. S. (2000). Treatment of children and adolescents. In E. B. Foa, T. M. Keane, & M. J. Friedman (Eds.), *Effective treatments for PTSD: Practice guidelines from the International Society for Traumatic Stress Studies* (pp. 106–138). New York: Guilford Press.

Datta, P. C., & Wallace, J. (1996). *Enhancement of victim empathy along with reduction in anxiety and increase of positive cognition of sex offenders after treatment with EMDR.* Paper presented at the annual conference of the EMDR International Association, Denver, CO.

de Roos, C., Greenwald, R., de Jongh, A., & Noorthoorn, E. (2004, November). *A controlled comparison of CBT and EMDR for disaster-exposed children.* Poster session presented at the annual meeting of the International Society for Traumatic Stress Studies, New Orleans, LA.

Deblinger, E., & Heflin, A. H. (1996). *Treating sexually abused children and their nonoffending parents: A cognitive behavioral approach.* Thousand Oaks, CA: Sage.

Devilly, G. J., & Spence, S. H. (1999). The relative efficacy and treatment distress of EMDR and a cognitive behavior trauma treatment protocol in the amelioration of posttraumatic stress disorder. *Journal of Anxiety Disorders, 13*(1–2), 131–157.

Foa, E. B., & Meadows, E. A. (1997). Psychosocial treatments for posttraumatic stress disorder: A critical review. *Annual Review of Psychology, 48,* 449–480.

Gil, E. (1991). *The healing power of play: Working with abused children.* New York: Guilford Press.

Greenwald, R. (1993). Treating children's nightmares with EMDR. *EMDR Network Newsletter, 3*(1), 7–9.

Greenwald, R. (1994). Applying eye movement desensitization and reprocessing (EMDR) to the treatment of traumatized children: Five case studies. *Anxiety Disorders Practice Journal, 1,* 83–97.

Greenwald, R. (1995). Eye movement desensitization and reprocessing (EMDR): A new kind of dreamwork? *Dreaming, 5,* 51–55.

Greenwald, R. (1996a). The information gap in the EMDR controversy. *Professional Psychology: Research and Practice, 27,* 67–72.

Greenwald, R. (1996b). Psychometric review of the Problem Rating Scale. In B. H. Stamm (Ed.), *Measurement of stress, trauma, and adaptation* (pp. 242–243). Lutherville, MD: Sidran.

Greenwald, R. (1998). Eye movement desensitization and reprocessing (EMDR): New hope for children suffering from trauma and loss. *Clinical Child Psychology and Psychiatry, 3,* 279–287.

Greenwald, R. (1999). *Eye movement desensitization and reprocessing (EMDR) in child and adolescent psychotherapy.* Northvale, NJ: Aronson.

Greenwald, R. (2000). A trauma-focused individual therapy approach for adolescents with conduct disorder. *International Journal of Offender Therapy and Comparative Criminology, 44,* 146–163.

Greenwald, R. (2002). Motivation–adaptive skills–trauma resolution (MASTR) therapy for adolescents with conduct problems: An open trial. *Journal of Aggression, Maltreatment, and Trauma, 6,* 237–261.

Greenwald, R. (2005). *Child trauma handbook.* New York: Haworth Press.

Greenwald, R. (in press). *EMDR: A trauma-informed treatment approach.* New York: Haworth Press.

Greenwald, R., & Rubin, A. (1999). Brief assessment of children's posttraumatic symptoms: Development and preliminary validation of parent and child scales. *Research on Social Work Practice, 9,* 61–75.

Hyer, L., & Brandsma, J. M. (1997). EMDR minus eye movements equals good psychotherapy. *Journal of Traumatic Stress, 10,* 515–522.

Ironson, G., Freund, B., Strauss, J. L., & Williams, J. (2002). Comparison of two treatments for traumatic stress: A communitybased study of EMDR and prolonged exposure. *Journal of Clinical Psychology, 58,* 113–128.

Jaberghaderi, N., Greenwald, R., Rubin, A., Zand, S. O., & Dolatabadi, S. (2004). A comparison of CBT and EMDR for sexually abused Iranian girls. *Clinical Psychology and Psychotherapy, 11,* 358–368.

James, B. (1989). *Treating traumatized children: New insights and creative interventions.* Lexington, MA: Lexington Books.

Kavanagh, D. J., Freese, S., Andrade, J., & May, J. (2001). Effects of visuospatial tasks on desensitization to emotive memories. *British Journal of Clinical Psychology, 40,* 267–280.

Lee, C., Gavriel, H., Drummond, P., Richards, J., & Greenwald, R. (2002). Treatment of PTSD: Stress inoculation training with prolonged exposure compared to EMDR. *Journal of Clinical Psychology, 58,* 1071–1089.

Lipke, H. (1995). Eye movement desensitization and reprocessing (EMDR): A quantitative study of clinician impressions of effects and training requirements. In F. Shapiro, *Eye movement desensitization and reprocessing: Basic principles, protocols, and procedures* (pp. 376–386). New York: Guilford Press. (Original work published 1994)

Lovett, J. (1999). *Small wonders: Healing childhood trauma with EMDR.* New York: Free Press.

Pellicer, X. (1993). Eye movement desensitization treatment of a child's nightmares: A case report. *Journal of Behavior Therapy and Experimental Psychiatry, 24,* 73–75.

Power, K. G., McGoldrick, T., Brown, K., Buchanan, R., Sharp, D., Swanson, V., & Karatzias, A. (2002). A controlled comparison of eye movement desensitisation and reprocessing versus exposure plus cognitive restructuring, versus waiting list in the treatment of posttraumatic stress disorder. *Clinical Psychology and Psychotherapy, 9,* 299–318.

Puffer, M. K., Greenwald, R., & Elrod, D. E. (1998). A single session EMDR study with twenty traumatized children and adolescents [Electronic version]. *Traumatology, 3*(2). Retrieved from www.fsu.edu/~trauma/v3i2art6.html

Rubin, A., Bischofshausen, S., ConroyMoore, K., Dennis, B., Hastie, M., Melnick, L., Reeves, D., & Smith, T. (2001). The effectiveness of EMDR in a child guidance center. *Research on Social Work Practice, 11,* 435–457.

Scheck, M. M., Schaeffer, J. A., & Gillette, C. S. (1998). Brief psychological intervention with traumatized young women: The efficacy of eye movement desensitization and reprocessing. *Journal of Traumatic Stress, 11,* 25–44.

Shapiro, F. (1989). Efficacy of the eye movement desensitization procedure in the treatment of traumatic memories. *Journal of Traumatic Stress, 2,* 199–223.

Shapiro, F. (1991). Eye movement desensitization and reprocessing: A cautionary note. *The Behavior Therapist, 14,* 188.

Shapiro, F. (2001). *Eye movement desensitization and reprocessing: Basic principles, protocols and procedures* (2nd ed.). New York: Guilford Press.

Soberman, G. B., Greenwald, R., & Rule, D. L. (2002). A controlled study of eye movement desensitization and reprocessing (EMDR) for boys with conduct problems. *Journal of Aggression, Maltreatment, and Trauma, 6*, 217–236.

Stickgold, R. (2002). EMDR: A putative neurobiological mechanism of action. *Journal of Clinical Psychology, 58,* 61–75.

Sweet, A. (1995). A theoretical perspective on the clinical use of EMDR. *The Behavior Therapist, 18,* 5–6.

Taylor, S., Thordarson, D. S., Maxfield, L., Fedoroff, I. C., Lovell, K., & Ogrodniczuk, J. (2003). Comparative efficacy, speed, and adverse effects of three PTSD treatments: Exposure therapy, EMDR, and relaxation training. *Journal of Consulting and Clinical Psychology, 71,* 330–338.

Taylor, T. L., & Chemtob, C. M. (2004). Efficacy of treatment for child and adolescent traumatic stress. *Archives of Pediatric and Adolescent Medicine, 158,* 786–791.

Tinker, R. H., & Wilson, S. A. (1999). *Through the eyes of a child: EMDR with children.* New York: Norton.

PART III

ISSUES AND PROPOSALS FOR COLLABORATION BETWEEN CHILD WELFARE AND MENTAL HEALTH

CHAPTER 14

The View from the Child Welfare System

VINCENT J. FONTANA
MAYU P. B. GONZALES

The 21st century promises to be one that will pose a great many challenges and problems for those professionals concerned with the welfare of children and families. According to former U.S. Surgeon General David Satcher (U.S. Department of Health and Human Services, 1999), approximately 25% of children in the United States have a mental health problem that affects their functioning at home and school. Melnyk et al. (2002) stated that 70% of children and teens affected by mental health problems do not receive any treatment. Today the provision of mental health services represents one of the largest health problems facing foster children in particular. Over 400,000 children in the U.S. foster care system have significant and often unmet health care needs. Only about 25% of children in foster care receive the mental health services they require at any given time (Myers, 2004). There is therefore a critical need for the development of innovative, multidisciplinary, community-based approaches that are effective in the treatment and management of the mental health of foster children.

This chapter reviews the interrelationship between child welfare and mental health—a relationship that is critical to providing high-quality, effective mental health care to children in need. Barriers that must be recognized and overcome in the provision of mental health services in the child welfare system are discussed. There are many apparent impediments that should be removed, and a variety of innovative treatment and prevention contemporary modalities that must be implemented. To improve mental health services within the child welfare system, efforts must be made to achieve the following goals proposed by former Surgeon General Satcher (U.S. Department of Health and Human Services, 2002):

1. Develop, disseminate, and implement scientifically proven prevention and treatment services.
2. Improve the assessment of and recognition of mental health needs in children at risk.
3. Eliminate racial/ethnic and socioeconomic disparities in access to children's mental health care services.
4. Improve the infrastructure for children's mental health services, including support for scientifically proven interventions across professions.
5. Increase access to and coordination of high-quality mental health care services.
6. Train front-line providers to recognize and manage mental health care issues.
7. Monitor the access to and the coordination of multidisciplinary, high-quality mental health care services.

HISTORICAL OVERVIEW

From a historical perspective, the beginnings of mental health services in America coincide with the colonial settlement of the United States. Individuals with mental health problems were cared for at home, and were usually kept in seclusion because of their families' feelings of stigma and shame regarding mental illness. With urbanization, colony (and later state) governments confronted a problem that had been largely the responsibility of families. The governments' response was to build institutions, known at that time as "asylums." In the mid-18th century, Virginia was the first colony to build an asylum for mentally ill individuals, which it constructed in its capital at Williamsburg. If not cared for at home or in asylums, those with mental illness were likely to be found in jails, almshouses, workhouses, and other institutions. Grace Abbott (1938) wrote that almhouses were built as towns increased in size, forcing urban children to live among the elderly, the mentally ill, and the disabled. Almshouses increased in number in the first decades of the 19th century; in 1823, a New York City almshouse was home to more than 500 children. Almhouses persisted into the 20th century (Meyers, 2004), even though in 1856, a New York State committee concluded that for children, almshouses were "the worst possible nurseries." In an article in the *North American Review*, Henry Smith Williams (1897) wrote that if the objective was to ensure dependent orphaned children would become paupers, vagabonds, and criminals, then this throwing them in the almshouse would be ideal. Eventually, separate institutions were created for children with blindness, mental retardation, and mentally illness or psychological problems.

An era of "moral treatment" was introduced from Europe at the turn of the 19th century. The first reformers, including Dorothea Lynde Dix, campaigned across the United States to convince the public that mental illness could be better treated by removing individuals to an asylum to receive a mix of somatic and psychosocial treatments in a controlled environment. Largely through her efforts, 32 public and private asylums were created in the United States. As the "moral treatment" period progressed, almost every state had an asylum dedicated to the early treatment of mental illness, to restore mental health and to keep patients from becoming chronically ill.

Shortly after the Civil War, the failures of the promise of early treatment were recognized, and asylums were now built for untreatable, chronic patients. The quality of care deteriorated in public institutions, where overcrowding, poor care, and underfunding ran rampant. A new reform movement, devoted to "mental hygiene," began late in the 19th century. The child guidance movement, which focused on improving treatment of children, paralleled the mental hygiene movement. A corresponding child guidance movement began in 1922. The movement focused on improving the treatment of children by establishing child guidance in an effort to prevent mental illness, treat maladjustment and behavior or emotional problems in school age children (Horn, 1989).

The reformers of the "mental hygiene" period called for bringing the new science of psychiatry to patients in smaller hospitals and clinics associated with medical schools. However, these treatments were not effective, either. In fact, they were no more successful in preventing patients from becoming chronically ill in the early 20th century than early treatment had been in the early years of the 19th century. Hospitals were providing custodial care, but in the process they neglected or abused the patients. By the middle of the 20th century, a new movement called "community mental health" came into being. Since long-term institutional care in mental hospitals had been neglectful, ineffective, and even harmful, "community care" and "deinstitutionalization" led to dramatic declines in the length of hospital stays and increased the discharge of many patients into the community. However, all this was done with little evidence of effectiveness of treatments and with inadequate human support systems to serve the hundreds of thousands of individuals with disabling mental illness who returned to the community. The special needs of individuals with severe and persistent mental illness were not being met. A fourth reform era (beginning in 1975), called the "community support" movement, grew directly out of the "community mental health" movement. This new reform movement viewed mental illness as a social welfare problem.

The mental health system has changed over time under the influence of a wide array of factors, including reform movements and their ideologies, social values, economic considerations, financial incentives based on who pays for what kind of services, and advances in care and methods of treatment. A growing body of literature now questions the effectiveness of presently existing traditional mental health services for children and their families. This neglect of children's basic mental health care needs is a result of inadequacies in the child welfare system, as well as inadequacies in the general health care system.

THE IDEAL OF PREVENTION

For most mental health problems, primary prevention is far better than treatment with questionable outcomes. Identifying these problems in their early stages; bringing them to the attention of families; and implementing effective health care management, assurance, and guidance can make children's lives better and longer. Unfortunately, there are barriers to these efforts. In particular, major barriers to providing health and mental health care for children in the child welfare system exist within the system itself. Our present child welfare system is not friendly to preventive efforts, and the value of prevention lacks political support and public recognition. Many children have become ill or even died after placement because the children's health care needs were not recognized early, and treatment was delayed or not given. In addition, frequent moves among foster homes contribute to the fragmentation and inadequacies of health and mental health care. It is crucial to recognize these children's mental health deficiencies, to provide early intervention, and to prevent the problems from getting worse. In the process the children should be provided every opportunity to achieve their fullest potential.

A variety of factors create barriers to formulating appropriate treatment care plans for children in the child welfare system. Information about health care services children have received and their mental health status before placement is often hard to obtain. In part, this is because children have had erratic contact with a number of health care providers before placement. Social workers often lack medical information about the types of health care services that children in foster care have received, and are therefore unable to effectively monitor compliance or quality of care delivered. Social workers are also often unable to obtain or review a child's health history in detail with the birth parents at the time of placement. Foster care parents often have been given limited training in health care issues or the means for accessing the health care system. The complicated untreated physical and mental health conditions that children bring with them when entering foster care often make taking care of these children very difficult and challenging for child welfare agencies.

It is important that mental disorders be evaluated in a multidisciplinary manner within the context of the family, peers, school, home, and community. Following the evaluation, services must be coordinated with primary care physicians, mental health professionals, social agencies, and schools. The American Academy of Pediatrics (AAP) Committee on School Health (2004) has emphasized the importance of enhanced collaboration and communication with school mental health service professionals in strengthening the medical home-based model of care and improving the mental health of children. Risk-assessment and treatment programs for individual children can prevent recognizing and identifying the broad family and parental conditions that are contributing to the suffering of these children.

More and more special programs are being designed for at-risk children. These approaches are necessary, but they are not enough. I remember (Fontana & Moolman, 1991) one young mother who pulled me up short and made me consider where she had come from and how she felt.

> Diane was about 19, and her little girl was 3. The two of them were participating in the temporary shelter program at the New York Foundling Hospital, in which abusive mothers and their children stayed with us for several months or a year while the mothers learned some of the basics of parenting. Our mistake with Diane was that we kept focusing on the child's needs and overlooking her concerns.
>
> Diane had originally come in after having seriously abused her child. After several weeks of doing very well with us, she and the little one were allowed to go home for a weekend, and when they came back the child had a bruise over one eye. I became involved when the social worker told me about the bruise and indicated that perhaps the mother was responsible for it.
>
> I took mother and child into my office, sat the child down on my lap, and started questioning Diane in what I thought was my most tactful manner. She said that the child had fallen down. I must have looked skeptical, because she started crying. The child got off my lap and, in a classic case of role reversal, put her arm around Diane and said, "Mommy, Mommy, don't cry, Mommy. Everything will be all right." And that was when Diane really broke down. Between sobs she said, "I'm sick and tired of all you damn people worrying about the kid. I didn't do it, I didn't hurt her! She fell down! A few years

> ago I was the one who was abused, and you were all concerned about me, but now I don't matter to you at all. Don't you *know* I can't take care of the kid unless you first take care of me? If I don't have my head straight, how can I possibly take care of her?"
>
> She was right. We had stopped taking care of her. Barely 16 when she'd had the child, she was still a child-mother herself, and she still needed our concern. She reminded me forcefully that we must always reach out to the parent in order to help the child.

Troubled parents need parenting, too; they need tender loving care, or they won't be able to give it. Unless we address the multiple troubling influences on families, we can easily see that we will continue to be faced with the prospect of thousands of children growing up unloved, unhappy, maltreated, and deprived. Their existence cannot be undone. There are remedies to their problems, however, and there are ways our child welfare system can help diminish the national and social neglect of our children, especially those in foster care.

CHALLENGES FOR THE FUTURE

Children don't exist in a vacuum. Several years ago, Marram, Barrett, and Bevis (1979) described total patient care as the oldest model of patient care delivery. Treatment and prevention programs that are intended to address the needs of at-risk children, without efforts to change the behavior of their adult caretakers, seem unlikely to succeed. Parents are a vital factor in mental health treatment for children. All efforts must be taken to ensure parental *involvement* in the intervention services, not solely parental *consultation*. Treating today's children means helping today's parents by enhancing the families' strengths, addressing families' problems, promoting family stability, building parenting competence, and training parents in sharing responsibilities for preventing illness and promoting good health.

Particularly promising efforts to achieve parental competence are home visitation programs. In some parts of the United States, "healthy families" prevention programs connect paraprofessionals with new parents. Visits by paraprofessionals or nurses are made to all new parents during pregnancy and after delivery. The home visits continue during the first months and in most cases during the first 3 years of "imprinting." These visits are complemented by an array of medical, child development, and social services. Daro and McCurdy (1996) and Constantino (2001) have demonstrated the effectiveness of home visitations as a public health intervention capable of reducing rates of child abuse and neglect, as well as of improving long-term parent–child relationships.

Some form of visiting nurse program has been in effect in Great Britain for close to 140 years and has been universal since the beginning of the 20th century. It is hoped that in the near future every community in the United States will have its own home visitor program and its own drop-in family center—one that serves all health functions, from routine checkups to providing any medical and mental health services required for the well-being of children and families.

Once a child is unfortunate enough to enter the foster care system, that child deserves not ordinary but extraordinary care. Children who come into foster care with a multiplicity of health problems are fragile and may also have special mental health needs that must be recognized and treated. First and foremost, they must be assured safety and protection from any further abuse and neglect. They are usually depressed, have low self-esteem, and lack much capacity for self-control. They have fears of being punished, neglected, or abandoned. They need nurturance, love, and the experience of feeling part of a family in order to achieve their full potential and live future healthy, productive lives.

Halfon, Mendoca, and Berkowitz (1995) have demonstrated that children in placement are susceptible to multiple and extensive emotional and behavioral disorders. Compared with children from the same socioeconomic background, children in foster care have much higher rates of serious emotional and behavioral problems, chronic physical disabilities, birth defects, developmental delays, and poor school achievement. Most of these children enter foster care in a poor state of health. Their poor health reflects exposure to poverty, poor or no prenatal care, prenatal infections, prenatal maternal substance abuse, HIV, family violence, and parental mental illness. Unfortunately, there are multiple and serious barriers to the provision of high-quality care for these children, as noted earlier. Health care for children in placement is often compromised by lack of health insurance; insufficient funding for mental health services; poor planning; lack of available health services; prolonged waits; and the lack of coordination, communication, and cooperation of services among health and child welfare professionals. In addition, families often deny that their children have physical or mental health problems, or have difficulty discussing these issues with their primary care providers because of fears of associated stigma (Schneid, 2003).

A report by the Commission on Children at Risk (2003)—a group of 33 pediatricians, research scientists, and mental health professionals—presented scientific evidence, largely in the field of neuroscience, that the human child is "hardwired to connect." The basic needs for "connection," "bonding," or "attachment" are essential to health and to human development. The clinical importance of these bonds was not fully appreciated until Bowlby (1940), introduced the concept of attachment in his seminal report on the effects of maternal deprivation. Children who have been abused and neglected, and who have been separated from their primary caretakers, often develop serious emotional problems that interfere with the attachment bond. Attachment is the deep and critical connection established between a child and caregiver in the first year of life. It influences every component of the human existence: mind, body, emotional relationships, and values. A disrupted connection or attachment not only leads to emotional and social problems, but also results in biochemical effects in the developing brain.

Bruce Perry (2004) has reported that brain development is dependent in great part on an individual's connection to other human beings. Most growth activity in the human brain occurs during the first 3–4 years of life. Infants require consistent connections with loving, sensitive caregivers for the healthy development of their brains. Abuse, neglect, and other adverse environmental factors can cause neurological damage that interferes with children's future ability to reason, to feel, and to regulate their emotions and behavior. We must understand the importance of infant attachment for child brain development. This points to a new direction—a biopsychosociocultural model for child development. This new model is intended to deepen our understanding of both childhood crisis and the practical help that can be provided by youth professionals, policy makers, and others working to improve the lives of children. In addition, more attention should be paid to a child's moral, spiritual, and religious needs. Some studies (Garbarino, 1999) suggest that children feel more grounded and are less prone to engage in antisocial behavior when they have a religious/moral foundation.

The unmet needs of child mental health services are prevention, early intervention, and relationship-based treatment. Those of us who have labored in the child welfare system for many years are aware of the numerous challenges encountered in navigating the multiple systems involved in the care and treatment of children with medical and mental health disorders. Many children in foster care are not receiving the mental health services they need, and many more are receiving inappropriate care. This absence of high-quality mental health interventions for children in child welfare programs often results in foster care disruption, accompanied by chronic health problems and repeated hospitalizations. Bernal (2003) has demonstrated that children with behavioral disorders generate higher overall general health care costs than those without behavioral disorders.

To achieve any amount of success in mental health care for children in foster care, we must develop an individualized health care plan for each child and integrate the health care plan into the child welfare plan. In 1993, the AAP adopted the policy statement "The Pediatrician and the New Morbidity." The statement focused on the significance of mental health programs for children and adolescents. In 2001, the AAP published another statement with a renewed commitment to the psychosocial aspects of pediatric care. In this second statement, the AAP has recommended that specialized health programs provide the overall case management that is imperative for improving both the physical and mental health of children. As repeatedly emphasized in this book, the child welfare system must recognize the interdependence of mental health and physical health. Rubin et al.'s (2004) study demonstrated the interdependence of mental health and the global health of children in foster care.

Children and families with mental health problems require and deserve professional and human support services in a comprehensive, culturally competent, coordinated, community-based, family-driven system of care. The system must be directed by the reality that helping children involves helping their parents through intensive interventions, including parent treatment and parent–child relationship therapy, in addition to providing human support services with prevention-oriented strategies. This goal assumes collaborative multidisciplinary planning, professional training in skills and competencies, and funds to support direct and preventive services and research. Pediatric health care professionals also need to be partners with others in the areas of risk assessment, prevention, and treatment of psychosocial disorders (Melnyk, 2003). Pediatricians need to partner with others to remain relevant to the health of children (Haggerty, 1995).

Regardless of the particular health care delivery model employed, we must advocate for integrating community-based systems of care with services that are client-centered and family-empowering. Each type of service alone has its limitations, but together they constitute an integrated, fully informed approach that spans the entire spectrum of mental and physical health. The particular health care services provided should include initial health screening, comprehensive medical and dental assessment, developmental and mental health evaluation, and ongoing primary care and monitoring of health status.

SUMMARY AND CONCLUSION

In summary, as child care professionals, we must advocate for the rights and needs of children in the child welfare system, and must work toward bringing about desperately needed systematic changes that can help these children function more adequately on both personal and social levels.

We must recognize the unmet medical and mental health needs of the abused, neglected, and abandoned children who enter foster care in a traumatized state, and must arrange to meet these needs in an integrated fashion within the social service system of child welfare agencies. In particular, we must prevent any additional abuse and neglect of foster children by an unresponsive and inadequate child welfare system.

We must advocate for the provision of high-quality, multidisciplinary medical and mental health services to our foster children with special needs. We must also insist on greater accountability for the delivery of these services, including an increased focus on outcome and quality indicators. We need specialized medical and mental health child and family human support programs sponsored by local, state, and federal governments at all levels of society. We need more crisis nurseries, more shelters, more day care centers, more parent aid groups, more parent helplines and parent education–both in the community and in our elementary schools.

Today, much of the dysfunction in family units and much of the damage inflicted on neglected foster children can be attributed to our vast, overwhelmed, and sometimes uncaring bureaucratic child care systems. We cannot continue to blame government for all of our social problems; however, we must recognize and acknowledge the general public's apathy and lack of concern about the crucial issues in the field of foster care. The public must recognize the bureaucratic budgetary problems professionals confront in providing therapeutic special services to treat, protect, and stabilize the innocent victims of child maltreatment who enter our foster care system.

I have always been aware of and admire the recognition professionals give to child maltreatment, and the broad mandate and responsibilities they assume in the protection, welfare, and health of children. Indeed, it is this professional concern that has led to the development of preventive and treatment programs for child abuse in the United States. I suggest that these dedicated professionals must now target quite deliberately the dramatic, critically important problems of the child welfare system and of children in out-of-home care. We are entering the 21st century with great changes in family ecology, in children, and in the communities we serve. As part of our work, we must carefully analyze and assess which of our existing programs and which of our interventions have truly bettered the lives of foster children. Whenever possible, we must offer empirical research demonstrating that such programs and interventions have indeed been effective, and then advocate that these services be adequately funded by federal, state, and local governments.

If we are to protect, preserve, and extend the gains that have been made in the prevention and treatment of child abuse and neglect during the last half century, our most important task is to provide healing to the innocent victims of abuse and neglect, especially those placed in the foster care system. Finally, foster care should not be a poor system for poor children, but a high-quality health care system that provides for and enforces a child's permanency plans.

REFERENCES

Abbot, G. (1938). *The child and the state.* Chicago: The University of Chicago Press.

American Academy of Pediatrics (AAP). (2001). The new morbidity revisited: A renewed commitment to the psychosocial aspects of pediatric care. *Pediatrics, 108*, 1227–1230.

American Academy of Pediatrics (AAP), Committee on School Health. (2004). School-based mental health services. *Pediatrics, 113*(6), 1839–1845.

Bernal, P. (2003). Hidden morbidity in pediatric primary care. *Pediatric Annals, 23*, 412–418.

Bowlby, J. (1940). The influence of early environment in the development of neurosis and neurotic character. *International Journal of Psycho-Analysis, 21*, 154–178.

Commission on Children at Risk. (2003). *Hardwire to connect: The new scientific case for authoritative communities.* New York: Institute for American Values.

Constantino, J. N. (2001). Supplementation of urban home visitation with series of group meetings for parents and infants: Results of a randomized controlled trial. *Child Abuse and Neglect, 25*, 1571–1581.

Daro, D., & McCurdy, K. (1996). Intensive home visitation: A randomized trial, follow-up and assessment study of Hawaii's healthy start program. Washington, DC: National Center on Child Abuse and Neglect, U.S. Department of Health and Human Services.

Fontana, V. J., & Moolman, V. (1991). *Save the family, save the child: What we can do to help children at risk.* New York: Dutton.

Garbarino, J. (1999). *Lost boys: Why our sons turn violent and how we can save them.* New York: Free Press.

Haggerty, R. J. (1995). Child health 2000: New pediatrics in the changing environment of children's needs in the 21st century. *Pediatrics, 96*, 804–812.

Halfon, N., Mendonca, A., & Berkowitz, G. (1995). Health status of children in foster care: The experience of the center for the vulnerable child. *Archives of Pediatric and Adolescent Medicine, 149*, 386–392.

Horn, M. (1989). *Before it's too late: The child guidance movement in the United States, 1922–1945.* Philadelphia: Temple University Press.

Marram, G., Barrett, M. W., & Bevis, E. O. (1979). *Primary nursing: A model for individualized patient care* (2nd ed.). St. Louis, MO: Mosby.

Melnyk, B. M. (2003). Mental health knowledge, worries, needs, and screening practices. *Journal of Pediatric Health Care, 17*(Suppl.).

Melnyk, B. M., Feinstein, N. E., Tuttle, J., Modewhauer, Z., Herendeen, P., & Veenema, T. G. (2002). Mental health worries, communication, and needs in the year of the U.S. terrorist attack: National KYSS Survey Findings. *Journal of Pediatric Health Care, 16*(5), 222–234.

Myers, J. E. B. (2004). *A history of child protection in America.* Philadelphia: Xlibris.

Perry, B. (2004, April 15). *Using principles of neurodevelopment to help traumatized and maltreated children*. The James R. Dumpson Colloquium in Child Welfare, Fordham University, Tarrytown, NY.

Rubin, D. M., Alessandrini, E. A., Feudtner, C., Mamdell, D. S., Locallo, A. R., & Hadley, T. (2004). Placement stability and mental health costs for children in foster care. *Pediatrics, 113*(5), 1136–1341.

Schneid, J. (2003). Recognizing and managing long term sequlae of childhood maltreatment. *Pediatric Annals, 36*, 391–401.

Smith Williams, H. (1897). What shall be done with dependent children? *North American Review, 164*, 404–405.

U.S. Department of Health and Human Services. (1999). *Mental health: A report of the Surgeon General*. Washington, DC: Author.

U.S. Department of Health and Human Services. (2002). *Report of the Surgeon General's conference on children's mental health: A national agenda*. Washington, DC: Author.

CHAPTER 15

The View from the Mental Health System

MARILYN B. BENOIT

The plight of children in the child welfare system of the United States of America should sound major alarm bells for our politicians, legislators, and policy makers at the federal, state, and local levels. By far too many of those children are "graduating" into the juvenile justice system and becoming teenage parents, victims of violence, and members of the homeless population. Child welfare has, in the past, focused mainly on the physical needs of children in out-of-home care, but the Child Welfare League of America (CWLA) has now taken the position that it is very important to address the mental health needs of these children as well. To address that commitment, the CWLA has incorporated a Behavioral Health Division as well as a Mental Health Advisory Board into its national organization. More recently, in 2001, CWLA and the American Academy of Child and Adolescent Psychiatry (AACAP) established a national collaboration with more than 50 child-serving agencies, specifically to address the mental health needs of children in the foster care system. Burns et al. (2004) concluded from a national survey of youth in child welfare that "routine screening for mental health need and increasing access to mental health professionals for further evaluation and treatment should be a priority for children early in their contact with the child welfare system" (p. 960).

The need for collaboration between mental health and child welfare services has been highlighted by the Pew Commission on Children in Foster Care (2004), and by the landmark publication *From Neurons to Neighborhoods* (Committee on Integrating the Science of Early Childhood Development, 2000). The Pew Commission made recommendations and set guidelines for practice in child welfare. Its report described its recommended policy and federal financing changes to improve the safety, placement permanence, and well-being of children in foster care. The report acknowledges that foster children are at higher-than-average risk for mental health and behavioral problems, as well as school failure. The science of early childhood trauma is developing in tandem with brain research, which is gaining tremendous ground and providing us with formidable insights into the workings of the human brain. The publication *From Neurons to Neighborhoods* has served as a major stimulus to change our thinking about the role of the brain physiology in emotions and behaviors. It is no longer acceptable to think about our children in the child welfare system as "bad seeds," and essentially to "write them off" as not worthy of our interventions. Now that we have a better understanding of the impact of trauma on brain development, we are obligated to do research and to design interventions that will either remediate, or at the very least minimize, the neuropsychiatric sequelae of childhood trauma. By definition, the children who are removed from their homes into the child welfare system are victims of some type of maltreatment trauma. Then the additive trauma of separation from their families is imposed upon these victimized children. Trauma in early childhood causes deviations in cognition, emotions, self-regulation, and behaviors. Adaptive functioning is compromised by such deviation. The degree of this compromise is determined by a confluence of many variables, which are now discussed further.

RISK FACTORS FOR PSYCHIATRIC ILLNESS IN THE CHILD WELFARE POPULATION

The concept of risk factors that can be cumulative and make a youngster more susceptible to psychiatric illness is well recognized in the mental health community. Using this concept, one can readily conclude that the child welfare population, as a group, is highly vulnerable. The risk factors begin with teenage pregnancy, which is associated with higher-risk births by reason of low birth weight, absent or poor prenatal care, poor emotional support, poverty, and poor education. The literature also shows that minority populations, especially, (African Americans and Hispanics) are overrepresented in the child welfare population (U.S. Department of Health and Human Services, 2004; see also Ortiz Hendricks & Fong, Chapter 8, this volume). It is not that race and ethnicity per se put children at risk, but that in the United States, race and ethnicity covary with many other negative socioeconomic factors that are more directly related to risk. This research shows as well that in the African American population, 80% of the children who are referred to child welfare are offspring of parents who are involved in drug and/or alcohol misuse. Domestic violence (spousal or partner) is also highly correlated with child maltreatment. Thus we see that a socioecological system that is toxic to development can preexist and set the stage for increased risk of neglect and abuse. The issue of risk factors is further complicated by the many mediating variables over the life trajectories of traumatized children that can alter risk for psychiatric morbidity.

Bowlby (1973) stated that early disruption of attachment is a primary form of trauma, which makes the infant more vulnerable to subsequent traumas. Research on rat pups and their mothers (Sanchez, Ladd, & Plotsky, 2001) has shown that separation from mothers during an early sensitive stage of development can lead to an altered response to stress. Rat research has also shown that the nurturing experience with the rat mother prior to a separation experience can alter the recovery period from stress. More nurturing rats (i.e., ones with high rates of licking and grooming offspring) produced less anxious and more resilient offspring (Champagne, Francis, Mar, & Meaney,2003). It is well recognized that youth in the child welfare system frequently have their placements disrupted, often because foster parents are unable to care for them as a result of their serious emotional and behavioral problems. The paradoxical reality is this: Traumatized children have emotional and behavioral problems related to their trauma, and those problems make their management quite challenging and often lead to further disruptions of stability, which the children so desperately need in order to remediate their emotional and behavioral problems (Harden, 2004).

CRITICAL IMPORTANCE OF GOOD EARLY ATTACHMENT

The percentage of young children coming into foster care, primarily because of neglect, has been increasing; the 0–5 age group currently accounts for approximately 25% of the children in care. For such young children the issue of the nature of their attachment is of significant importance. Boris et al. (2004) studied attachment disorders in some diverse high-risk groups (children in Head Start, children living in homeless shelters, and maltreated children) and found that the maltreated children were significantly more likely to meet criteria for one or more attachment disorders. The nature of a child's early attachment experience is one of the major predictors of emotional and social well-being as the child develops. The evolving field of attachment research (both behavioral and neuroscientific) is providing us with increasing insights into the critical role of the child's cumulative attachment experiences with the primary caretaker. Those experiences influence the development of regulatory processes within the brain of the developing child. It is interesting that the attachment outcome is highly correlated with the ability of the mother (or other primary attachment figure) to have her own coherent life narrative. For example, a mother whose brain is on and off drugs/alcohol will lose continuity of her own experience of herself, and therefore cannot provide the developing child with continuity of nurturing care and attention. If one considers that a mother who is addicted to drugs and/or alcohol has a primary attachment to the substance that gratifies the pleasure center of the brain, then that mother is less likely to derive pleasure from the caretaking of a dependent and demanding infant, and thus her attachment to the infant will be compromised. It should not be surprising, therefore, that children who are neglected and/or abused are more likely to have attachment difficulties, and consequently problems with self-regulation. These can play out as behavioral problems reflected in poor bladder and bowel control, poor control of aggression, poor mood and affect modulation, or difficulty settling into a predictable circadian rhythm (with sleeping and eating difficulties). The Center for the Vulnerable Child in Oakland, California, has a pilot program that has been informed by their research. The program, called Services to Enhance Early Development (SEED), is designed to provide early assessments of young children entering foster care and to work on establishing positive, stable relationships as soon as possible. A similar program, Starting Young, has been implemented at the Medical College of Pennsylvania. Ultimately, it is the establishment of an enduring, stable relationship that will be the most important agent of healing for traumatized children.

Psychoanalytic thinking conceptualizes the mother as the primary auxiliary ego of the developing child, functioning as an external regulator until such time as the child is able to identify with the mother and "internalize" his or her own controls and regulation. Now we understand that the dyadic, interpersonal experiential environment actually stimulates the development of the neural circuitry, and hence the neuroregulatory infrastructure of the developing brain (Siegel, 1999). The child will work to preserve its attachment (even a highly ambivalent or disorganized one), resorting to negative behaviors if those are the behaviors that are reinforced within the attachment relationship. For example, a neglected child who gets beaten for nagging at the mother will continue to nag, because that behavior receives attention from the critically important person in his or her life. Once this behavior is learned, it may then be generalized to other domains (e.g., the classroom, the playground).

The issue of moral development is too often neglected. Moral development also occurs within the context of an attachment relationship and is important in the internalized regulation of morally driven behavior. For the most part, children wish to please the adults to whom they are emotionally connected. They therefore ascertain right and wrong and ultimately make moral judgments based on their experience (rather than on what they are told) within their important attachment relationships. It is my clinical opinion that we should focus more on addressing the moral developmental line of all children (Coles, 1997) and its association with behavioral regulation, and that we should specifically examine how this develops in our foster care population.

REPEATED LOSSES AND DEPRESSION

The chronic sense of loss experienced by youth in the child welfare system makes them vulnerable to depression. As discussed by Webb (Chapter 2, this volume), these children's losses are not limited to the object loss of their primary caregivers, but extend more deeply to their psychological identities—their sense of self, which can help them to organize their lives and develop a sense of personal competency and agency. Poor self-esteem develops when children feel that they are not worthy enough for their parents to stick around. Children are often unable to understand the circumstances leading to their removal from their parents' homes, and often blame themselves for the separation. Internalized blame, shame, and guilt, combined with profound real losses, make children very vulnerable to depression. Brown, Cohen, Johnson, and Smailes (1999) found that both dysthymia and major depression were more common in adolescents with a history of maltreatment, the odds being 3.4 to 4.5 times greater for that population. Children who get into behavioral difficulties and have crises while in care have often experienced repeated losses of foster homes, schools, neighborhoods, and the people with whom they are involved, and such experiences further exacerbate their profound sense of loss. Such children may believe that they can never be worthy of others' investing in them, leading to a profound sense of hopelessness.

Some standard questions that I pose when I am evaluating youngsters probe their expectations of whether they can expect adults to meet their needs. It is not unusual for the responses to reveal a sense that adults cannot be counted upon, and that they must either have to turn to their own individual resources or be left to the whims of fate. One child indicated that he would depend upon his bookbag as a resource, rather than a single person! With attachment and dependency being major issues for this youngster, one can quickly imagine how challenging he would be in a foster care home. Rubin et al. (2004) studied 1,635 foster children in placement and found that 41% had had more than three placements in the first year of foster care; this placement instability was associated with increased mental health and overall health care costs. The children with more placements had multiple mental health, developmental, and general health problems. Similarly, the Pew Commission on Children in Foster Care (2004) reported that the average foster child had three placements.

POSTTRAUMATIC STRESS DISORDER AND DISRUPTIVE BEHAVIORAL SYMPTOMS

Given the various traumas they have experienced (i.e., neglect, physical abuse, sexual abuse, and the witnessing of violence), children in the child welfare system are more prone to suffer from symptoms of posttraumatic stress disorder (PTSD). These symptoms include hypervigilance; flashbacks of the trauma; nightmares; intrusive thoughts that interfere with daily functioning; avoidance of any person, thing, or place that may trigger traumatic memories; emotional numbing; and dissociation. Some youth may not meet full diagnostic criteria for PTSD (American Psychiatric Association, 2000), but nonetheless may be chronically disturbed by specific traumatic stress related symptoms. They may remain hypervigilant and overreactive to minor insults that they perceive as major assaults. One young man was referred for physically assaulting an adult for apparently no reason. He later revealed that that person looked at him in the same manner that his parent had looked at him prior to physically abusing him. Ford et al. (2000) found that "children with ODD [oppositional defiant disorder] had more historical exposure to maltreatment, more severe current hyperarousal symptoms, worse overall psychopathology, and poorer social competence" (p. 212). Their research found an increased rate of PTSD symptoms for children with comorbid ODD and attention-deficit/hyperactive disorder (ADHD). These findings concur with my own clinical experience.

Dissociation is an effective defense mechanism used in the face of traumatic experiences over which one has no control. Some refer to this as "compartmentalization," and some maltreated youth call it "checking out." With dissociation, one's psychic world becomes fragmented, and there is a lack of continuity of the self through various experiences. Former President Bill Clinton, who witnessed serious domestic violence and alcohol abuse in his family of origin, described in his personal memoir, *My Life* (Clinton, 2004), how he came to live "parallel lives" in order to survive the trauma of his early environment. Fortunately for him, he had significant and enduring attachment figures in his life who functioned as protective factors: his grandparents and his mother. This fact, combined with his superior intellect and a deep involvement with religion, contributed to the resilience that he demonstrated in coming from such humble and troubled beginnings to become the president of the United States.

Unfortunately, most of the children in foster care are not as lucky to have such protective factors. Instead, the child welfare system, which was created with the intent to protect children, imposes upon them further trauma with the frequent disruptions in placement that they must endure. The federal government (see U.S. Department of Health and Human Services, 2004) has recently completed state-by-state evaluations of children's well-being in the child welfare system. As of 2003, *not a single state* had met standards to be rated as being in compliance with meeting the criteria for "child well-being." If one considers "well-being" as a global measure of children's adaptive functioning, and reflective of their state of mental health, it is time to sound the alarm on the malfunctioning of the system that is supposed to help restore children to stability.

LIVING WITH CHRONIC ANXIETY

Living in a traumatizing environment creates a breeding ground for anxiety. It is not only the inflicted trauma itself (be it sexual abuse, physical abuse, neglect, or witnessing of violence) that is stress-inducing; the accompanying feelings of impotence, unpredictability, and general lack of mastery over one's very personal world also produce a chronic state of anxiety. For anxious children, academic learning can present a significant challenge. If their cognitive functioning is further compromised by learning disabilities, below-average intellect, or an understimulating environment, these children can fall behind academically. Without appropriate special education and psychotherapeutic intervention, school success may be elusive. In addition, pervasive and persistent anxiety can be masked by interpersonal behavioral difficulties, which can include both verbal and physical aggression. Although psychotherapeutic interventions should include behavioral management techniques, it is important that the underlying anxieties be recognized, validated, labeled, and addressed.

THE NEUROSCIENCE OF MALTREATMENT

The information gained from the past two decades of brain research has provided us with new insights into the working of the traumatized brain. One of the most revealing findings is related to the effect of chronic stress on the developing brain. Traumatized children are more likely to be hypervigilant as a protective mechanism to allow them to identify threats in their environments. This hypervigilance leaves them in a chronic state of heightened physiological arousal that is maladaptive in typical social settings. They are therefore more likely to respond to everyday nonthreatening events as threats, to respond with a "flight-or-fight" response that is socially inappropriate or frankly abusive, and to get into serious trouble as a result. Pollack's (2003) research has shown that abused children have a heightened physiological response to an angry face, and that once this response is triggered, they do not easily dampen it down; instead, they take this affective response into their subsequent task. This certainly argues for the concept of taking a "time out" when there is affective flooding in these children, rather than expecting them to make a transition easily into another activity. This research finding definitely correlates with my own clinical experience, and reinforces the concept that interventions have to be highly individualized for traumatized children, whose affective storms can be triggered by events that may go unregistered in the brains of nontraumatized children.

Research has shown that the recovery profile of brain-based stress hormones in traumatized individuals is different from that of nontraumatized persons. We also know that in chronic stress situations, cortisol (one of the stress hormones) can be neurotoxic, and research findings indicate that a part of the brain that plays a role in memory development (the hippocampus) can show neural degeneration under chronic stress experiences. I have had the experience of managing a residential treatment center for maltreated children, and it was striking that almost all the children had a similar finding of short-term memory problems on formal psychological testing.

Ongoing research is examining the interactive effects of stress and various aspects of brain development. Critical questions relate to the developmental timing of specific brain functions: how they unfold during typical development, and then how both internal and external factors may influence that development. Interdisciplinary, longitudinal research on developmental psychopathology that explores a wide range of mechanisms–genetic, neuroendocrine, neuroimmunological, familial, and environmental (including infectious agents toxic, electrochemical, electromagnetic, and nutritional) factors–is essential to our understanding and development of targeted treatment interventions for our foster care population.

TREATMENT INTERVENTIONS

The mental health treatment of children in foster care is in great need of an overhaul. Care is fragmented–provided in a "hit-or-miss" manner, with little attempt to discern outcomes in any systematic manner. Treatment is generally not based on any evidence as to what works for which children under what circumstances. There is no consensus on how much treatment is necessary, or on who should participate in the treatment intervention. Mental health costs for the foster care population are estimated at $2.4 billion, and Rubin et al. (2004) reported that 10% of the population used up 83% of the funding. One has to conclude that the high-end mental health utilization includes inpatient acute hospitalization and longer-term residential treatment. I am aware of no research that has determined that inpatient and residential treatments result in significantly improved and sustained outcomes for the majority of youth who utilize such care. In contrast, multisystemic therapy (Henggeler, 1998), which is community-based, intensive, and comprehensive, has been rigorously tested and proven to be effective.

Although there are evidence-based treatment interventions available for a number of mental health problems, very little is known about treatments specifically targeted to the needs of children in foster care. As noted at the beginning of this chapter, the AACAP and the CWLA have established a collaboration of national stakeholders in foster care. The group has been meeting since 2001, with the expressed goal of addressing treatment interventions and policy actions that would improve mental health treatments for children in the foster care system. The group first established fundamental values and principles that would guide all the subsequent work. In a systematic manner, it then developed a "first-responders" document to guide the initial contact with a child who is being removed from the parental home. The group strongly believes that the initial trauma of the forced removal and separation can be minimized by sensitive first-contact handling. With a focus on prevention and intervention, the group considers the first 30 days to be an opportunity for the caseworkers, social workers, and foster parents to become aware of critical mental health issues for the child, and to be responsive to his or her needs in a manner that will minimize mental health sequelae. The AACAP and the CWLA have also prepared a joint policy statement on the mental health and substance use evaluation of foster children (AACAP & CWLA, 2003). At this writing, this document can be accessed at the websites of both organizations.

The issue of the use of psychotropic medications for the treatment of emotional and behavioral disorders in foster children remains controversial and intense. It is confounded by racial issues, because African American and Hispanic children are overrepresented minorities within the child welfare system, as noted earlier. Some advocates argue that these specific populations are overmedicated by European American physicians, and that the children are more likely to receive medication alone and not to receive adjunctive therapies. This concern over medication has reached the level of the courts in many states, where specific permission from the courts has to be received before certain medications can be used. Although the overt intent is to protect foster children from medical abuses, the result in many cases is to introduce a barrier to timely care for some children, who have an appropriately diagnosed psychiatric disorder for which medication treatment is appropriate. I once had the unfortunate experience of having a hypomanic youngster who needed urgent intervention with antimanic medication. The request was sent to the agency for approval, but it took several weeks before this approval was given. Meanwhile, the youngster proceeded to become very manic, highly impulsive, and dangerously out of control, requiring emergency psychiatric hospitalization. Balanced thinking is needed to protect children, and at the same time to ensure that they receive appropriate and timely medical/psychiatric care, rather than disputes that do not work in children's best interests. As of this writing this issue is being played out in an increasing number of sites around the United States.

A specific category of foster care, called "therapeutic foster care" or "treatment foster care," is intended for those children who have been specifically identified as having special mental health needs. However, the AACAP and CWLA (2003) have stated–and I agree–that *all* foster care should be "therapeutic" to these already traumatized children (see also Lyons, 2004). In the current system, a variety of mental health and other supportive services may be accessed by foster families who sign up to provide "therapeutic foster care." They are also paid a higher rate to care for the children, because of the increased demands on the foster parents' time and personal investment. The training is specialized to help foster parents handle the serious emotional and behavioral problems with which the children present. Therapeutic foster care was intended to decrease the placement of children in psychiatric hospitals and in residential facilities. Multisystemic therapy (Henggeler, 1998) is one successful model that has been used and has popularized the use of wraparound interventions. This model emphasizes the use of (1) comprehensive services that are monitored for quality assurance, (2) qualified personnel with good training, and (3) interventions that are ecologically sound. For example, Milwaukee Wraparound has a very successful record with careful and sustained implementation. Not all agency programs that profess to use the model demonstrate this degree of follow-through, however, because the fidelity of the implementation may fall short. Unfortunately, the interpretation of how a particular service should be implemented may deviate substantially from the model that was deemed efficacious and effective. Another effective treatment approach has been described by Chamberlain (1994). This model provides ongoing professional consultation to foster parents who have been trained and receive teaching and supervision to reinforce positive relationships and prosocial skills in their foster children. The successful "ingredients" that good programs appear to share are as follows:

- They are individualized.
- They are strengths-based.
- They are child-focused.
- They are family-centered.
- They are part of a community systems-of-care continuum.
- They are culturally sensitive.
- They are not too difficult to implement.

Cohen, Deblinger, Mannarion, and Steer (2004), in a randomized, controlled multisite clinical trial, reported on the efficacy and effectiveness of short-term (12 weeks) trauma-focused cognitive-behavioral therapy for children ages 8–14 who had experienced sexual abuse, with resulting PTSD and related emotional and behavioral difficulties. At a 1-year followup, the treated children showed fewer symptoms of depression and greater improvement in social competence than subjects who were treated with nonspecific therapies. Parent treatment was a necessary component of the intervention.

Brown (2003) has reviewed the emerging literature on efficacious treatments for children who have been physically abused. Findings indicate that cognitive-behavioral therapy that consistently includes the caregivers shows efficacy. Unfortunately, at this time, children who are receiving various psychotherapies may be treated by providers without much experience and supervision. Often, too, the foster parents are not included in the therapeutic interventions. A common tale is that the agency driver drops off the foster child at the therapist's clinic or office. As emphasized in the description of efficacious and effective therapies above, the involvement of the caregiver is an essential part of the treatment interventions. Parent training as an isolated module of intervention is insufficient. The inclusion of home-based therapies is becoming more popular, but it is my own belief that the use of manualized and empirically driven therapies has a better track record of success.

Similarly, mentorship has been shown to be a useful adjunctive intervention for troubled youth. A mentor should be committed to staying with a child over time, developing a sustained relationship, and being a consistent and predictable person who assists through transitions that are imposed upon the child, often by the system itself. I was dismayed to learn that one mentoring organization used by a child welfare agency deliberately and systematically changed mentors monthly, because the director did not want the children to "get attached!"

SUMMARY

It is encouraging that different groups are publicly addressing the issue of maltreatment and its potentially devastating mental health sequelae for the more than 500,000 children who are in the U.S. child welfare system. The federal government (U.S. Department of Health and Human Services, 2004) recently completed 3 years of evaluation of states' programs, and it was appalling to learn that not a single state met the criteria for successfully addressing the "well-being" of the children and youth in the child welfare system. Included among the "well-being" criteria was attention to the mental health needs of these children. Because excellent research continues to inform us of the brain effects of maltreatment, we must make some long-term commitments to providing the best mental health care, based on the best available scientific information, for this most vulnerable sector of our population of children. There is a critical need for longitudinal studies that are also developmentally designed, so that we can better target specific treatments and "treatment doses" to specific groups of maltreated children. Our country has a moral obligation to address the needs of its children, so that we can provide the necessary mental health interventions that will enable them to prosper as contributing members of the society. It is the hope of the AACAP/CWLA collaboration to work with the National Institute of Mental Health to craft a long-term research agenda to address this need.

REFERENCES

American Academy of Child and Adolescent Psychiatry (AACAP) & Child Welfare League of America (CWLA). (2002). *AACAP/CWLA policy statement on mental health and substance use screening and assessment of children in foster care*. Available at www.aacap.org and www.cwla.org

American Psychiatric Association. (2000). *Diagnostic and statistical manual of mental disorders* (4th ed., text rev.). Washington, DC: Author.

Boris, N. W., Hinshaw-Fuselier, S. S., Smyke, A. T., Scheeringa, M. S., Heller, S. S., & Zeanah, C. H. (2004). Comparing criteria for attachment disorders: Establishing reliability and validity in high-risk samples. *Journal of the American Academy of Child and Adolescent Psychiatry, 43*, 568–577.

Bowlby, J. (1973). *Attachment and loss. Vol. 2. Separation, anxiety and anger.* London: Hogarth Press and Institute of Psychoanalysis.

Brown, E. (2003). Child physical abuse: Risk for psychopathology and efficacy of interventions. *Current Psychiatry Reports, 5*, 87–94.

Brown, J., Cohen, P., Johnson, J. G., & Smailes, E. M. (1999). Childhood abuse and neglect: Specificity of effects on adolescent and young adult depression and suicidality. *Journal of the American Academy of Child and Adolescent Psychiatry, 38*, 1490–1496.

Burns, B. J., Phillips, S. D., Wagner, H. R., Barth, R. P., Kolko, D. J., Campbell, Y., & Landsverk, J. (2004). Mental health need and access to mental health services by youths involved with child welfare: A national survey. *Journal of the American Academy of Child and Adolescent Psychiatry, 43*, 960–970.

Chamberlain, P. (1994). *Family Connections: A treatment foster care model for adolescents with delinquency*. Eugene, OR: Castalia.

Champagne, F. A., Francis, D. D., Mar, A., & Meaney, M. J. (2003). Variations in maternal care in the rat as a mediating influence for the effects of environment on development. *Physiology and Behavior, 79*, 359–371.

Clinton, B. (2004). *My life*. New York: Knopf.

Cohen, J. A., Deblinger, E., Mannarion, A. P., & Steer, R. A. (2004). A multi-site, randomized controlled trial for children with sexual abuse-related PTSD symptoms. *Journal of the American Academy of Child and Adolescent Psychiatry, 43*, 393–402.

Coles, R. (1997) *The moral intelligence of children: How to raise a moral child.* New York: Random House.

Committee on Integrating the Science of Early Childhood Development. (2000). *From neurons to neighborhoods: The science of early childhood development* (J. P. Shonkoff & D. A. Phillips, Eds.). Washington DC: National Academy Press.

Ford, J. D., Racusin, R., Ellis, C. G., Daviss, W. B., Reiser, J., Fleischer, A., & Thomas, J. (2000). Child maltreatment, other trauma exposure, and posttraumatic symptomatology among children with oppositional defiant and attention deficit hyperactivity disorders. *Child Maltreatment, 5*, 205–217.

Harden, B. J. (2004). Safety and stability for foster children: A developmental perspective. *Future Child, 14*, 31–47.

Henggeler, S. W., & Cunningham, P. B. (1998). *Multisystemic treatment of antisocial behavior in children and adolescents.* New York: Guilford Press.

Lyons, J. S., & Rogers, L. (2004). The U.S. Child Welfare System: A de facto public behavioral health care system. *Journal of the Academy of Child and Adolescent Psychiatry, 43*, 971–973.

Pew Commission on Children in Foster Care. (2004). *Fostering the future: Safety, permanence and well-being for children in foster care.* Washington, DC: Author.

Pollack, S. D. (2003). Experience dependent affective learning and risk for psychopathology in children. *Annals of the New York Academy of Sciences, 1008*, 102–111.

Rubin, D. M., Alessandrini, E. A., Feudtner, C., Mandell, D. S., Locallo, A. R., & Hadley, T. (2004). Placement stability and mental health costs for children in foster care. *Pediatrics, 113*, 1336–1341.

Sanchez, M. M., Ladd, C. O., & Plotsky, P. M. (2001). Early adverse experience as a developmental risk factor for late psychopathology: evidence from rodent and primate models. *Development and Psychopathology, 13*, 419–449.

Siegel, D. J. (1999). *The developing mind: Toward a neurobiology of interpersonal experience.* New York: Guilford Press.

U.S. Department of Health and Human Services, Children's Bureau, Administration for Children and Families. (2004). *Child and family services reviews.* Available at www.acf.hhs.gov/programs

PART IV

APPENDIX

CHILD-RELATED AND TRAUMA-RELATED PROFESSIONAL ORGANIZATIONS

Many of these organizations have national and regional conferences at which presentations feature current research, policy ,and practice. Some also offer specialized training and certifications (see "Training Programs and Certifications," below).

American Academy of Child and Adolescent Psychiatry
3615 Wisconsin Avenue, NW
Washington, DC 20016-3007
Phone: 202-966-7300
Fax: 202-966-2891
www.aacap.org

American Academy of Experts in Traumatic Stress
368 Veterans Memorial Highway
Commack, NY 11725
Phone: 631-543-2217
Fax: 631-543-6977
www.aaets.org

American Academy of Pediatrics
141 Northwest Point Boulevard
Elk Grove Village, IL 60007-1098
Phone: 847-434-4000
Fax: 847-434-8000
www.aap.org

American Association of Suicidology
5221 Wisconsin Avenue, NW
Washington, DC 20008
Phone: 202-237-2280
Fax: 202-237-2282
www.suicidology.org

American Medical Association
515 North State Street
Chicago, IL 60610
Phone: 312-464-5000
Toll free: 800-621-8335
www.ama-assn.org

American Professional Society on the Abuse of Children
P.O. Box 30669
Charleston, SC 29417
Phone: 843-764-2905
Toll free: 877-402-7722
Fax: 803-753-9823
www.apsac.org

American Psychiatric Association
1000 Wilson Boulevard, Suite 1825
Arlington, VA 22209-3901
Phone: 703-907-7300
www.psych.org

American Psychological Association
750 First Street NE
Washington, DC 20002-4242
Phone: 800-374-2721, 202-336-5510
www.apa.org

American Red Cross
National Headquarters
2025 E Street NW
Washington, DC 20006
Phone: 202-303-4498
www.redcross.org

Annie E. Casey Foundation
701 St. Paul Street
Baltimore, MD 21202
Phone: 410-547-6600
www.aecf.org

Association for Play Therapy, Inc.
2060 North Winery Avenue, Suite 102
Fresno, CA 93703
Phone: 559-252-2278
Fax: 559-252-2297
www.iapt.org

Association for Traumatic Stress Specialists
7701 North Lamar Boulevard, Suite 504
Austin, TX 78752
Phone: 512-300-2877
Fax: 512-300-2878

Child Welfare League of America
440 First Street NW, Suite 310
Washington, DC 20001-2085
Phone: 202-638-2952
Fax: 202-638-4004
www.cwla.org

Children's Group Therapy Association
P.O. Box 521
Watertown, MA 02172
Phone: 617-894-4307, 617-646-7571
Fax: 617-894-1195
www.cgta.net

International Society for Traumatic Stress Studies
60 Revere Drive, Suite 500
Northbrook, IL 60062
Phone: 847-480-9028
Fax: 847-480-9282
www.istss.org

National Association of Social Workers
750 First Street NE, Suite 700
Washington, DC 20002-4241
Phone: 800-638-8799, 202-408-8600
www.naswdc.org

NATIONAL CHILD WELFARE RESOURCE CENTERS

These federally funded centers provide information on best practices to promote permanency planning for children and youth. This is a selected list of centers in different parts of the United States.

ARCH National Respite Network and Resource Center
Chapel Hill Training–Outreach Project, Inc.
800 Eastowne Drive, Suite 105
Chapel Hill, NC 27514
Phone: 919-490-5577
Fax: 919-490-4905
www.archrespite.org

"Friends" National Resource Center for Community-Based Family Resource and Support Programs
Chapel Hill Training Outreach Project
800 Eastowne Drive, Suite 105
Chapel Hill, NC 27514
Phone: 800-888-8879
jldenniston@intrex.net

National Center for Children Exposed to Violence
Yale Child Study Center
P.O. Box 207900
New Haven, CT 06520-7900
Phone: 203-785-4608
Toll-free: 877-496-2238
www.nccev.org

National Resource Center on Child Maltreatment
Child Welfare Institute
1349 W. Peachtree Street NE, Suite 900
Atlanta, GA 30309-2956

National Resource Center on Child Welfare Training and Evaluation
University of Louisville Kent School of Social Work
Louisville, KY 40292
Phone: 502-852-6402
Fax: 502-852-0422
www.louisville.edu/kent

National Center for Children in Poverty
Joseph L. Mailman School of Public Health of Columbia University
215 West 125th Street, 3rd floor
New York, NY 10027
Phone: 646-284-9623
www.nccp.org

Research and Training Center on Family Support and Children's Mental Health
Portland State University
P.O. Box 751
Portland, OR 97207-0751
Phone: 503-727-4040
Fax: 503-725-4180
www.rtc,pdx.edu

Zero to Three: National Center for Infants, Toddlers, and Families
2000 M Street NW, Suite 200
Washington, DC 20036
Phone: 202-638-1144
www.zerotothree.org

TRAINING PROGRAMS AND CERTIFICATIONS

Play Therapy as a Method for Helping Children and Youth

A comprehensive directory of play therapy training programs may be obtained for a fee from the Center for Play Therapy, Denton, TX 76203. The programs listed here represent a small selection of those available in different parts of the United States.

Boston University School of Social Work
Postgraduate Certificate Program in Advanced Child and Adolescent Psychotherapy
Candace Saunders, LICSW, Director
264 Bay State Road
Boston, MA 02215
Phone: 617-353-3756
Fax: 617-353-5612

California School of Professional Psychology
Alliant University
Dr. Kevin O'Connor, Director
5130 East Clinton Way
Fresno, CA 93727
Phone: 559-456-2777 ext. 2273
Fax: 559-253-2267

Center for Play Therapy
Dr. Sue Bratton, Director
P.O. Box 311337
University of North Texas
Denton, TX 76203
Phone: 940-565-3864
Fax: 940-565-4461
www.centerforplaytherapy.org

Play Therapy Training Institute
Dr. Heidi Kaduson and Dr. Charles Schaefer, Directors
P.O. Box 1435
Hightstown, NJ 08520
Phone: 609-448-2143
Fax: 609-448-1665
www.ptti.org

Post-Master's Certificate Program in Child and Adolescent Therapy
Dr. Nancy Boyd Webb, Director
Fordham University Graduate School of Social Service
Tarrytown, NY 10591
Phone: 914-332-6008
Fax: 914-332-7101
www.fordham.edu

Reiss–Davis Child Study Center
Director of Training
3200 Motor Avenue
Los Angeles, CA 90034
Phone: 310-836-1223

Trauma/Crisis/Mental Health Counseling

American Academy of Experts in Traumatic Stress
368 Veterans Memorial Highway
Commack, NY 11725
Phone: 631-543-2217
www.aaets.org

American Association of Suicidology
5221 Wisconsin Avenue, NW
Washington, DC 20008
Phone: 202-237-2280
Fax: 202-237-2282
www.suicidology.org

ChildTrauma Academy
5161 San Felipe, Suite 320
Houston, TX 77056
Phone: 281-932-1375
Fax: 713-481-9821
www.ChildTrauma.org

Child Trauma Institute
P.O. Box 544
Greenfield, MA 01302-0544
Phone: 413-774-2340
www.childtrauma.com

EMDR International Association
P.O. Box 141925
Austin, TX 78714-1925
Phone: 512-451-5200
www.emdria.org

National Institute for Trauma and Loss in Children
900 Cook Road
Grosse Pointe Woods, MI 48236
Phone: 313-885-0390
Toll free: 877-306-5256
www.tlcinst.org

Animal-Assisted Therapy

Delta Society
875 124th Avenue NE
Suite 101
Bellevue, WA 98005
Phone: 425-235-1076

Mercy College
Animal Assisted Therapy Facilitation Certificate Program
555 Broadway
Dobbs Ferry, NY 10522
Phone: 914-693-4500
www.mercy.edu

People, Animals, Nature (PAN), Inc.
1820 Princeton Circle
Napierville, IL 60665
Phone: 630-369-8328
www.pan-inc.org
[E-learning course in animal-assisted therapy]

CHILD-RELATED AND TRAUMA-RELATED PROFESSIONAL JOURNALS

Child Abuse and Neglect
Elsevier Science, Inc.
360 Park Avenue South
New York, NY 10010-1710
Phone: 212-989-5800
Fax: 212-633-3990
www.elsevier.com

Child and Adolescent Social Work Journal
Kluwer Academic Publishers
P.O. Box 358
Accord Station
Hingham, MA 02018-0358
Phone: 781-871-6600
Fax: 781-681-9045
www.kluweronline.com

Child and Family Behavior
Haworth Press, Inc.
10 Alice Street
Binghamton, NY 13904
Phone: 800-429-6784
Fax: 800-895-0582
www.haworthpressinc.com

Child: Care, Health and Development
Blackwell Publishing
350 Main Street
Malden, MA 02148
Phone: 781-388-8200
Fax: 781-388-8210
www.blackwellpublishing.com

Child Development
c/o Society for Research in Child Development
3131 South State Street, Suite 202
Ann Arbor, MI 48108-1623
Phone: 734-998-6524
www.scrd.org

Child Psychiatry and Human Development
Kluwer Academic Publishers
P.O. Box 358
Accord Station
Hingham, MA 02108-0358
Phone: 781-871-6600
Fax: 781-681-9045
www.kluweronline.com

Child Study Journal
State University of New York College at Buffalo
Educational Foundations Department
Bacon Hall 306
1300 Elmwood Avenue
Buffalo, NY 14222-1095
Phone: 716-878-5302
Fax: 716-873-5833
www.buffalostate.edu/~edf/csj.htm

Child Welfare (formerly *Child Welfare Quarterly*)
P.O. Box 2019
Annapolis Junction, MD 20797-0118
Phone: 800-407-6273
www.cwla.org

Children and Youth Care Forum
Human Sciences Press, Inc.
233 Spring Street
New York, NY 10013-1578
Phone: 212-807-1047
Fax: 212-463-0742
www.cyc-net.org

Children and Youth Services Review
Elsevier Science, Inc.
360 Park Avenue South
New York, NY 10010-1710
Phone: 212-633-3730
Fax: 212-633-3680
www.elsevier.com

Children's Health Care
Lawrence Erlbaum Associates
10 Industrial Avenue
Mahwah, NJ 07430
Phone: 201-258-2200
www.erlbaum.com

Early Child Research Quarterly
Ablex Publishing Corporation
355 Chestnut Street
Norwood, NJ 07648
Phone: 201-767-8450
Fax: 201-767-6717

Gifted Child Quarterly
National Association for Gifted Children
1707 L Street NW, Suite 550
Washington, DC 20036
Phone: 202-785-4268
www.nagc.org

Journal of Abnormal Child Psychology
Kluwer Academic Publishers
P.O. Box 358
Accord Station
Hingham, MA 02108-0358
Phone: 781-871-6600
Fax: 781-681-9045
www.kluweronline.com

Journal of the American Academy of Child and Adolescent Psychiatry
Lippincott Williams & Wilkins
351 West Camden Street
Baltimore, MD 21201
Phone: 410-528-4200
Fax: 410-528-4312
www.jaacap.com

Journal of Child and Adolescent Group Therapy
Kluwer Academic Publishers
P.O. Box 358
Accord Station
Hingham, MA 02108-0358
Phone: 781-871-6600
Fax: 781-681-9045
www.kluweronline.com

Journal of Child and Youth Care (formerly *Journal of Child Care*)
Department of Human Services
Malaspina University-College
900 Fifth Street
Nanaimo, British Columbia V9R5S5, Canada
Phone: 250-753-3245
www.uofcpress.com

Journal of Child Psychology and Psychiatry and Allied Disciplines
Blackwell Publishing
350 Main Street
Malden, MA 02148
Phone: 781-388-8200
Fax: 781-388-8210
www.blackwellpublishing.com

Journal of Clinical Child and Adolescent Psychology
Lawrence Erlbaum Associates
10 Industrial Avenue
Mahwah, NJ 07430
Phone: 201-258-2200
www.jccap.net

Journal of Family Violence
Kluwer Academic Publishers
P.O. Box 358
Accord Station
Hingham, MA 02018-0358
Phone: 781-871-6600
Fax: 781-681-9045
www.kluweronline.com

Journal of Traumatic Stress
Kluwer Academic Publishers
P.O. Box 358
Accord Station
Hingham, MA 02018-0358
Phone: 781-871-6600
Fax: 781-681-9045
www.kluweronline.com

Psychoanalytic Study of the Child
Yale University Press
P.O. Box 209040
New Haven, CT 06520-9040
Phone: 203-432-0960
Fax: 203-432-0948
www.yale.edu/yup/books/083718.htm

Trauma and Loss: Research and Interventions
National Institute for Trauma and Loss in Children
900 Cook Road
Grosse Pointe Woods, MI 48236
Phone: 313-885-0390, 877-306-5256
www.tlcinst.org

Trauma, Violence and Abuse
Sage Publications Ltd.
6 Bonhill Street
London, EC2A 4PU, UK
Phone: +44 (0)20 7374 0645
Fax: +44 (0)20 7374 8741
www.sagepub.co.uk

ADDITIONAL TRAUMA RESOURCES

Children's Defense Fund
25 E Street NW
Washington, DC 20001
Phone: 202-628-8787
www.childrensdefensefund.org

Child Witness to Violence Project
Boston Medical Center
91 East Concord Street, 5th Floor
Boston, MA 02118
Phone: 617-414-4244
www.bostonchildhealth.org

Federal Emergency Management Agency (FEMA)
500 C Street SW
Washington, DC 20472
Phone: 202-566-1600, 800-480-2520
www.fema.gov

Index